Oxford Handbook of

Musculoskeletal Nursing

Published and Forthcoming Oxford Handbooks in Nursing

Oxford Handbook of Musculoskeletal Nursing, 2nd edition
Edited by Susan M. Oliver OBE

Oxford Handbook of Cancer Nursing, 2nd edition
Edited by Mike Tadman, Dave Roberts, and Mark Foulkes

Oxford Handbook of Learning and Intellectual Disability Nursing, 2nd edition
Edited by Owen Barr and Bob Gates

Oxford Handbook of Adult Nursing, 2nd edition
Edited by Maria Flynn and Dave Mercer

Oxford Handbook of Midwifery
Janet Medforth, Susan Battersby, Maggie Evans, Beverley Marsh, and Angela Walker

Oxford Handbook of Mental Health Nursing
Edited by Patrick Callaghan and Helen Waldock

Oxford Handbook of Children's and Young People's Nursing
Edited by Edward Alan Glasper, Gillian McEwing, and Jim Richardson

Oxford Handbook of Nurse Prescribing
Sue Beckwith and Penny Franklin

Oxford Handbook of Cardiac Nursing
Edited by Kate Johnson and Karen Rawlings-Anderson

Oxford Handbook of Primary Care Nursing
Edited by Vari Drennan and Claire Goodman

Oxford Handbook of Gastrointestinal Nursing
Edited by Christine Norton, Julia Williams, Claire Taylor, Annmarie Nunwa, and Kathy Whayman

Oxford Handbook of Respiratory Nursing
Terry Robinson and Jane Scullion

Oxford Handbook of Nursing Older People
Beverley Tabernacle, Marie Barnes, and Annette Jinks

Oxford Handbook of Clinical Skills in Adult Nursing
Jacqueline Randle, Frank Coffey, and Martyn Bradbury

Oxford Handbook of Emergency Nursing
Edited by Robert Crouch, Alan Charters, Mary Dawood, and Paula Bennett

Oxford Handbook of Dental Nursing
Kevin Seymour, Dayananda Samarawickrama, Elizabeth Boon and Rebecca Parr

Oxford Handbook of Diabetes Nursing
Lorraine Avery and Sue Beckwith

Oxford Handbook of Women's Health Nursing
Sunanda Gupta, Debra Holloway, and Ali Kubba

Oxford Handbook of Perioperative Practice
Suzanne Hughes and Andy Mardell

Oxford Handbook of Critical Care Nursing
Sheila Adam and Sue Osborne

Oxford Handbook of Neuroscience Nursing
Sue Woodward and Cath Waterhouse

Oxford Handbook of Musculoskeletal Nursing

SECOND EDITION

EDITED BY

Susan M. Oliver OBE

Independent Nurse Consultant;
Former Chair of the RCN Rheumatology Forum and Chief Nurse Advisor for the Past Chair of European League Against Rheumatism (EULAR) Health Professional Standing Committee, UK

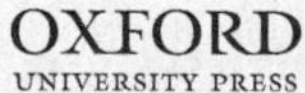
OXFORD
UNIVERSITY PRESS

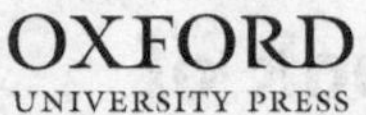

Great Clarendon Street, Oxford, OX2 6DP,
United Kingdom

Oxford University Press is a department of the University of Oxford. It furthers the University's objective of excellence in research, scholarship, and education by publishing worldwide. Oxford is a registered trade mark of Oxford University Press in the UK and in certain other countries

First Edition published in 2009
Second Edition published in 2020

Impression: 1

Published in the United States of America by Oxford University Press
198 Madison Avenue, New York, NY 10016, United States of America

British Library Cataloguing in Publication Data

Data available

Library of Congress Control Number: 2019949830

ISBN 978–0–19–883142–6

Printed in Great Britain by
Ashford Colour Press Ltd, Gosport, Hampshire

Forewords

Although we live in a digital era with easy access to information, often we find that we are uncertain of where to access quick evidence-based guidance. Access to timely, precise, systematic, and accurate information remains very important, especially in the healthcare context, when mobile phones and computers can be a huge barrier to the comprehensive and emphatic approach to care.

The way this handbook is organized facilitates quick overviews of the subject under consideration, with very useful summary text boxes, red flags, and images, practical and real 'frequently asked questions'. It also provides clear indications for the essentials of physical and clinical examination, complementary examinations, and assessments, never losing the focus on the psychosocial dimension and patient-centred care. Essential topics for patient education, useful clinical and patient-reported measurements, and guidance for more detailed readings are provided in an elegant manner. Both pharmacological and non-pharmacological approaches are presented with a good balance.

I truly found this an extremely valuable tool to empower nurses, not only for those in the field of rheumatology, but also for those working in other clinical contexts, which include primary and community healthcare, occupational health units, medical and surgical wards, perioperative, urgency and intensive care units, nursing homes, among others. The intuitive interconnection between contents makes this guide both straightforward while providing a holistic perspective. It surely deserves to be available on the bookshelf of all health units.

Ricardo J. O. Ferreira
Registered nurse, researcher, and PhD student,
Rheumatology Outpatient Department,
Coimbra Hospital and University Centre (CHUC), Portugal;
Chair Elect of European League Against
Rheumatism Health Professional Standing Committee

Rheumatic musculoskeletal diseases impose significantly upon global health. Comprising more than 200 varied conditions, these diseases afflict millions of people and lead collectively to substantial disability, co-morbidity, loss of quality of life, and reduction in life expectancy. These are, however, exciting times in our discipline. The last decade witnessed a revolution in the management of rheumatic musculoskeletal diseases with the advent of novel therapeutics, built on unprecedented understanding of pathogenesis and advances in the application of modern molecular medicine techniques. In parallel, the clinical approach to care of patients has been transformed by the recognition of the merits of early interventions, remission-targeted strategies, and especially the optimal use of the multidisciplinary team. In this respect, nurses have never played a more important role, operating at the centre of complex therapeutic teams, yet retaining the essential compassion and communication skills that define optimal care. This remarkable volume provides necessary background matched with pragmatic guidance that will support the delivery of such outstanding nursing care in the enthralling years yet to come, as we seek to transform the lives of our patients. I commend it to you with my highest enthusiasm!

Iain B. McInnes CBE, FRCP, PhD, FRSE, FMedSci
Muirhead Professor of Medicine and
Versus Arthritis Professor of Rheumatology,
University of Glasgow; President of EULAR 2019–2021

It was a pleasure and a privilege to be involved in the development of this important publication. Rheumatology specialist nurses remain a pivotal part of the multidisciplinary team by delivering the highest quality care to patients in increasingly pressurized environments. Therefore, the need for accessible, evidence-based, and up-to-date clinical resources has never been higher. The content and scope of information provided in this handbook is an invaluable asset for all of us to support our roles and the care of our patients.

I would like to take the opportunity to thank my Royal College of Nursing Rheumatology Forum colleagues who have also contributed to the text and the expertise and rigour that they have provided to ensure this is a 'must have' guide for all nurses working within the field of rheumatology and musculoskeletal conditions.

Louise Parker RN, BSc (Hons) MSc, NIP
Lead Nurse, Rheumatology & Connective Tissue Disease,
Royal Free London NHS Foundation Trust; Chair,
Royal College of Nursing Rheumatology Forum

I met Sue when Hong Kong started to develop rheumatology nursing after the UK model in 2007. Sue was always passionate in promoting rheumatology nursing and helped conduct the first rheumatology training class for nurses and many more since then. Sue's passion extended beyond Hong Kong and she was one of the core working group members for the development of the Asia Pacific League Against Rheumatisim (APLAR) web-based rheumatology nurse training programme known as ASia-Pacific Initiative for Rheumatology Nurse Education (ASPIRE). Currently, we have rheumatology nurses serving our patients in some parts of Asia including Australia, Hong Kong, Japan, China, India, and so on. However, rheumatology nursing development is still in a rudimentary phase in some parts of Asia. I am particularly thrilled that Sue managed to have this book available for the development of musculoskeletal nursing across the globe, in particular, Asia Pacific countries, which account for more than half of the world's population. This book is carefully and specifically designed to provide a straightforward go-to book for nurses in all care settings to empower nurses, in order for patients to gain access to the right care. I am confident that this book can be a practical and user-friendly resource to extend the role of the nurse in all healthcare settings worldwide.

Lai-Shan Tam, MD
Professor Head, Division of Rheumatology,
Department of Medicine and Therapeutics,
The Chinese University of Hong Kong, Hong Kong

There are often many more issues facing a rheumatology patient than the management of pain and it is imperative those involved in their care understand this and appreciate that concerns, symptoms, and problems may change over time and do not begin and end with swollen joints. This book will arm nurses with the knowledge they need to make a real difference to the lives of the patients they treat. Whether working in a rheumatology setting or not, with around 10 million people in the UK alone thought to have some form of arthritis, there is no doubt all nurses will treat patients with a rheumatological condition during their career. Being informed and able to treat these patients with understanding and confidence can, in my opinion, be as efficacious as the drugs they may be administering.

Dr Natalie Williams, PhD and person with rheumatoid arthritis

Preface

I am excited and hopeful that this second edition of the *Oxford Handbook of Musculoskeletal Nursing* will be used by nurses in a range of healthcare settings across the world. In the 1970s and 1980s, Europe and America recognized the need for nurses to extend their roles to optimize care. Increasingly, healthcare services have come to recognize the need to develop and enhance the role of the nurse. As such, nurses will play an increasing role in care of those with musculoskeletal conditions (MSCs).

The focus of the handbook is to provide precise core information and references for many of the most common MSCs that nurses in all care settings are likely to see.

The last 10 years have resulted in many developments within the field of rheumatology and MSCs. This edition offers guidance on the individual conditions, examination techniques, investigations, treatment, as well as management and monitoring approaches. In recent years, there has been an increasing number of new therapies, extending the range of treatment options, particularly within the field of biologic therapies for immunologically driven diseases. Nurses will come across individuals who are being treated with these therapies and will need to be informed about how to best manage the screening and support the patient, while maintaining a vigilant eye on potential side effects.

As we strive to support nurses to advance their practice, this edition offers guidance on the principles of carrying out nurse-led consultations and other roles that were previously considered the domain of the doctor, such as physical examination. The demands of preparing and monitoring patients for treatments have now become an integral aspect of advanced nursing practice. Whatever the care setting, this edition offers guidance for those who are supporting patients in the clinic, community, or ward-based care. References and key links are offered for those who wish to delve further into the issues or require further guidance.

MSCs is a term that covers a wide range of conditions, some may be mild and self-limiting while others may be life-threatening, or at least have a significant impact on the individual's quality of life. One of the challenges has been to make sense of what MSCs encompass and what is the difference between MSCs and rheumatology. The term MSCs refers to all conditions that affect muscles, bones, and joints. It describes not only long term conditions such as those that are usually seen within the field of rheumatology (e.g. rheumatoid arthritis), but also includes self-limiting conditions that will frequently be seen in general practice (e.g. tennis elbow) and those seen in orthopaedics (e.g. joint replacement surgery). In preparing this second edition, our aim has been to offer both the basic principles of musculoskeletal nursing and guidance on aspects of advanced practice.

In many parts of the world there is insufficient training and education to prepare the undergraduate nurse to support people with MSCs. There are country differences in the way services are offered and in the design and funding of healthcare systems. Some countries face financial, legal, or political barriers to developing a full multidisciplinary approach to care. In recent years, this appears to be changing as we all face the new challenges in the provision of healthcare for the future. Over the last 10 years I have been encouraged to see how much rheumatology nursing is developing internationally and have been especially enthused to see expertise grow across areas such as the Asia Pacific region. When meeting with nurses across the world, I have been saddened to see how few resources are available for nurses to become empowered and enable them to specialize within the field of musculoskeletal care. My hope is that this book may be a useful tool for those nurses as they advance their practice.

In the current climate, with the growing elderly and chronic disease populations, there is a vital need for prompt and effective approaches to inform and empower individuals to manage their mild short-term complaints, but also to know how and when to seek prompt healthcare support. Equally, when individuals are diagnosed and require ongoing treatment, they need to be able to actively engage in the decision-making process with their healthcare team. Nurses play a vital role in aiding the patient to optimize their care while working in collaboration with the wider healthcare team. A central aspect of nursing models of care applies a holistic approach with the focus on enabling patients to participate in shared decision-making. Nurses can find information on how to implement holistic and patient-centred approaches while also understanding factors that may impact the patient's life, such as fertility, pregnancy, and relationships, or achieving symptom control and effective pain management. Advanced practice often involves additional roles such as joint injections, physical examinations, monitoring blood results, and emergency and rapid access care, all of which are discussed in a clear and concise way.

Acknowledgements

A personal thanks to all those contributors to both the original edition and this second edition. Without their support and professionalism, I would have found the second edition impossible to achieve. My thanks also to Sylvia Warren at Oxford University Press for always providing prompt and decisive guidance and cheerfully so.

My long-suffering family deserve significant recognition: my husband Mike and our grown-up children, Daniel, Andrew, and Rebecca, who have always inspired and encouraged me to strive and achieve despite the challenges to relaxation and time out from our family life.

Finally, I would like to give a very humble thanks to specifically my nursing colleagues nationally and internationally as well as all health professionals within the field of rheumatology—throughout my career I have enjoyed an inspiring and rewarding career with a wonderfully talented and resourceful group of professionals.

Contents

Contributors

Julian Barratt *(Chapter 6)*
Head of Post-Registration Education, Insititute of Health, University of Wolverhampton, Wolverhampton, UK

Alice Berry *(Chapters 2, 11, and 19)*
Research Fellow, Department of Health and Applied Sciences, University of the West of England, Bristol, UK

Ailsa Bosworth *(Chapter 22)*
Chief Executive, National Rheumatoid Arthritis Society, Maidenhead, Berkshire, UK

Patricia Cornell *(Chapters 4 and 16)*
Rheumatology Nurse Consultant, AbbVie; Honorary Senior Rheumatology Practitioner, Poole Hospital NHS Trust, Poole, UK

Maureen Cox *(Chapter 7)*
Former Clinical Governance and Risk Practitioner NOTSS Division, John Radcliffe University Hospital, Oxford, UK

Ian Giles *(Chapter 14)*
Professor of Rheumatology, Centre of Rheumatology Research, University College London, London, UK

Diane Home *(Chapters 16 and 18)*
Nurse Consultant Rheumatology, West Middlesex Hospital, Middlesex, UK

Dawn Homer *(Chapters 12 and 21)*
Rheumatology Nurse Consultant, Modality Partnership, Community Rheumatology Service, Birmingham, UK

Alison Leary *(Chapter 23)*
Chair of Healthcare and Workforce Modelling, London South Bank University, London, UK

Polly Livermore *(Chapter 4)*
Paediatric Rheumatology Matron/NIHR Clinical Nursing Research Fellow, Great Ormond Street Children's Hospital NHS Foundation Trust,, London, UK

Janice Mooney *(Chapters 5 and 17)*
Senior Fellow, Higher Education Academy and Course Director Masters in Advanced Clinical Practice, School of Health and Social Care, University of Staffordshire, Staffordshire, UK

Daniel James Murphy *(Chapters 4 and 6)*
GP Principal, Honiton Surgery
Staff Grade Rheumatologist, Royal Devon & Exeter Hospital
Versus Arthritis MSK Champion
Devon, UK

Mwidimi Ndosi *(Chapters 20 and 23)*
Senior Lecturer in Rheumatology Nursing, University of the West of England, Bristol, UK

Michael H. Oliver *(Chapters 13 and 17)*
Consultant Physician, (retired) North Devon District Hospital, Devon, UK

Susan M. Oliver *(Chapters 1, 4, 8, 11, 12, 13, 17, 18, and 24)*
Independent Nurse Consultant; Nurse Consultant and Former Chair of the RCN Rheumatology Forum and Chief Nurse Advisor for the National Rheumatoid Arthritis Society, Devon, UK

Louise Parker *(Chapter 5)*
Lead Nurse, Rheumatology and Connective Tissue Disease, Royal Free London NHS Foundation Trust, London, UK

Yeliz Prior *(Chapters 11 and 19)*
Senior Research Fellow, School of Health and Society, Advanced Clinical Specialist Occupational Therapist, Mid Cheshire NHS Foundation Trust Hospitals, Crewe, UK

Donna Lorraine Rowe *(Chapter 3)*
Service Delivery Lead/Specialist Nurse, National Osteoporosis Society, Camerton, Bath, UK

Sarah Ryan *(Chapters 9, 10, and 15)*
Professor Rheumatology Nursing, Midlands Partnership NHS Foundation Trust, Haywood Hospital, Staffordshire, UK

Liz Smith *(Chapter 4)*
Lead Nurse, Nottingham Children and Young Peoples' Rheumatology Service, Nottingham Children's Hospital, Nottingham, UK

Catharine Thwaites *(Chapter 17)*
Keele University School of Nursing and Midwifery, Staffordshire, and Stoke on Trent Partnership NHS Trust, Staffordshire, UK

Nicola Walsh *(Chapters 2, 11, and 19)*
Professor of Musculoskeletal Health and Knowledge Mobilisation, Faculty of Health and Applied Sciences, University of the West of England, Bristol, UK

Richard Watts *(Chapters 5 and 17)*
Consultant Rheumatologist, Ipswich Hospital NHS Trust, Ipswich, and Honorary Professor at University of East Anglia, Ipswich, Suffolk, UK

Symbols and abbreviations

💣	controversial topic
➲	cross-reference
❗	warning
►	important
►►	don't dawdle
🖱	website
☎	telephone
↓	decreased
↑	increased
♂	female
♀	male
1°	primary
2°	secondary
~	approximately
≈	approximately equal to
∴	therefore
ACJ	acromioclavicular joint
ACR	American College of Rheumatology
ACS	acute compartment syndrome
ADL	activity of daily living
ALP	alkaline phosphatase
ALT	alanine transaminase
ANA	antinuclear antibody
ANCA	antineutrophil cytoplasmic antibody
aPL	antiphospholipid antibodies
APS	antiphospholipid syndrome
AS	ankylosing spondylitis
AxSpA	axial spondyloarthritis
AZA	azathioprine
bDMARD	biologic disease-modifying antirheumatic drug
BMD	bone mineral density
BMI	body mass index
BNF	*British National Formulary*
BSPAR	British Society of Paediatric and Adolescent Rheumatology
BSR	British Society for Rheumatology
CBT	cognitive behavioural therapy
CCP	cyclic citrullinated peptide
cDMARD	conventional disease-modifying antirheumatic drug
CMC	carpometacarpal
CMP	clinical management plan
COPD	chronic obstructive pulmonary disease
COX	cyclooxygenase
CPPD	calcium pyrophosphate deposition
CRP	C-reactive protein
CTD	connective tissue disease
CTS	carpal tunnel syndrome
DAS	disease activity score
DH	Department of Health
DIP	distal interphalangeal
DMARD	disease-modifying antirheumatic drug

DVT	deep venous thrombosis
DXA	dual-energy X-ray absorptiometry
EA	enteropathic arthritis
ED	emergency department
EGPA	eosinophilic granulomatosis with polyangiitis
EMS	early morning stiffness
ENT	ear, nose, and throat
EPP	Expert Patient Programme
ERP	enhanced recovery programme
ESR	erythrocyte sedimentation rate
EULAR	European League against Rheumatism
FBC	full blood count
GCA	giant cell arteritis
GP	general practitioner
GPA	granulomatosis with polyangiitis
Hb	haemoglobin
HCP	healthcare professional
HCQ	hydroxychloroquine
HLA	human leucocyte antigen
HQIP	Healthcare Quality Improvement Partnership
HRCT	high-resolution computed tomography
HRT	hormone replacement therapy
IA	intra-articular
ICP	integrated care pathway
Ig	immunoglobulin
IJD	inflammatory joint disease
IL	interleukin
ILAR	International League of Associations for Rheumatology
IM	intramuscular
IV	intravenous
JIA	juvenile idiopathic arthritis
L	litre(s)
LFT	liver function test
LTC	long-term condition
MCP	metacarpophalangeal
mcg	microgram(s)
MDT	multidisciplinary team
mesna	2-mercaptoethane sulfonate
MI	myocardial infarction or motivational interviewing
min	minute(s)
mL	millilitre
MMF	mycophenolate mofetil
MPA	microscopic polyangiitis
MPO	myeloperoxidase
MRI	magnetic resonance imaging
MRSA	methicillin-resistant *Staphylococcus aureus*
MSC	musculoskeletal condition
MTP	metatarsophalangeal
MTX	methotrexate
NCD	non-communicable disease
NHS	National Health Service

NOS	National Osteoporosis Society
NRAS	National Rheumatoid Arthritis Society
NSAID	non-steroidal anti-inflammatory drug
NYHA	New York Heart Association
OA	osteoarthritis
OT	occupational therapist
PAH	pulmonary arterial hypertension
PE	pulmonary embolism
PFT	pulmonary function test
PH	pulmonary hypertension
PIP	proximal interphalangeal
PMR	polymyalgia rheumatica
PPI	proton pump inhibitor
PRCN	paediatric rheumatology clinical nurse specialist
PsA	psoriatic arthritis
PSA	prostate-specific antigen
PSV	primary systemic vasculitis
PT	physiotherapist
PTH	parathyroid hormone
PV	plasma viscosity
RA	rheumatoid arthritis
RBC	red blood cell
RCN	Royal College of Nursing
ReA	reactive arthritis
RF	rheumatoid factor
RICE	rest, ice, compression, and elevation
RNS	rheumatology nurse specialist
ROAM	range of active movement
ROM	range of motion
SAS	sulfasalazine
SD	standard deviation
SE	self-efficacy
sec	second(s)
SIGN	Scottish Intercollegiate Guidelines Network
SLE	systemic lupus erythematosus
SLR	straight leg raising
SOB	shortness of breath
SpA	spondyloarthritis
SPC	Summary of Product Characteristics
SS	Sjögren's syndrome
SSRI	serotonin-specific reuptake inhibitor
SUA	serum uric acid
TB	tuberculosis
TCA	tricyclic antidepressant
TENS	transcutaneous electrical nerve stimulation
THR	total hip replacement
TKR	total knee replacement
TNFα	tumour necrosis factor alpha
tsDMARD	targeted synthetic disease-modifying antirheumatic drug
U&Es	urea and electrolytes

ULT	urate-lowering therapy
UN	United Nations
US	ultrasound or United States
VAS	visual analogue scale
VZ	varicella zoster
WBC	white blood cell
WHO	World Health Organization

Part I

Musculoskeletal conditions and their management

Chapter 1

Introduction

Musculoskeletal conditions

There are >200 musculoskeletal conditions (MSCs) that affect all age groups from the very young to the elderly. MSCs are common and are generally referred to by the public as 'arthritis'—a term referring to disorders of the muscles, joints, bones, or connective tissues (Figs. 1.1 and 1.2).

MSCs are also the major cause of morbidity throughout Europe, substantially affecting health and quality of life and causing significant costs to health and society. MSCs as a group are estimated to cause 21.3% of total years lived with disability (YLDs) in the world, behind mental and behavioural problems.

Key facts about MSCs

- Pain is the predominant feature and the main reason for seeking medical advice.
- Currently, individuals experiencing musculoskeletal symptoms constitute up to 30% of general practitioner (GP) consultations.
- Each year in England and Wales, 20% of the general population see a GP about a musculoskeletal problem. These costs are compounded by the further £5 billion pounds per year spent on treating musculoskeletal problems.[1]
- Some MSCs can be mild and self-limiting; others can involve ongoing treatment with cytotoxic therapies and significant reductions in life expectancy or affect long-term functional ability.
- Affect all ages but become increasingly common with ageing. The number of people aged >60 years is set to double by 2050.
- One-quarter of adults in Europe are affected by longstanding musculoskeletal problems.
- The prevalence of MSCs varies by age and diagnosis and between people across the globe, yet it is calculated that 20–33% of people internationally live with a painful MSC.[2]
- Numbers are set to rise with ↑ elderly and obese populations.
- Evidence suggests that soft tissue and back disorders represent the most common types of patient self-reported pain and limited activity in the young and middle aged.

The major MSCs that present a significant burden are outlined in ➲ Table 1.1, p. 6.

The UK General Household Survey (GHS) has highlighted the significant unmet needs of individuals with joint pain as high levels of self-reported joint pain are noted yet there continues to be the mistaken belief that 'nothing can be done' and thus many individuals fail to seek medical advice. There will be an ↑ need for specialist expertise in managing the MSCs where the prevalence ↑ with age (e.g. osteoarthritis (OA), gout, and osteoporosis). Nurses and allied healthcare professionals play an essential role:

- Providing key information and support to patients.
- Enhancing self-management principles to enable individuals to manage their symptoms effectively.

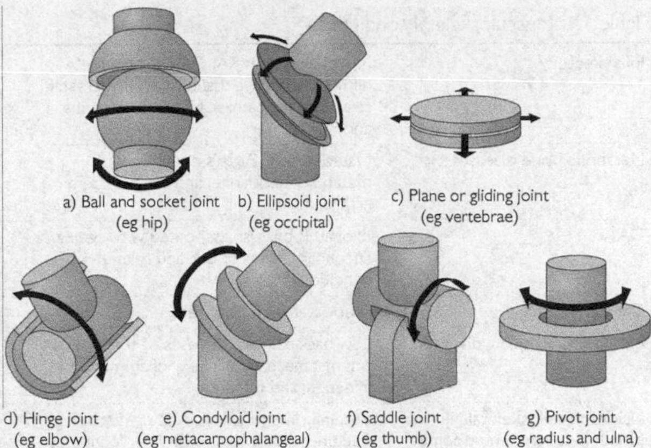

Fig. 1.1 Types of joints. These figures represent the different types of joints found in the body. For example, panel (a) shows a ball and sock joint—as seen in the hip. It is important to have a sound knowledge of the type of joints involved in a specific condition, allowing for clarity about the range of movements possible.

Reproduced with permission of Clinical Skills Ltd.

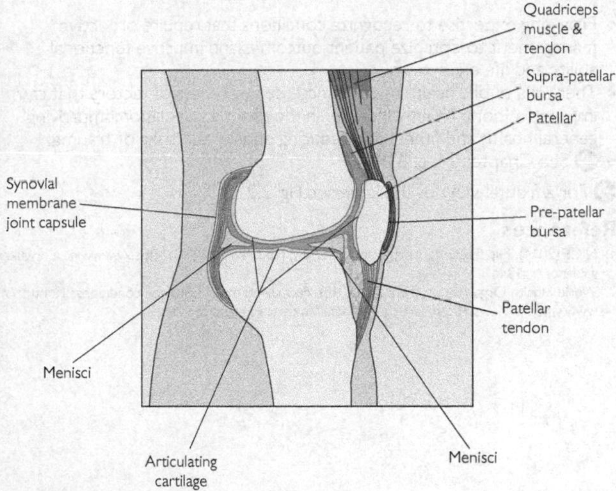

Fig. 1.2 Joint capsule with surrounding tissues.

Reproduced with permission of Clinical Skills Ltd.

Table 1.1 Musculoskeletal conditions

Inflammatory	Most common is RA. Others include JIA, diffuse connective tissue disorders, crystal-related arthropathies, infectious arthritis, and PsA
Metabolic bone diseases	Osteoporosis, Paget's disease, metabolic, endocrine, and other systemic arthropathies
OA	Idiopathic but also associated with ageing. Secondary forms of OA and related conditions
Osteoporosis	Associated with fractures
Back pain and spinal disorders	Low back pain and diseases of the spine, trauma, mechanical injury, inflammation, infection, and tumours
Major musculoskeletal injuries including severe limb trauma	Resulting in permanent disability including fractures, blood vessels, and nerve injuries
Occupational musculoskeletal injuries	Work-related injuries: repetition, direct pressure, high force, vibration, or prolonged constraint on posture
Sports injuries	Physical activity or sports-related injuries

- Providing expertise to recognize conditions that require proactive management to optimize patient outcomes and improve functional ability and life expectancy.
- There is a public health need to increase awareness of factors that can improve a 'bone healthy lifestyle' in the general population, improving general health and fitness and reducing obesity and risks of trauma.
- ➲ See Chapter 24, p. 639.

➲ For a frontal view of the knee see Fig. 2.2, p. 9.

References

1. NICE (2014). Hip fracture: management (CG124) [updated 2017]. https://www.nice.org.uk/guidance/cg124
2. World Health Organization (February 2018). Fact sheet: musculoskeletal conditions. http://www.who.int/news-room/fact-sheets/detail/musculoskeletal-conditions

Classifying joint diseases

The way differing MSCs present, which group of tissues and structures are affected, and the persistence of the symptoms all add up to the complexity of diagnosis and management.

Joint diseases can be classified as:

- Inflammatory diseases: e.g. rheumatoid arthritis (RA), ankylosing spondylitis (AS), psoriatic arthritis (PsA), and juvenile idiopathic arthritis (JIA).
- Connective diseases: e.g. systemic lupus erythematosus (SLE) and systemic sclerosis.
- Metabolic bone disorders: e.g. osteoporosis and associated fragility fractures.
- OA and related disorders.
- Non-inflammatory joint pain/soft tissue syndromes:
  - Mild self-limiting conditions (e.g. tennis elbow).
  - Acute or chronic.
  - Mono (single joint) or poly (many joints).
- Back pain or spinal conditions.
- Major trauma to joints and surrounding tissues (requiring surgical or medical management).
- Sports or occupational injuries: e.g. trauma, sports injuries, mechanical disorders, occupational, or changes as a result of destructive joint diseases.

There are a variety of ways of classifying MSCs and referral pathways to diagnosis and treatment are usually based upon early decisions about patients potentially requiring surgery (orthopaedic) or medical management (rheumatology). These referral pathways and management approaches have not always served patients well; e.g. a patient may ultimately require knee replacement but may wish initially to consider a conservative route of weight reduction and adaptations, walking aids, etc. There is now an increasing emphasis on incorporating the two disciplines more closely to improve patient flows and ultimately pathways of care using the term 'musculoskeletal'.

There is also recognition that the prevalence and incidence of MSCs is set to rise. The focus on management should be that of:

- Rapid proactive management for mild self-limiting conditions.
- Prompt referral for those who have conditions that require specialist advice and treatment.
- Encouragement of patient self-management principles.

A clear diagnosis is essential; however, from the nursing perspective, clarity needs also to focus on the consequences for the patient. This should include how best to support the individual in understanding their condition and how best to manage the problem in the context of the individual's daily life. Individuals should be supported to enable them to be active participants in decisions about their treatment including self-management principles.

➲ Also see 'Education, social, and psychological issues', Chapter 10, pp. 336–339.

Website resources

Patient information websites

- AbilityNet information on computing and disability: http://www.abilitynet.org.uk
- Arthritis and Musculoskeletal Alliance (ARMA)—umbrella body for >30 support groups providing guidance on standards of care for those with MSCs: http://www.arma.uk.net
- Benefit enquiries: http://www.dwp.gov.uk
- BMJ Best Practice http://www.bestpractice.bmj.com
- Citizen's Advice: http://www.citizensadvice.org.uk
- Community Legal Service Direct for guidance on work-related issues: http://www.clsdirect.uk
- Department of Health: http://www.dh.gov.uk/
- Disabled Living Foundation advice on equipment and aids/advice: http://www.dlf.org.uk/
- Family Planning Association: http://www.fpa.org.uk
- Patient UK—information on all conditions: http://www.patient.co.uk
- National Institute for Health and Care Excellence: http://www.nice.org.uk
- Reach Volunteering—volunteering in the community: http://www.reach-online.org.uk
- Royal British Legion—financial, social, and emotional support for former service people and their dependants: http://www.britishlegion.org.uk
- Versus Arthritis for leaflets or website access: https://www.versusarthritis.org.

Patient organizations

- Antiphospholipid syndrome: http://www.aps-support.org.uk
- BackCare: http://www.backcare.org.uk
- British Sjögren's Syndrome Society: http://www.bssa.uk.net
- Carers UK: http://www.carersuk.org
- Fibromyalgia Association UK: http://www.fmauk.org
- Lupus UK: http://www.lupusuk.org.uk
- Myositis UK: http://www.myositis.org.uk
- National Ankylosing Spondylitis Society: http://www.nass.co.uk
- National Rheumatoid Arthritis Society: http://www.nras.org.uk
- Patient experiences of conditions: http://www.healthtalk.org
- Royal Osteoporosis Society: http://www.theros.org.uk
- Scleroderma and Raynaud's UK: http://www.sruk.co.uk
- The British Pain Society: http://www.britishpainsociety.org

Employment information

- Acas: http://www.acas.org.uk
- College of Occupational Therapists: http://www.cot.org.uk
- Equality and Human Rights Commission: https://www.equalityhumanrights.com

- HM Courts and Tribunals Service: 🔗 http://www.gov.uk/government/organisations/hm-courts-and-tribunals-service
- Job Centre Guide: 🔗 http://www.https://www.gov.uk/contact-jobcentre-plus

Assessment tools

- EuroQuol: 🔗 http://www.euroqol.org
- Fatigue Tool (FACIT): 🔗 http://www.facit.org
- Low Back Pain Tool. The Chartered Society of Physiotherapy (LBP tools): 🔗 http://www.csp.org.uk
- Short Form 36 and Sickness Impact Profile: 🔗 http://www.rand.org

Chapter 2

Osteoarthritis

Overview

Introduction

OA is a common MSC that is characterized by changes to the structure of a joint and the joints affected. OA can develop in any joint and is most commonly referred to as a syndrome of joint pain and changes in functional ability impacting the individual's quality of life. Joint changes are slowly progressive and will result in changes to synovial joints including changes to subchondral bone, loss of articular cartilage, formation of osteophytes, and thickening of the joint capsule (Figs. 2.1 and 2.2). This can result in malalignment of normal joint anatomy.

Higher numbers of ♀ populations have severe OA. Generalized and nodal OA is more common in postmenopausal ♀ but can occur in those in their 40s.

Estimates of OA prevalence vary depending upon how OA is defined (clinically or radiographically) but there are 8.75 million people in the UK affected by OA, and worldwide figures suggest that OA is the fifth most common form of disability.[1]

Figures are set to rise due to:

- ↑ growing elderly and chronic disease populations.
- ↑ obesity.
- ↓ physical activity.
- ↑ prevalence of multimorbidities.

As the world's population continues to age, it is estimated that OA might affect at least 130 million individuals around the globe by 2050.[2]

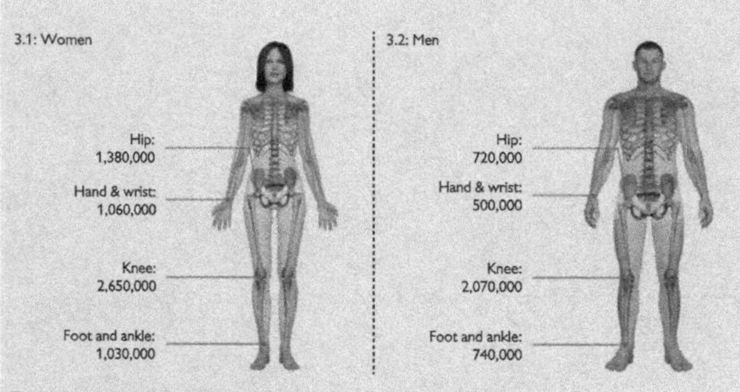
3.1: Women
Hip: 1,380,000
Hand & wrist: 1,060,000
Knee: 2,650,000
Foot and ankle: 1,030,000
3.2: Men
Hip: 720,000
Hand & wrist: 500,000
Knee: 2,070,000
Foot and ankle: 740,000
This schematic shows the estimated number of women and men in the UK who have sought treatment for osteoarthritis in four regions of the body which are often affected.*
*Based on 7 year consultation prevalence in general practice, see Annex I for methods.

Fig. 2.1 OA in four regions of the body.

Reproduced from: *Osteoarthritis in General Practice* July 2013 ARUK with kind permission from Versus Arthriti.

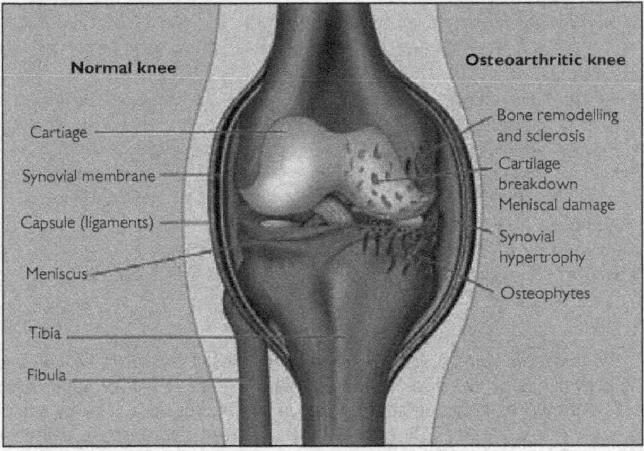

Fig. 2.2 Normal joint and OA changes in the knee.
Reproduced with permission from *Practice Nursing* (2008).

Box 2.1 Causes of osteoarthritis

Causes of OA can be attributed to:

- 1° idiopathic.
- 1° to:
  - Local mechanical causes—post trauma, sports injury (e.g. rugby player).
  - Metabolic or systemic predisposition (e.g. familial OA).
  - Pre-existing joint disease (e.g. RA or gout).
  - Haemochromatosis.
  - Hypermobility.

Box 2.2 Signs on examination

- Mild cool effusions—non-inflammatory.
- Restricted, painful ranges of motion (ROMs).
- Crepitus on movement.
- Stiffness of joint on movement —'gelling'.
- Tenderness on palpation around joint margin of affected joint.
- Changes at joint margins, e.g. 'squaring' of OA of the base of the thumb or presence of bony changes/thickening of joint on palpation.

Box 2.3 Symptoms of osteoarthritis

The key symptom related to OA is that of joint pain usually in association with:

- Activity and relieved when the joint is rested—particularly in early phases of OA.
- In lower limbs, joint pain may be exacerbated by weight bearing.
- Pain is often accompanied by stiffness (lasting <30 min) after periods of prolonged rest or inactivity. Often referred to as 'gelling'.

In addition, individuals may:

- Complain of 'crepitus' (grating sound) on movement.
- Report changes in functional ability—↓ in ROM and ↓ joint stability.

It is less common to see OA changes in those <40 years of age and the prevalence of OA does ↑ with age. Approximately half of adults aged >50 years will have radiographic evidence of OA, yet not all will be symptomatic. For example, 25% of individuals X-rayed demonstrate evidence of knee OA but only 13% are symptomatic. See Box 2.1 for causes of OA.

Approximately 4.7 million people over the age of 45 have symptomatic knee OA, and 2.12 million have hip OA.[3]

References

1. Murray CJ, Vos T, Lozano R, et al. (2012). Disability-adjusted life years (DALYs) for 291 diseases and injuries in 21 regions, 1990–2010: a systematic analysis for the Global Burden of Disease Study 2010. *Lancet* 380:2197–223.
2. Maiese K (2016). Picking a bone with WISP1 (CCCN4): new strategies against degenerative joint disease. *J Transl Sci* 1:83–5.
3. Arthritis Research UK (2013). *Osteoarthritis in General Practice: Data and Perspectives.* Chesterfield: Arthritis Research UK.

Further reading

Clunie GPR, Wilkinson N, Nikiphorou E, Jadon D (eds) (2018). *Oxford Handbook of Rheumatology*, 4th edn. Oxford: Oxford University Press.

Hochberg M, Gravallese E, Silman A, et al. (eds) (2018). *Rheumatology*, 7th edn. Philadelphia, PA: Elsevier Inc.

Clinical features and investigations

OA is a heterogeneous group of conditions sharing common features (such as anatomical changes) yet functional impairment, pain, and stiffness vary significantly and do not necessarily correlate with radiological damage.

The features of OA can be categorized as:

- Nodal generalized OA (tends to affect small joints).
- Erosive OA (uncommon): episodes of inflammation and erosive changes on X-ray.
- Large-joint OA.

In OA, the most common joints affected are:

- Distal and proximal joints of the fingers and thumb (Fig. 2.3):
  - Changes at base of thumb (carpometacarpal (CMC)).
  - Proximal interphalangeal (PIP) joints (Bouchard's nodes can sometimes be palpated).
  - Distal interphalangeal (DIP) joints (Heberden's nodes can sometimes be palpated).
- The weight-bearing lower limbs:
  - Hip and knee.
  - Feet (commonly hallux valgus (bunion)).
- Spine (facet joints).

Signs and symptoms

SeeBoxes 2.2 and 2.3.

Diagnosis and investigations

OA is chiefly a clinical diagnosis requiring a thorough musculoskeletal examination, history taking, and patient-reported symptoms (➔ see 'Assessing pain', p. 292). The presence of joint pain for most days of the previous month is used in many diagnostic criteria.[1]

Where diagnosis is in doubt, or in complex cases, further investigations may include:

- Radiological or magnetic resonance imaging (MRI) investigations.

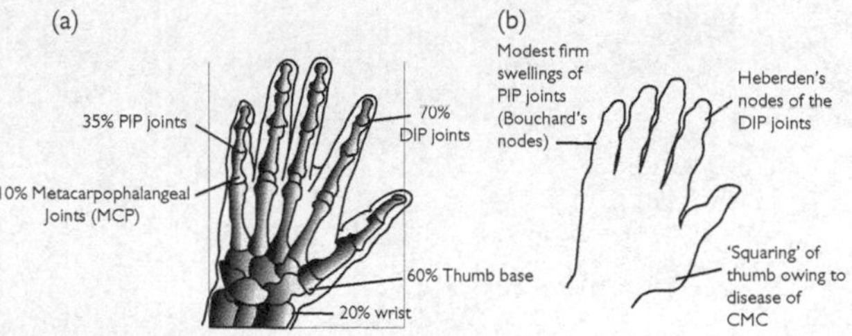

Fig. 2.3 The osteoarthritic hand. (a) Joint involvement. (b) Fingers and thumb affected by OA.

- Synovial fluid analysis, e.g. to exclude gout.
- Evidence of mechanical problems, e.g. true 'locking of joint' or loose bodies—may require referral.
- Blood tests for evidence of inflammatory markers—erythrocyte sedimentation rate (ESR), C-reactive protein (CRP)—or urate.
- 2° OA as a result of other conditions, e.g. haemochromatosis or Wilson's disease.

Reference

1. Arden N, Cooper C (eds) (2006). *Osteoarthritis Handbook*. London: Taylor and Francis.

Further reading

National Institute for Health and Care Excellence (NICE) (2014). *Osteoarthritis: Care and Management in Adults*. Clinical Guideline 177. London: NICE. https://www.nice.org.uk/guidance/cg177

Hip and knee

Weight-bearing joints affected by OA commonly result in significant disability. Hip and knee OA show variable outcomes and rates of progression. Hip OA tends to show the worst overall outcome of the major sites affected by OA.

Diagnostic features for peripheral joint OA

- Persistent joint pain worse with activity.
- Age ≥45 years.
- Morning stiffness lasting no more than 30 min—'gelling'.
- Absence of raised inflammatory markers—ESR, CRP, plasma viscosity (PV).

In addition, the most common problems related to hip and knee OA include:

- Pain on walking/using stairs/prolonged standing.
- Getting in and out of buses or cars/getting up from low chairs/toilets.
- Adjusting footwear.

Hip OA

In the UK, 2.1 million people have sought treatment for hip OA.

The course of the disease varies with most of those affected demonstrating slow progression, while some cases show rapid deterioration (Box 2.4).

Knee OA

In the UK, 4.72 million people have sought treatment for knee OA, and 14 million people in the US have symptomatic knee OA.

The knee is complex with two joints (tibiofemoral and patellofemoral sharing a joint cavity) but three compartments (medial and lateral tibiofemoral and patellofemoral). Obesity is an important contributing factor in OA of the knee. The subtle changes in load bearing of the joint may be as a result of underlying disorders of the anatomy. If there are varus or valgus deformities, the load distribution of the joint will be altered and will result in different stresses to the joint (Fig. 2.4).

The most common presentation for symptomatic knee OA is combined tibiofemoral and patellofemoral changes including irregularly distributed loss of cartilage, sclerosis of subchondral bone, and osteophytes. The predisposing factors for 2° knee OA fall into two groups:

- Young ♂ with isolated knee OA—usually due to previous trauma or surgical interventions, e.g. meniscectomy.
- Middle aged (predominantly ♀) with generalized OA.

Obesity is strongly associated with OA of the knee; see Box 2.4. The core management principles for OA are outlined in ➔ 'Advice and general management issues', p. 22.

Further reading

Hochberg M, Gravallese E, Silman A, et al. (eds) (2018). *Rheumatology*, 7th edn. Philadelphia, PA: Elsevier Inc.

Box 2.4 Signs, symptoms, and investigations for hip and knee osteoarthritis

Signs and symptoms for hip OA

- Pain and stiffness of hip particularly on activity (walking)—reports of pain in buttock, groin, front of thigh, or in the knee (20%).
- Changes in gait (antalgic gait)—Trendelenburg sign (tipping of pelvis before walking).
- Loss of internal rotation ↑ pain.
- Crepitus may be audible.
- Joint swelling cannot be detected on examination.
- X-ray is not indicated routinely but if done must be standing anterior–posterior view.

Specific investigations for hip OA

X-ray to:

- Examine degree of damage.
- Confirm diagnosis or identify contributing factors, e.g. susceptibility following trauma, avascular necrosis.

Signs and symptoms for knee OA

- Pain and stiffness on mobilizing or weight bearing.
- Crepitus may be audible.
- Joint changes may be palpable around the joint margin—osteophytes.
- Later stages may show signs of muscle wasting and valgus or varus deformity.
- Pain on climbing stairs or sensation of 'giving way'.
- Effusions may be present with 2° inflammatory process—aspirate from an OA joint with mild or no inflammation is viscous with a low cell count, unlike inflammatory fluid which has a high cell count and is non-viscous.

Specific investigations for knee OA

- Crepitus or bony swelling may be present on joint margins.

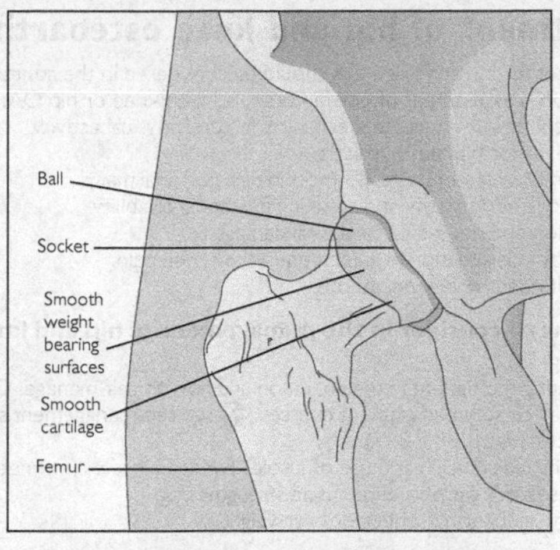

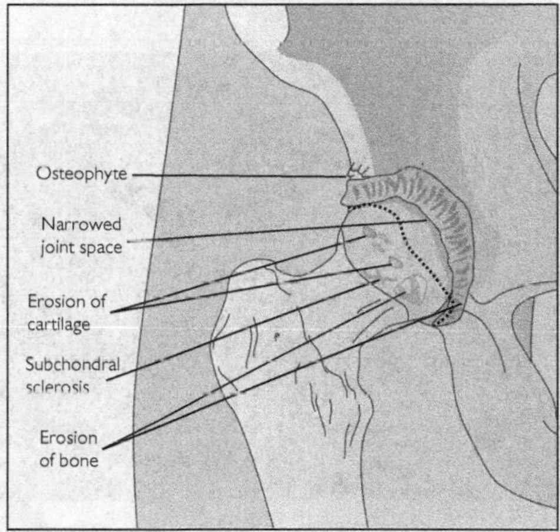

Fig. 2.4 OA of the hip.

Reproduced with permission of Clinical Skills Ltd.

Treatment of hip and knee osteoarthritis

Treatment for hip and knee OA should be considered in the context of:

- A tailored assessment of risk factors relating to knee or hip OA:
  - Knee: obesity, adverse mechanical factors, physical activity.
  - Hip: as for hip plus dysplasia.
- General risk factors: age, co-morbidities, polypharmacy.
- Level of pain intensity and resulting functional disability.
- Location and degree of structural damage.
- Signs of inflammation, e.g. joint effusion in knee pain.
- Patient needs and expectations.

Options to consider in the management of hip and knee OA

- See Fig. 2.5.
- Educating the patient in the condition and how to self-manage. Consider referral for self-management courses (➔ see self-management sections, Chapter 19, pp. 343–347).
- Walking aids (sticks) and use of insoles (wedged insoles for knee).
- Exercises, e.g. aerobic and muscle strengthening.
- Weight reduction if obese or overweight.

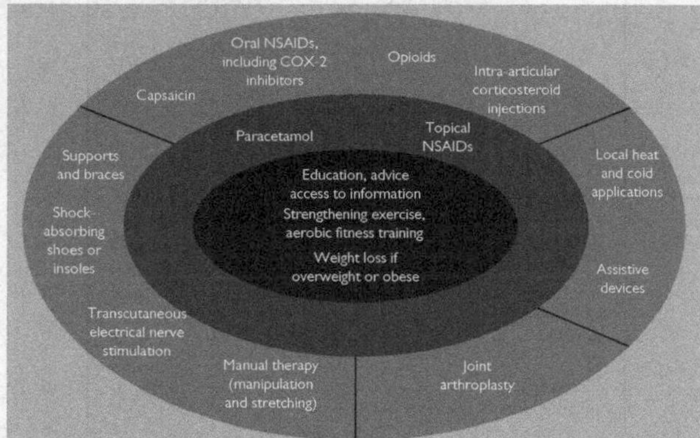

Fig. 2.5 Treatments for OA in adults. The core treatments (centre) should be considered first for every person with OA. If further treatment is required, consider the drugs in the second circle before the drugs in the outer circle. The outer circle shows other treatments to be considered if there is persistent pain or disability.

Reproduced from Conaghan P. Dickson J. and Grant R. (2008) Care and management of osteoarthritis in adults: summary of NICE guidance, *The BMJ* (2008)336:502 with permission from the British Medical Journal Publishing Group.

- Analgesia:
  - First-choice paracetamol for long-term pain relief but as part of a comprehensive treatment package (regular dosing regimen to maximum indicated doses). Refer to the *British National Formulary* (*BNF*).[1]
  - Consider topical NSAIDs or capsaicin (knee).
  - Additional pain relief may be required. This treatment option must be based upon a patient-centred risk assessment and contraindications/ cautions and patient choice. Consider:
    —Non-steroidal anti-inflammatory drugs (NSAIDs) may be indicated for short-term pain relief. Prescribe at lowest effective dose for shortest duration. Refer to the *BNF*.[1]
    —Compound analgesia or opiates may be indicated for some patients.
- Self-management aids (thermotherapy, walking aids, footwear, pacing, and muscle strengthening exercises) (➔ see self-management sections, Chapter 10, pp. 343–347).
- Intra-articular (IA) steroid injection for treatment if a 2° inflammatory component present:
  - Knee—particularly if signs of effusion.
  - Hip—injections should be guided by ultrasound (US) or X-ray.
- Joint replacement surgery for those who have symptomatic and radiographic evidence and where pain, stiffness, and reduced function impact quality of life and fail to respond adequately to non-surgical treatments.
- Knee: a knee brace may reduce pain and improve function.
- Hip: manual therapies (stretching of shortened muscles).

Reference

1. Joint Formulary Committee (2019). *British National Formulary*, 78th edn. London: British Medical Association and Royal Pharmaceutical Society of Great Britain. https://bnf.nice.org.uk/

Hand, wrist, foot, and ankle osteoarthritis

Hand and wrist OA

Symptomatic hand and wrist OA affect 1.6 million people in the UK, and 1 in 12 people in the US have hand OA.

Many people fail to seek medical advice yet the impact and associated disability are significant, affecting many activities related to dexterity and hand function (➲ see functional issues sections, pp. 308 and 361). Over 600,000 ♀ of working age have sought treatment for hand and wrist OA.

The prevalence of hand OA is higher in ♀ and ↑ with age yet has a good prognosis. Hand OA is associated with knee OA and obesity. Hallmarks of OA include nodes which may be initially painful (active) but usually settle with bony overgrowth (osteophytes) (➲ see Fig. 2.3, p. 15):

- Heberden's nodes—DIP swelling on superior-lateral margins of joint.
- Bouchard's nodes—PIP swelling on superior-lateral margins of joint.

Poorly localized pain and tenderness around the wrist may be related to thumb OA. Crepitus may be present. In severe disease, deformities and 'squaring off of the base of thumb' can be seen. The loss of movement and joint deformity in the thumb and digits required particularly for pinch grip may create functional problems due to loss of manual dexterity. Loss of movement in the wrist and functional changes are similar to those outlined for the hand.

Hand and wrist OA core treatment issues

- Refer to core management advice on all OA treatments.
- Core treatment should be provided to those presenting with symptomatic OA of the hand or foot.

Treatment should be individualized and considered in the context of:

- Patient anxieties, needs, and expectations.
- Level of pain, impact on functioning, and quality of life.
- Type of OA—nodal, erosive, traumatic.
- Localization.
- Severity of structural damage.
- Additional risk factors—age, work-related issues, co-morbidities.
- See Boxes 2.5 and 2.6.

Foot and ankle OA

In the UK, 1.8 million people have sought treatment for foot and ankle OA. Ankle involvement is uncommon (related to previous injury, e.g. previous fracture site); however, the forefoot is the main site for OA of the first metatarsophalangeal (MTP) joint. Hallux valgus (bunion) is extremely common in ♀ (Fig. 2.6). Relationship to generalized OA is unclear. The bunion is related to the use of modern footwear and is painful on walking or localized pressure.

➲ Also see 'Treatment options', p. 29.

Box 2.5 Hand- and wrist-specific treatment issues

- Education and advice on avoiding mechanical aggravating factors.
- Strengthening and mobility exercise.
- Topical NSAID or capsaicin cream.
- Joint protection—based upon expert opinion and limited research evidence:
  - Referral to occupational therapist for joint protection and assistive devices, e.g. tap turners.
  - A wrist component to splints for base of thumb OA will improve efficacy.
- Local heat or cold applications (as an adjunct to treatments) encourage self-management strategies and can be safely used.
- Surgery may be beneficial for severe base of thumb OA if refractory to conventional treatment.

Box 2.6 Foot-specific treatment issues

- Advice on the use of insoles, and footwear with shock-absorbing properties —limited evidence but cost-effective.
- Topical NSAID or capsaicin cream.
- Referral for footwear advice may be appropriate depending upon functional issues and severity.
- Hallux valgus and hallux rigidus—surgery may be appropriate to correct deformities.

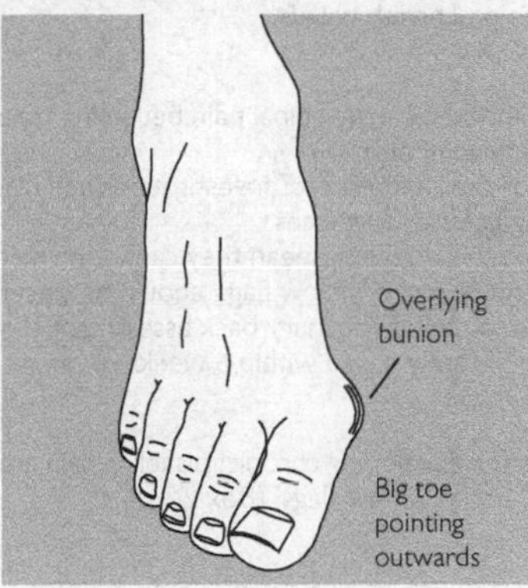

Example of bunion (hallux valgus) OA of foot.

Fig. 2.6 OA foot bunion (hallux valgus).

Reproduced with kind permission from the Arthritis Research Campaign (ARC).

Further reading

Arthritis Foundation. What is osteoarthritis? https://www.arthritis.org/about-arthritis/types/osteoarthritis/what-is-osteoarthritis.php

Neck and spine

Joints of the spinal column may show many of the changes evident in peripheral joints. If symptoms are not due to serious pathology, pain in spinal joints can be managed in the same way as peripheral joint pain.

Prevalence of spinal (back and neck) pain

- Back and neck pain are very common, about 60–80% of people will get spinal pain at some time in their life.
- Often starts for no apparent reason, or after everyday activities, e.g. gardening, poor sitting or sleep postures, and working environment.
- Recovery (or lack of) is unpredictable.
- <5% of people with spinal pain have a diagnosable condition, such as irritation of a nerve root (radicular pain) or spinal stenosis.
- Very few (<1%) have a serious medical problem.

Natural course of spinal pain

- Most spinal pain resolves within 6–8 weeks.
- Most people have long-term episodic periods of relatively little or no pain interspersed with acute 'flares' of pain.
- 15–20% develop chronic, disabling pain.

Examination and investigations

- Rarely establish a clear-cut cause of the pain.
- This often results in multiple, inconsistent, false diagnoses, inappropriate advice, anxiety, and undermining confidence in management and reinforcing unhelpful health beliefs.

Management

Reducing the likelihood of acute spinal pain becoming chronic and disabling is a key aim of management.

- Be honest about the limitations of investigations and diagnosis.
- Avoid confusing pseudo-diagnoses.
- Reassure people this does not mean they cannot be helped.

Individuals with one or more 'yellow flags' should be closely monitored and referred (ideally to a multidisciplinary back assessment clinic) if their symptoms have not significantly eased within 6 weeks of presentation.

Yellow flags

The main reasons for developing chronic, disabling pain are the presence of psychological and social 'yellow flags' (Box 2.7).

Red flags

People who present with a 'red flag' (Box 2.8) should be closely assessed and, if necessary, referred for investigation to eliminate serious pathology.

Box 2.7 'Yellow flags' for the risk for developing chronic pain and disability

- Belief that pain and activity are harmful.
- 'Sickness behaviours'—extended rest, fear avoidance.
- Low or negative moods, social withdrawal.
- Treatment that does not fit best practice—extended bed rest, opiate use.
- Problems with insurance claims and accident compensation.
- History of back pain, time-off, or other claims.
- Problems at work or poor job satisfaction.
- Heavy work or unsociable hours.
- Overprotective family or lack of support.

Box 2.8 'Red flags'—if present consider referring for investigation

- Age <20 or >55 years.
- Systemically unwell.
- Weight loss.
- Persistent night pain (lying more than sitting)—indicator to consider malignancy.
- Cancer, steroids, HIV, or other significant past history.
- Widespread neurology (>one nerve root) or progressive motor weakness in the legs or gait disturbance.
- Cauda equina syndrome—indicators might include radicular pain, sensory loss, difficulty with micturition, faecal incontinence, and saddle anaesthesia.
- Thoracic pain.
- Violent trauma—e.g. fall from a height or road traffic accident.
- Constant, progressive, non-mechanical pain—capsular pattern.
- Persisting, severe restriction of lumbar flexion or structural deformity.
- Inflammatory disorders (e.g. AS)—pain worse at night, often accompanied by early morning stiffness (EMS).

Management of osteoarthritis spinal pain

Encouraging people to stay active is of the utmost importance. Consider:

- Advice to rest completely or take more than a few days off work ↑ the chance of long-term disability.
- People might take things easier for a day or two, but even during this time they must be encouraged to be gently active.
- Challenge fear-avoidance beliefs and behaviours that lead to muscle weakness, joint damage and pain, ↓ activity, disability, and dependency.
- Advise about changing lifestyle to include participation in regular exercise and physical activity.
- Teaching 'rest–activity cycling' (interspersing bouts of exercise and activity with short rests).
- Suggest ways people can protect their back in the work/home environment provides control and avoids exacerbating their pain.
    - Apply heat (place a hot-water bottle wrapped in a towel on back for 5–10 min, or take a hot bath) before or after exercise or unavoidable activities that ↑ pain (e.g. gardening, work).
    - Empathetically explore psychological and social factors (e.g. relationships, work problems) that might contribute to the problem.

Advice and general management issues

Overview

OA is a heterogeneous condition. Radiological evidence of OA may be evident, yet the individual may be symptom free. OA presents a significant health burden with prevalence set to rise. It is essential for practitioners in all care settings to provide, at the minimum, core information and support to those presenting with symptomatic OA. Pain is the predominant feature and is usually the driver for seeking a medical consultation.

Presentation in the clinical setting can vary significantly, from individuals presenting with OA of the base of the thumb, with an insidious onset of pain and minor functional difficulties, right through to others presenting with severe and rapidly progressing joint pain that causes significant loss of function as a result of OA of the hip. There are a number of factors that need to be considered in the management of those with symptomatic OA. Management should be tailored according to:

- Disease presentation, severity, and treatment options.
- Impact of pain, stiffness, and functional changes to the individual.
- Psychological, social (including age, cultural background), and work-related issues.
- Prior understanding and knowledge of the condition and how to self-manage.
- Additional co-morbidities and the vulnerable—consider in treatment plan.

The evidence base behind treatment recommendations is usually based on studies and efficacy of one or two specific joint sites (often the knee joint); ∴ advice and evidence needs to be considered in the context of the specific joints (e.g. weight loss may not be appropriate for OA hand, although evidence suggests OA hand is linked to obesity). Expert opinion and systematic reviews of research evidence identify 'core' aspects of management that should be offered to every person presenting with signs of symptoms of OA.

Core treatment and patient-centred assessment

Decisions about core treatment and additional treatment needs must be considered following a thorough history taking and clinical examination, which should include a holistic assessment to identify the individual's specific anxieties, needs, and expectations in the context of their condition (Table 2.1). The benefits of a patient-centred approach include:

- The informed patient can consider their pathway of care applying self-management principles with the potential to enhance self-efficacy.
- Improvement in patient outcomes and reduction in resource inefficiencies (↓ referrals and investigations).
- Positive health-seeking behaviours will enable individuals to seek information on their condition, treatment options, and how to access services.

Supporting these principles, verbal information must be reinforced by providing written information. Equally, individuals should be offered a review of educational needs as well as a review of treatment benefits.

Table 2.1 Holistic assessment of osteoarthritis

Assessment	Consider	Effects on the individual	Consider
Disease	• Joint involved and severity of symptoms	• Joint abnormalities • ↓ muscle strength • ↓ functional ability	Confirmation of diagnosis Symptom control/ functional ability
Pain	• Pain score • Distribution and description of pain experienced • Duration of pain	• ↓ quality of life • Fatigue, disturbed sleep • Difficulties in work and activities of daily living (ADLs)	• Family responsibilities • ADLs • Work-related factors
Knowledge, expectations, attitudes, and beliefs	• Knowledge of condition • Patient expectations • Health beliefs and behaviours • Coping styles/ self-efficacy • Cultural factors	• Ability to undertake positive health-seeking behaviours • Fears and anxieties about limitations • Beliefs about medications	• Educational needs • Concordance • Prior experiences in relation to health and illness • Relationship/ support by significant family/ friends • Cultural and religious beliefs
Psychological	• Anxiety and depression • Coping styles • Self-image • Perceptions of chronic disease status	• Negative mood, fatigue • Negative coping styles • Poor self-esteem	• Tailored information giving • Support groups • Information sharing and education • Management of co-morbidities
Social	• Level of social need • Social support available—significant other	• Financial burden • Social isolation • Loss of independence	• Carer needs and abilities • Maintaining independence and functional ability • Community, voluntary, or social services support

Treatment options

There are pharmacological and non-pharmacological treatment options available for OA. A combination of these treatment modalities should be offered to individuals presenting with symptoms, in the context of the joints affected and tailored to specific needs following a full holistic, patient-centred assessment (Table 2.2) (➲ also see nursing issues sections, pp. 330 and 326; ➲ 'Patient-centred care', p. 332). The level of treatment required and support necessary will vary according to:

- Disease severity and functional loss.
- Impact on the individual's quality of life and activities of daily living (ADLs).
- Other compounding factors such as co-morbidities.

Core treatments—pharmacological

- Paracetamol (prescribed up to 4 g per day) should be regularly taken over 24 hours when pain relief is required. For those failing to achieve pain relief on paracetamol, check dose and frequency of administration (may be suboptimal).
- Topical NSAIDs (knee and hand) or topical capsaicin cream.
- Where topical NSAIDs and paracetamol are ineffective consider:
  - An alternative NSAID/cyclooxygenase (COX)-2 inhibitor (➲ see 'NSAIDs', p. 438), or
  - Addition of an opiate (rarely indicated in OA) after a thorough risk–benefit assessment of the patient has been made (caution in the elderly).

Core treatments—non-pharmacological

Individuals with symptomatic OA should be offered the following core advice and treatments:

- Information and education about the condition and how to self-manage symptoms including non-pharmacological advice and information on complementary therapies.
- Exercise advice—irrespective of age, co-morbidity, pain, or severity of condition. Exercises should include:
  - Local muscle-strengthening exercises above and below the affected joint, e.g. quadriceps for the knee.
  - General aerobic fitness.
- Consider referral to a self-management programme (e.g. expert patient programme (EPP)) if appropriate.
- Weight loss/support for weight loss.

Review of treatment

For those whose symptoms fail to be managed using core treatments, a prompt reassessment should consider additional treatment options available to the patient.

A review of the individual's holistic assessment should also consider building on information and education about the condition with the aim of enhancing self-efficacy. Building the individual's ability to understand and manage their condition is not a 'one-stop shop' but an ongoing programme of information giving, tailored to their specific needs.

Table 2.2 Holistic assessment of person with osteoarthritis

Social	Effect on life • ADLs • Family duties • Hobbies Lifestyle expectations
Health beliefs	Concerns Expectations Current knowledge of OA
Occupational	Ability to perform job: • Short term • Long term Adjustments to the home or workplace
Mood	Screen for depression Other current stresses in life
Quality of sleep	
Support network	Ideas, concerns, and expectations of the main carer How carer is coping Isolation
Other musculoskeletal pain	Evidence of a chronic pain syndrome Other treatable sources of pain
Attitudes to exercise	
Influence of co-morbidity	Interaction of two or more morbidities Falls Assessment of most appropriate drug therapy Understanding surgical options Fitness for surgery
Pain assessment	Self-help strategies Analgesics: • Drugs, doses, frequency, timing • Side effects

Data sourced from NICE (2014) Osteoarthritis: care and management Clinical guideline. Available from https://www.nice.org.uk/guidance/cg177.

Additional pharmacological and non-pharmacological treatment options

💣 The use of NSAIDs (traditional and the newer generation of COX-2 inhibitors) may be required for those who have pain unresponsive to core treatments.

The use of these therapies must be considered carefully in the context of:

- The individual's specific gastrointestinal (GI), renal, and cardiovascular risk factors.
- NSAIDs should be prescribed at the lowest possible effective dose for the shortest duration (e.g. to ease the pain during an exacerbation of symptoms). See Box 2.9 for NSAID prescribing advice.

In severe disease, NSAIDs may be required in addition to paracetamol or opiates.

IA joint injections

- For flare of joints—particularly if signs of inflammation (warm, effusion)—consider corticosteroid injections.

Non-pharmacological options as an adjunct to treatment

- Exercise.
- Weight loss if obese (weight-bearing joints).
- Use of aids and devices/walking aids/insoles—braces may be beneficial in the presence of varus deformity (knee)
    - Complementary and alternative therapies for pain relief: 💣
    - Fish oil supplements (omega-3 fatty acids) have shown some benefit for pain relief. Further research is required.

NICE no longer recommends glucosamine or acupuncture.[1] If patients elect to take these options, they should be informed of the limited evidence and advised not to stop any prescribed medication.

- Use of cold packs or hot packs for topical symptom relief.

Physiotherapy treatments

- Stretching and strengthening exercises (hip and knee).
- Land and water-based exercise is beneficial (hip and knee).

Surgical interventions

- For those whose symptoms impact significantly on their quality of life and fail to be adequately controlled using non-surgical management, referral should be considered for joint replacement surgery.
- 💣 If a clear history of mechanical 'locking' arthroscopy or debridement may be required:
    - Arthroscopic lavage and debridement is not considered necessary for the treatment of general symptoms related to OA.
- Osteotomy and joint-preserving procedures should be considered for young adults in the presence of dysplasia or valgus/varus deformity.

References

1. NICE (2014). *Osteoarthritis: Care and Management in Adults*. Clinical Guideline 177. London: NICE. https://www.nice.org.uk/guidance/cg177
2. Joint Formulary Committee (2019). *British National Formulary*, 78th edn. London: British Medical Association and Royal Pharmaceutical Society of Great Britain.

Further reading

Osthoff AKR, Niedermann K, Braun J, et al. (2018). 2018 EULAR recommendations for physical activity in people with inflammatory arthritis and osteoarthritis. *Ann Rheum Dis* 77:1251–60.

When to refer

OA is not one clearly defined disease but represents joint failure at a specific site, or sites, accompanied by the symptoms of pain, stiffness, and limited functional ability. In most cases of OA the deterioration is slow with gradual limitation as a result of the symptoms experienced. Approximately 80% of all hip and knee replacements are attributed to OA.

Symptoms may be constant or, more commonly, relapsing and remitting.

The first step in the pathway of care must include patient education about the condition and treatments available, encouraging the patient's ability to self-manage using a range of options that might include pharmacological and non-pharmacological pain-relieving strategies. The patient's reported symptoms, joint (or joints) involved, and length of time between relapsing and remitting symptoms will help inform the practitioner of treatment benefits.

In many cases, surgery may never be required although additional treatment options may be needed from time to time. For others, particularly those with OA in load-bearing joints such as the knees or hips, the condition can rapidly deteriorate with the accompanying changes in functional ability. It is therefore important to recognize when to refer patients who do not gain benefit from early treatment. Specific scoring systems have been developed to aid clinicians identify those who need to receive prompt surgery (➔ see Chapter 7, 'Elective orthopaedic surgery', Chapter 7, pp. 250–252).

Joint replacement surgery is expensive, although generally an effective intervention with improved postoperative outcomes.

Features that should prompt the nurse to consider referral for a medical/surgical opinion include:

- Joint pain that wakes the patient at night.
- Moderate to severe pain that is not effectively treated by pharmacological or non-pharmacological options.
- Moderate to severe functional impairment.
- Joint pain that places a significant burden on the patient, e.g. work limitations or loss of independence—inability to undertake ADLs effectively.
- Doubts about the diagnosis of OA or changes in symptoms, joints affected.
- Patients who may require psychological assessment, e.g.:
  - Inability to alter perceptions of pain despite treatment with a range of pharmacological options.
  - A patient who demonstrates anxiety, depression, or persistently rates pain as maximum score.

Integrated care pathways (ICPs) are often used to aid management and have particular value in surgical interventions such as total hip or knee replacements.

Factors that need to be considered prior to referral for a surgical intervention will include:

- Has the patient been offered other treatment options (pharmacological and non-pharmacological) without sufficient sustained benefit?
- General health and ability to undergo an anaesthetic.
- The patient's wish to undergo surgery.

Box 2.9 NSAIDs

Note: consider NSAIDs and COX-2 as a continuum of drugs within one class with differing side effect profiles (called NSAIDs). Refer to the *BNF*.[2]

All patients

- Consider prior treatments prescribed and side effects/benefits.
- Review renal function (urea and electrolytes (U&Es)).
- Prescriptions for NSAIDs should be at the lowest effective dose for the shortest duration. NICE recommends the co-prescription of a proton pump inhibitor (PPI) (including COX-2 inhibitors)[1] (➲ see 'NSAIDs and COX-2', p. 438).
- Review efficacy, health status, and treatment plan.
- Identify risk factors related to changes in treatment, e.g. risk of falls with opiates.

Assessment for NSAIDs

Risk factor:

- Age <65 years.
- No GI risk factors.
- No cardiovascular risk factors.
- No age-related or renal risk factors.

Prescribing plan: standard NSAID with PPI at lowest possible dose for shortest duration.

Risk factor:

- All age groups.
- GI risk factors and no cardiovascular risks.

Prescribing plan: all NSAIDs are recommended to be prescribed with a PPI (select appropriate therapy with a good GI profile + PPI).[2]

Risk factor: cardiovascular risk—on low-dose aspirin.

Prescribing plan: select other analgesia prior to NSAIDs (e.g. opiates).

Risk factor: renal insufficiency or frail elderly.

Prescribing plan: consider compound analgesics (e.g. co-codamol 8/500) or opiates (e.g. tramadol hydrochloride) or other pain-relieving strategies where appropriate (e.g. joint injections). *Caution*: opiates—lower doses in the elderly (opioid side effects).

- Absence of infections—particularly in or around surrounding tissues.
- The potential success of the proposed surgical intervention, e.g.:
  - Hip and knee replacement surgery will be negatively affected if the patient is obese or is unable to actively rehabilitate postoperatively.
  - Patient expectations and ability to rehabilitate need to be considered.

Equity of access for surgical interventions

Evidence has demonstrated that socially deprived groups and some ethnic groups or minority groups (e.g. visual impairment) may be less likely to receive total hip or knee replacements.

Lack of access may be related to:

- Lower expectations of treatment access.
- Anxiety in seeking a medical opinion.
- Experiencing difficulty in articulating their needs to healthcare professionals.
- Having other health/co-morbidity/risk factors that result in reduced referral for surgical opinion.

Frequently asked questions

I never really know what to do when someone comes into my clinic and starts talking about their joint pain. I worry it might be something serious like septic arthritis

Joint pain can cover a multitude of problems including acute conditions such as septic arthritis. The first thing to do is to take a good clinical history and examine the joint(s) affected and compare it against the unaffected joint. Patients with septic arthritis usually have severe pain and will not want you to touch the joint; they may have rapid and dramatic onset of pain, with a tender swollen joint that is warm/hot to touch—however, there are cases that don't always fit this criteria so if the patient presents with these described symptoms, until you have developed your knowledge of joint diseases, ensure your provisional diagnosis is confirmed by the GP/physician. If OA is confirmed, make sure you educate the patient about their condition and start the process of self-management.

What is the first thing I should think about when someone presents with newly diagnosed OA?

Undertake a patient-centred consultation (including an assessment of pain). You will then know how much of an issue the joint pain is to the patient and what they understand about their problems. Make sure you start the process promptly when giving information and, based upon the symptoms and joints affected, offer a number of practical tips (e.g. wearing 'sensible' shoes) as well as non-pharmacological options (pacing) and pharmacological support based upon what the patient has already tried. Check the dosages and frequency of self-medications.

It seems to me there still isn't enough evidence to support many of the complementary therapies patients take for their OA—should I advise them not to take them?

Most patient wish to explore the option of taking complementary therapies and this may enhance their own perception of self-efficacy. You may be asked your opinion of treatment options—the most important thing to say is that although the evidence may not be sufficient for us to recommend such treatments, if they are going to take them they need to ensure they evaluate them carefully in relation to cost and benefits achieved. Importantly, you must encourage an open and transparent relationship so that they will report what therapies they are taking.

How can we help patients with their pain when the risks of NSAIDs now mean they can only have these prescribed in the short term and at the lowest effective dose?

Pain relief is a basic human right and we must ensure patients do get effective treatment. However, we often fail to encourage patients to take their simple analgesia (at maximum prescribed dose on a regular dosing regimen) so we should apply these principles together with an objective assessment of pain (for instance, using a visual analogue scale). Paracetamol can be an effective treatment for many provided it is prescribed at maximum doses and taken at regular intervals to maintain therapeutic levels. NSAIDs do have an important place in the treatment plan, but they must be used with adjunct therapies that will help to moderate the symptoms and reduce reliance on NSAIDs. Remember, topical NSAIDs/capsaicin cream may be of value particularly for small joints. However, the ultimate point must be to ensure that patients who need additional pain relief have an opportunity to make a fully informed decision about their treatment options based upon their individual risk factors.

Which patients should I refer to a self-management programme?

In reality, all patients should have access to the same level of care, including self-management. However, it is helpful if you understand a little bit about the patient and their prior knowledge of the condition before asking them whether they would like to participate in a self-management programme. Key points to consider are:

- Able and willingness to attend a self-management course.
- Prior knowledge of the condition and treatment.
- Other co-morbidities/conditions/medications.
- Level of social support or other voluntary support accessed.
- Their health beliefs/behaviours.
- Prior history of concordance with treatments/attendance of programmes.
- The individual's ability and wish to socialize/interact within a group setting.

These points are not discriminatory but are of value in considering:

- Which individuals might gain the most benefit from the course.
- When the option would be most positively received by the patient.

Chapter 3

Osteoporosis

Overview

Definition

The World Health Organization (WHO, 2001) has defined osteoporosis as 'a progressive systemic skeletal disease characterized by low bone mass and micro-architectural deterioration of bone tissue, with a consequent increase in bone fragility and susceptibility to fracture'.

Clinical features

- Osteoporosis is largely asymptomatic until fractures occur.
- Hip and spine fractures are linked to ↑ mortality and all fractures may lead to disability and reduced quality of life.

Is osteoporosis an important problem?

In the UK, osteoporosis is estimated to affect 3 million people and results in >300,000 fractures each year, with the most common fractures occurring at the forearm, femoral neck, and vertebral body. Such fractures are associated with significant morbidity; the most serious consequences arise in patients sustaining hip fracture, with a significant ↑ in mortality to >25% in the first 12 months following a fracture.

- Health and social expenditure in the UK for the treatment of osteoporotic fractures is estimated to cost £1.5 billion/year. For example, osteoporotic fractures lead to 69,000 unplanned admissions/year, equating to 1.3 million bed days.
- With an ageing population and ↑ rates of fracture incidence, it is estimated that this figure could ↑ to £3 billion/year by 2021.

What happens during bone growth?

Bone mass and bone loss

- Bone is a dynamic tissue that undergoes constant remodelling throughout life; being metabolically active it is continually formed and resorbed by bone cells known as osteoblasts and osteoclasts. This remodelling allows the skeleton to:
    - ↑ in size during growth.
    - Respond to the physical stresses.
    - Repair structural damage due to fatigue or fracture.
- Up to 90% of an individual's bone mass is deposited during skeletal growth. This is followed by a phase of consolidation lasting for up to 15 years. Bone loss starts between the ages of 35 and 40 years in both sexes, with an acceleration of bone loss in ♀ in the decade following the menopause.

What are the important factors influencing bone mass and bone loss?

Heredity

Genetic factors account for as much as 80% of the variance in peak bone mass and also influence the rates of bone loss.

Activity

Activity is vital as the associated weight bearing and muscular activity stimulates bone formation and ↑ bone mass. Immobilization may result in rapid bone loss and a decline in activity with advancing age is likely to cause further bone loss.

Nutrition

- *Dietary calcium* intake is essential to ensure attainment of peak bone mass. The role of calcium and its effect on bone loss remains controversial but skeletal losses in older life may be accelerated by low-calcium diets and evidence suggests that low calcium intakes in childhood and adolescence are associated with an ↑ risk of osteoporosis in later life.
- Prolonged *vitamin D* deficiency in childhood delays puberty and is likely to ↓ bone mass in relation to height attained. With advancing age, vitamin D absorption is reduced due to impaired percutaneous absorption and impaired metabolism. Low vitamin D levels cause ↑ parathyroid hormone (PTH) levels which can lead to ↑ bone loss in the frail older person. People with low or no exposure to the sun, including for cultural reasons and those who are housebound, or who have darker skin have a higher risk of developing vitamin D deficiency.
- *Dietary intake* of protein, sodium, fluoride, caffeine, magnesium, vitamin K, and alcohol may also influence bone mass and bone loss, but their importance remains uncertain.

Body weight

Low body weight associated with amenorrhea and eating disorders may result in ↓ bone mass. Bone loss is more rapid in postmenopausal ♀ with low body weight as there is insufficient fat tissue to convert androgens to oestrogens.

Hormonal

Gonadal hormones are probably the most important determinants of skeletal mass in ♀. Delayed menarche and persisting amenorrhoea may account for an impaired bone mass. Loss of ovarian function at the menopause leads to ↑ bone loss. There is an association between hypogonadism, low body mass, and ↑ bone loss in ♂.

2° *causes*

Bone mass and bone loss are influenced by a large number of 2° causes, including:

- Medications, particularly oral glucocorticoids.
- Malabsorption disorders, e.g. coeliac disease.
- Renal disease.
- Cancer.

Further reading

NOS (2015). The Osteoporosis Agenda England. ℘ https://nos.org.uk/media/1959/agenda-for-osteoporosis-england-final.pdf

Diagnosis

Osteoporosis is often undetected as people are usually asymptomatic. However, an index of suspicion for osteoporosis should be considered in patients who might present regularly to their GP reporting back pain or complaining of a loss of height, or those who have been admitted to hospital with a low-impact fracture in sites such as the wrist, forearm, or neck of femur, or have identified risk factors such as:

- Genetic predisposition, particularly parental history of hip fracture <75 years.
- Persistent amenorrhoea (>6 months) or early menopause.
- Malabsorption disorders, such as coeliac disease.
- Endocrine disorders, such as parathyroid disease.
- Low body mass index (BMI <19 kg/m^2).
- Prolonged use of glucocorticoids (>3 months in duration or exceeding three courses in 12 months).
- Other factors including lifestyle issues, such as inadequate dietary calcium intake, smoking, excessive alcohol consumption, smoking, and lack of exercise.

Osteoporosis can be detected using:

- Dual energy X-ray absorptiometry (DXA) is the most widely used method of measuring bone mineral density (BMD).
- X-rays will detect fractures and may suggest osteoporosis but are too insensitive to measure BMD.

What is a DXA scan?

- A scan that uses minimal doses of radiation and is a quick, non-invasive procedure.
- Provides measurements of BMD at spine and hip and may also perform total body and vertebral fracture assessment.
- Confirms the diagnosis of osteoporosis and allows the most appropriate targeting of treatment.

BMD measurements are expressed in standard deviation (SD) units. They are then compared to a reference range of young healthy adults with average bone density. The difference between this average and the reported BMD is then given as a T-score (Box 3.1). A Z-score is also calculated, and this compares the reported BMD with an age-matched range, and is most commonly applied to those <40 years old.

Box 3.1 T-scores

- Between 0 and –1 SD: normal.
- Between –1 and –2.5 SD: osteopenia.
- Below –2.5 SD: osteoporosis.

Will blood tests diagnose osteoporosis?

- Biochemical tests will not diagnose osteoporosis.
- Biochemical tests may help to identify 2° causes of bone loss, e.g. untreated thyroid disease.
- Specific serum and urine markers can measure bone turnover and may be useful in indicating rapid bone loss and also response to treatment.

Osteoporosis in premenopausal women and in men

Osteoporosis in premenopausal ♀ may be as a result of low peak bone mass, ↑ bone loss, or a combination of the two. It may be attributable to an underlying cause but may also be idiopathic.

Common causes

- Menstrual factors include persisting amenorrhoea (>6 months) due to simple oestrogen deficiency or hypothalamic hypogonadism (related to either anorexia nervosa or exercise-induced amenorrhoea).
- The use of Depo-Provera®, particularly when commenced before skeletal maturity, may be associated with low BMD. May be reversible on cessation and restoration of normal menses.
- Underlying 2° causes include:
  - Inflammatory diseases, e.g. RA.
  - Endocrine disorders, e.g. thyrotoxicosis.
  - Conditions associated with malabsorption, e.g. coeliac disease.
- Glucocorticoid therapy is the most significant cause of drug-induced osteoporosis.
- Lifestyle factors such as:
  - Prolonged immobility—a potent cause of bone loss.
  - Dietary calcium intake in childhood and adolescence may also impact peak bone mass.
  - Limited data on the relevance of smoking or alcohol intake in premenopausal ♀.

Management

- Investigation for an underlying cause (about 50% of cases may be 2°). If a cause is identified this should be treated appropriately.
- Patient education to ↑ understanding of osteoporosis and ways to optimize bone health. Reassure that absolute fracture risk is probably low. Occupational assessment and advice may be required.
- Calcium and vitamin D supplements may be required if dietary intake is poor.
- Bisphosphonates are the only licensed therapies for glucocorticoid-induced osteoporosis in premenopausal ♀. Treatment must be made on an individual basis only if the benefit is felt to outweigh the potential risk, e.g. if the patient is at an unacceptably high current risk of fracture.
- ❗ Bisphosphonates should be avoided during pregnancy and lactation. Patient must be counselled on effective contraception to avoid pregnancy while taking treatment.
- Hormone replacement therapy (HRT) may be the optimal approach in hypogonadism.
- The use of teriparatide and strontium ranelate has not been evaluated in premenopausal ♀.
- Raloxifene should not be given to premenopausal ♀ as it may ↑ bone loss.

Osteoporosis in men

Up to 20% of symptomatic vertebral fractures, 25% of forearm fractures, and 30% of hip fractures occur in ♂. The lifetime risk for a 50-year-old white ♂ in the UK has been estimated to be 2% for the forearm, 2% for the vertebra, and 3% for the hip.

♂ with low-trauma fractures tend to have lower BMD, smaller skeletal size, and more disruption of trabecular architecture than ♂ control groups of the same age.

Causes

Major causes with strong evidence:
- Hypogonadism.
- Alcoholism.
- Oral glucocorticoids.
- Following organ transplant.

Other factors:
- Low BMI.
- Smoking.
- Physical inactivity.
- Poor dietary calcium intake.
- Impaired vitamin D production.
- 2° hyperparathyroidism.
- Malabsorption syndromes.

Management
- Use of DXA to confirm osteoporosis.
- Reference ranges for BMD measurements in ♂ are derived from a smaller sample size than ♀; there is a similar inverse relationship between BMD and fracture risk.
- Investigations to exclude 2° causes. In addition to routine biochemical investigations, testosterone and gonadotrophins should be checked and prostate-specific antigen (PSA) should be measured in those with vertebral fractures, to exclude possible malignancy.
- Advice on lifestyle measures to ↓ bone loss, including a balanced diet rich in calcium, weight-bearing exercise, smoking cessation, and moderation of alcohol intake.
- Bisphosphonates are the treatment of choice for most ♂, although alendronate is the only one licensed for idiopathic osteoporosis in ♂.
- Teriparatide is licensed for male osteoporosis but is recommended only when there is severe osteoporosis or intolerance of bisphosphonates.
- Testosterone treatment has shown beneficial effects in study populations but due to potential side effects and cardiovascular risk factor profiles it has not to date been used widely.

Osteoporotic vertebral and hip fractures

Vertebral fracture

Vertebral fractures commonly present in the lower thoracic or upper lumbar spine and can occur spontaneously or as a result of minimal trauma such as coughing.

The major features may include:

- *Acute back pain*: at the specific site of fracture and may also be referred around the body in a symmetrical fashion and can mimic chest or abdominal discomfort. Pain may be accompanied by paravertebral spasm and can persist for several weeks; during this time, back movements—particularly flexion—may be limited.
- *Chronic back pain*: residual pain persists in a proportion of patients requiring long-term management with analgesia, exercises, and various psychological support mechanisms.
- *Kyphosis and height loss* which may subsequently result in ↓ lung and abdominal volumes and skeletal disproportion.
- *Quality-of-life measures* have indicated a substantial reduction in quality of life following vertebral fracture, comparable with other major diseases. These include a decline in both physical and mental functions with several studies suggesting ↑ anxiety, depression, and impaired mobility.

Hip fracture

- Common complications in the peri- and postoperative phase include cardiac and thromboembolic events, pneumonia, sepsis, urinary tract infections, the development of pressure sores, dehydration, and confusion.
- Longer term there may be loss of function and independence.
- ~40% of patients are unable to walk independently 1 year after hip fracture and 60–80% may become limited in ADL.
- In the first year after hip fracture, ~27% of patients will require nursing home care and 30% will require additional home support.
- Hip fractures are also associated with ↑ mortality with most deaths occurring in the first days and months following the fracture.

Avoiding hip fractures

>95% of hip fractures occur in association with a fall and the highest risk of fracture is observed in those people who have osteoporosis and are also at the highest risk of falling.

How should falls be addressed?

- 30% of people aged >65 years fall each year and >50% of those living in long-term care fall every year, some repeatedly.
- Recurrent falls are associated with ↑ mortality, ↑ rate of hospitalization, curtailment of daily activities, ↑ fear of falling, and loss of confidence.
- Although estimates vary, ~25% of falls result in serious injury with 1 in 40 falls resulting in a fracture. Among older people, falling accounts for 95% of hip fractures.
- >400 potential risk factors for falling have been identified. The most important of these include those related to the environment, gait/

Table 3.1 Multifactorial risk assessment and interventions

Multifactorial risk assessment	Multifactorial interventions
• Falls history	• Strength and balance training
• Gait, balance, muscle weakness	• Vision assessment
• Osteoporosis risk	• Modification of medication
• Perceived functional ability	• Identify future risk
• Vision	• Participation in falls-prevention programme
• Cognition	• Prevention programmes
• Urinary continence	
• Home hazards	
• Cardiovascular examination	
• Medication	

balance disorders or weakness, dizziness and vertigo, use of assistive devices, impaired ADLs, chronic diseases, and polypharmacy.

Randomized controlled trials of falls prevention strategies have focused on both multifactorial and unifactorial approaches. It is likely that there are a number of approaches that should be applied to reduce the risks related to falls and osteoporotic fracture.

NICE guidelines[1] considered the use of multifactorial falls risk assessment; NICE does not recommend low-intensity or untargeted group exercises and unifactorial cognitive/behavioural interventions (Table 3.1).

Reference

1. NICE (2013). *Falls in Older People: Assessing Risk and Prevention*. Clinical guideline CG161. London: NICE.

Prevention of osteoporosis: lifestyle factors

- Nutritional factors are important to maintain skeletal integrity.
- Tobacco consumption may adversely affect bone density.
- Strongest evidence on beneficial effect of exercise on bone density is during childhood and adolescence. Exercise in later life may improve muscle tone, balance, and ↓ risks related to falls and related fractures.
- ➲ See 'Osteoporotic vertebral and hip fractures', p. 46.

What is important in the diet?

- Calcium intake is important during skeletal growth and peak bone mass development and higher intakes may also be effective in reducing bone loss in late postmenopausal ♀.
- Dairy products are the major sources of calcium and ideally dietary calcium intake should be maintained throughout life to help maintain skeletal integrity (Table 3.2).
- Vitamin D_3 is necessary for optimal absorption of calcium.
- Exposure to sunlight and subsequent cutaneous production of vitamin D_3 is the major source of this vitamin with only about 10% being derived from the diet.
- Vitamin D deficiency is common in various groups:
  - Frail elderly people with poor nutrition and limited exposure to sunlight. In this group, vitamin D deficiency may lead to impaired muscle strength which can ↑ the risk of falls.
  - ↑ skin pigmentation and ↓ sunlight exposure (due to strict dress codes) exposes infants, young children, and pregnant ♀ of Asian, African, and Afro-Caribbean origin to the risk of developing vitamin D deficiency.
  - Strict vegans and individuals with malabsorption syndromes or those who have undergone extensive gastric surgery may be at risk.
- Anticonvulsant therapy may lead to vitamin D deficiency syndrome.

Table 3.2 Calcium requirements: reference nutrition intake (RNI).

Age (years)	Daily intake (mg)
<1	525
1–3	350
4–6	450
7–10	550
11–18	1000 (♂); 800 (♀)
>19	700

- Low body weight. Bone loss is more rapid in postmenopausal ♀ with low body weight. Eating disorders leading to amenorrhea in young ♀ may also affect bone density. Foods rich in dietary alkali such as fruit, vegetables, beans, and nuts may also benefit bone health.
- Vitamins A, B, C, and K may contribute to bone health but many of the data on these individual nutrients are based on small studies only.
- Carbonated drinks or beverages containing caffeine may be detrimental to bone health but findings are not universal.
- Phytoestrogens are widely distributed within the plant kingdom and have oestrogen-like properties. High intakes of isoflavones and the lignans, which are found in soy products and grains, cereals, and linseed, may help to improve bone density although evidence is limited.

Does tobacco and alcohol affect bone density?

Smoking

- Smoking may affect several mechanisms that ↑ fracture risk.
- Current and past smoking may adversely affect BMD. ♀ smokers have an earlier menopause and ↑ rate of bone loss after menopause, suggesting that smoking may enhance oestrogen catabolism.
- Smokers are also thinner and ∴ have lower BMI, losing the protective effect of adipose tissue and impairing peripheral oestrogen metabolism.
- Current smoking is associated with a significantly ↑ risk of any kind of fracture in both ♂ and ♀ with the risk slowly ↓ on cessation of smoking.
- Bone loss is reported to be ↑ in ♂ smokers than in ♀ smokers perhaps due to higher exposure to cigarette smoking in ♂.

Alcohol

- Heavy alcohol consumption is associated with a ↓ in bone density and an ↑ fracture risk.
- A probable direct effect of ethanol on osteoblasts but in addition relative malnutrition, lack of exercise, and impaired vitamin D metabolism will ↑ the likelihood of osteoporosis and fractures.

Exercise

- Physical activity—particularly weight-bearing exercise—provides the mechanical stimuli or 'loading' important for the maintenance and improvement of bone health as well as enhancing gait, balance, coordination, proprioception, reaction time, and muscle strength in elderly people.
- Repetitive (e.g. jumping) or resistance exercise (e.g. weight training) can produce the necessary loading to provide mechanical stimuli.
- Activity needs to be within safe limits but must be more than just customary attempts if it is to produce improvements, e.g. extra walking, at a normal pace, >10 min daily has failed to ↑ BMD at vulnerable sites for fracture.
- Exercise benefits to bone are doubled if activity is commenced before or at puberty (e.g. in gymnastics, tennis, and jumping).

- In adulthood, exercise appears to largely preserve bone but does not add new bone. In the immediate postmenopausal years it is unlikely that exercise will balance the effect of oestrogen deficiency.
- Exercise can reduce the risk of falls in the elderly.
- It is unclear how long benefits of young adulthood exercise will be sustained in advancing years. Evidence supports benefit of earlier sports activities producing lasting benefits until the late 60s but only if activity at a lower level is sustained.

Further reading

NOS (2015). Vitamin D and bone health: a practical clinical guideline for management in children and young people. https://theros.org.uk/media/2074/vitamin-d-and-bone-health-children.pdf

Providing education and support

Where can education have an impact?

- Knowledge and ability to explain issues related to osteoporosis and prevention.
- Guiding on the results of DXA scans and effect on lifestyle and treatment.
- Providing advice on treatment options leading to adherence.

Outline the evidence on the role of diet and exercise

At a population-based level, the role and importance of dietary calcium intake and exercise are the major preventive options that have been addressed across various age groups.

- ♀ adolescents have heard about osteoporosis and may have some limited knowledge about dietary calcium intake and exercise but have little concept about types of calcium-rich foods and the specific types of weight-bearing activity required for skeletal preservation. ♀ of this age believe they are unlikely to develop osteoporosis and that it is less serious than heart disease and breast cancer. Health information is commonly sought from brochures, magazines, and the media, suggesting a preference for this source rather than from a healthcare professional.
- In evaluating the impact of osteoporosis knowledge and preventive behaviour in older ♀, there is greater recognition of the condition and a trend towards ↑ dietary calcium intake and weight-bearing activity following education-based programmes.

DXA scans

It has been suggested that information on and explanation of DXA results may influence health-related behaviours with respect to relevant lifestyle changes and also adherence to treatments.

- Several studies have shown that those who understand their DXA results—particularly when they are low—are more likely to be prescribed medication and are more likely to continue treatment on a long-term basis.
- In contrast, those who were either uncertain of their DXA results or thought it did not show osteoporosis were less likely to continue treatment.

Adherence with treatment

Despite studies showing that osteoporosis treatments are generally well tolerated and associated with significant efficacy benefits, adherence to therapies on a long-term basis remains inconsistent.

Factors affecting adherence include:

- Understanding of disease.
- Severity of symptoms.
- Complexity and duration of treatment regimens.
- Immediacy of beneficial effects.

- Perceived or actual side effects.
- Use of concomitant medications.
- 'The Adherence Gap: Why Osteoporosis Patients Don't Continue with Treatment' is a European survey that has highlighted reasons why patients fail to continue with bisphosphonate therapy.[1]
- ♀ report side effects and inconvenience of medication as the most common reasons for discontinuing therapy.
- Physicians attribute non-adherence to lack of patient understanding only.
- 27% of ♀ felt their risk of fracture was the same whether or not they took treatment; 20% were unaware of treatment benefits; and a further 17% did not believe their treatment had any benefit at all.
- This survey suggests that although advice is given it is not always interpreted in the correct manner. Factors that may explain this include a lack of communication skills of both doctor and patient, use of inappropriate terminology, inadequate emphasis on, and repetition of, key features, and diminished motivation.

Education

In a clinical setting, most patient education should ideally take place on an individualized basis, with the emphasis on verbal communication.

Patient information leaflets and booklets from various sources including the Royal Osteoporosis Society (ROS) and pharmaceutical companies provide written information on osteoporosis. Most of these are reasonably composed and have undergone some form of scientific ratification but there have been few attempts to analyse their educational value and effect on relevant behavioural change.

The role of the Royal Osteoporosis Society

The ROS is a major national charity whose membership comprises people with osteoporosis, their families and carers, and clinical and research professionals. Its activities include:

- Providing information via a comprehensive range of leaflets, newsletters, public meetings, and a helpline staffed by nurse specialists.
- Fundraising activities.
- Media communication.
- Political lobbying.
- Organizing an international conference every 2 years, funding research projects, and supporting studentships.
- Supporting >100 patient groups across the UK, assisted by 1000 volunteers.

References

1. International Osteoporosis Foundation (2005). The Adherence Gap: Why Osteoporosis Patients Don't Continue with Treatment. https://www.iofbonehealth.org/sites/default/files/PDFs/adherence_gap_report_2005.pdf
2. Royal Osteoporosis Society: ℜ https://theros.org.uk

Treatment for osteoporosis

What drugs are commonly used?

There are a number of agents that have been shown to prevent bone loss and reduce fracture incidence in postmenopausal ♀ and ↑ evidence to suggest that some of these have similar effects in ♂ (Boxes 3.2 and 3.3).

- Bisphosphonates: alendronate, etidronate, risedronate (all given orally); ibandronate, given orally and intravenously. Zoledronic acid is an annual infusion.
- HRT.
- Raloxifene.
- Teriparatide.
- Denosumab.

For detailed drug information, see ℘ http://www.bnf.nice.org.uk.

The bisphosphonates, HRT, and raloxifene slow down bone resorption while strontium has both an antiresorptive effect and stimulates bone formation. Teriparatide is an anabolic agent that stimulates bone formation and leads to large ↑ in bone mass.

► Calcium + vitamin D recommended in all cases unless clinicians are confident that ♀ have an adequate dietary calcium intake and are vitamin D replete.

Issues related to treatment

Although antifracture efficacy is proven, use of therapy in the clinical setting is not always straightforward for varied reasons. Adherence to osteoporosis therapies is generally poor. Of patients taking a once-daily bisphosphonate, 77% stop treatment within a year with almost two-thirds of patients taking a once-weekly preparation also failing to adhere to treatment. Non-adherence has significant repercussions on prognosis with evidence showing a greater fracture reduction in those who adhere to therapy compared to those who do not.

Treatment is long term; therapies do not provide symptomatic improvement and side effects may present. These include:

- Bisphosphonates may cause upper GI symptoms and the dosing instructions may be difficult to follow.
- Strontium is taken as granules dissolved in water, recommended at bedtime. It may be associated with diarrhoea, nausea, and headache, particularly in the first few months. Early trials suggested a possible unexplained small ↑ in the risk of venous thromboembolism.

Box 3.2 1° **prevention of osteoporotic fragility fractures in postmenopausal ♀**

- ♀ aged 70+ who have one or more clinical risk factors for fracture or medical conditions suggestive of low BMD. In ♀ aged 75+, DXA may not be required:
  - Treat with alendronate.
- ♀ aged <70 with medical conditions suggestive of low BMD and at least one clinical factor suggestive of ↑ fracture risk and a T-score <–2.5 SD:
  - Treat with alendronate.

Table 3.3 Osteoporosis assessment questionnaires

Name	Administration	Number of questions	Domains
OFDQ	Interview	69	General health, back pain, ADLs, socialization, depression, confidence
OPAQ	Self-administer	67	Physical function, emotional status, symptoms, social interaction
OPTQOL	Interview	33	Physical activity, adaptations, fears
OQLQ	Interview	30	Physical function, ADLs
Quallefo-41	Self-administer	41	Pain, physical function, social function, general health perception, mental function
QUALIOST	Self-administer	23	Physical function, emotional status

OFDQ, Osteoporosis Functional Disability Questionnaire; OPAQ, Osteoporosis Assessment Questionnaire; OPTQOL, Osteoporosis Targeted Quality of Life Questionnaire; OQLQ, Osteoporosis Quality of Life Questionnaire; Qualleffo-41, Quality of Life Questionnaire of the International Osteoporosis Foundation; QUALIOST, Questionnaire Quality of Life in Osteoporosis.

The role of the nurse in osteoporosis

All nurses should be able to identify key resources to inform the patient about the lifestyle factors, disease-specific issues, and treatment options. Depending upon the local resources, nurses should look for links with:

- GPs, community pharmacists, and physiotherapists.
- Community falls services, if appropriate.
- Social care if appropriate.
- Patient support groups and telephone advice lines.
- 2° care services.
- Voluntary organizations that may offer local exercise or education classes.

See Table 3.4.

Table 3.4 The nurse's role across different specialties

Practice nurse	• Risk assessment • Health promotion • Treatment issues • Education about the disease • Identification of those at an elevated risk of osteoporosis
District nurse	• Nursing care of frail elderly • Link with residential/nursing care • Falls prevention • Treatment issues • Education of teams and patients
Health visitor	• Health promotion across lifespan • Encourage bone healthy lifestyle
Orthopaedic nurse in trauma wards and fracture clinic	• Acute fracture management of in- and outpatients • Rehabilitation • Falls prevention • 2° prevention of fracture including early identification of those 'at risk' of osteoporosis • Liaise with community services
Rheumatology nurse in outpatients and in ward	• Risk assessment • Health promotion • Treatment issues • Use of intravenous (IV) bisphosphonates/ corticosteroids • Identification of those 'at risk'
Care of the elderly nurse in hospital and nursing home	• Nursing care of frail elderly • Rehabilitation • Falls prevention • Treatment issues

Continued

Table 3.4 *Contd.*

Nurses in other specialities, e.g. endocrinology, oncology	• Risk assessment • Awareness of specialist therapy on bone health (e.g. glucocorticoids and aromatase inhibitors)
Osteoporosis specialist nurse	• Risk assessment • Clinical assessment • Interpretation of DXA results • Possible DXA scanning role • Initiation and monitoring of treatment • Wide-based educational role for healthcare professionals, patients, and general public
Community specialist bone health service	• Identification, assessment, treatment, and management of those with, or at an ↑ risk of, osteoporosis and fragility fracture • Patient education • Accessible specialist nursing service providing support and advice to patients, carers, and healthcare professionals

➲ See also Chapter 21, 'Specialist nursing support—the role and nurse prescribing', pp. 613–619 and ➲ Chapter 10, 'Holistic and patient-centred care', pp. 329–350.

Frequently asked questions

Is loss of height something I should take note of when I see patients I think might be at risk of osteoporosis?

Loss of height >4 cm might indicate that a vertebral fracture has occurred. If several vertebrae are crushed, there may also be curvature of the spine.

If someone has been diagnosed as having osteoporosis, should we discuss their dietary intake and lifestyle choices?

All patients diagnosed with osteoporosis should be encouraged to maintain a well-balanced diet, incorporating 1000 mg calcium daily, essential vitamins B, C, and K, and also minerals such as magnesium. Regular helpings of dairy produce and fruit and vegetables will provide these essential nutrients. All guidance offered should be supported by written information.

Is there a good source of information on dietary advice that I can use to help people understand their calcium and vitamin D intake?

The Food Standards Agency[1] is an excellent source of information; just type in 'osteoporosis' in their website search box and a range of options are available to print off for the patient. You may also find your own organization has a dietician who may be able to provide additional information. The ROS and WHO[3] are also good sources of information.

How can I encourage concordance with bisphosphonates—so many people struggle with taking them?

Providing sufficient information on the benefits is really important particularly if they have few symptoms. Patient-orientated information, both verbal and written, given on initial diagnosis and subsequently reiterated on review visits will be helpful. Some people struggle with remembering a treatment that is once a week. There are plenty of practical tips such as encouraging them to take the medication on the day that has more of a routine. Magnetic fridge timers are available that can be programmed to sound an alarm once a week.

IV zoledronic acid is an extremely viable alternative to oral medication and eliminates GI disturbances which are frequently associated with bisphosphonate use.

I see a lot of patients who have, over a year, quite a high dose of steroids, for example, regular Depo-Medrone® injections—shouldn't they be on bone protection?

The guidelines recommend that patients receiving regular doses >7.5 mg for >3 months, or prescribed >more than three episodes in 12 months, should be receiving bone-sparing treatment. Research is ongoing at the present time to review the impact of lower doses (2.5–7.5 mg daily), and the possible long-term potential impact of inhaled steroids.

References

1. Food Standards Agency (UK): http://www.food.gov.uk
2. ROS: https://theros.org.uk
3. WHO (2004). Diet, nutrition and the prevention of chronic diseases. Report of the joint WHO/FAO expert consultation. WHO Technical Report Series, No. 916 (TRS 916). M http://www.who.int/dietphysicalactivity/publications/trs916/en/gsfao_osteo.pdf

Chapter 4

Inflammatory joint diseases

Overview

Inflammatory joint diseases are conditions that have an underlying inflammatory component that may be driven by a faulty autoimmune response by the body, often resulting in the body's tissues being attacked by the body's own immune responses. Examples of such conditions include:

- AS.
- PsA.
- RA.
- JIA.
- Connective tissue diseases.
- Crystal-related arthropathies.

These inflammatory conditions are understood to:

- Target specific joints and/or surrounding tissues.
- Have a genetic predisposition—although this does not provide the complete picture to causality.

Prompt diagnosis is essential to differentiate between acute, mild self-limiting conditions from those that can rapidly result in life-threatening, multisystem disorders. Evidence related to inflammatory (polyarticular) joint diseases (IJDs) such as RA demonstrates that prompt aggressive and proactive treatment improves long-term outcomes. This is referred to as the 'window of opportunity' and requires a 'treat to target' approach to management.[1] ➲ Also see 'Pharmacological management', Chapter 16, pp. 445–452.

On initial presentation, it can sometimes be difficult even to the trained eye to detect swelling and tenderness on palpation of the joints (Box 4.1). ➲ Also see 'Assessing the patient', p. 289.

Box 4.1 Index of suspicion for inflammatory joint disease requiring referral

- Joint pain.
- Report of joint stiffness >30 min in the morning.
- Presence of inflammation (joint swelling) in more than two joints—beware of swollen ankles (oedema).
- Hand or foot pain with positive MCP or MTP 'squeeze test'
- Relationship between joint pain and symptoms related to movement—stronger relationship more likely to be OA.
- Presence of fatigue—if associated with poor sleep and widespread pain consider fibromyalgia.
- Raised inflammatory markers (CRP, ESR) and rheumatoid factor (RF) positive (absence of RF positive does not preclude diagnosis or referral) Anti-cyclic citrullinated peptide antibodies (anti-CCP) similar sensitivity to RF but ↑ specificity.

❶ Individuals presenting with a monoarthritis, particularly if accompanied by red, hot swollen, and tender joint—consider septic arthritis (emergency treatment required).

Key points to consider

- Short-term symptom relief may be achieved by steroids or NSAIDs.
- Initially, signs and symptoms may be sudden or insidious.
- Early presentation of IJD may not fit any classical diagnostic group but early assessment and treatment is paramount.
- Regardless of diagnosis/prognosis indicators, all patients presenting with joint pain should receive appropriate treatment and advice on managing their symptoms.

➲ Also see 'Classifying joint disease', pp. 7–9; ➲ 'Psoriatic arthritis', p. 95; ➲ 'Ankylosing spondylitis', p. 93; ➲ 'Rheumatoid arthritis', p. 64.

Reference

1. NICE (2018). RA in adults: diagnosis and management: evidence C: treat to target (NG100). https://www.nice.org.uk/guidance/ng100/evidence/evidence-review-c-treattotarget-pdf-4903172320

Further reading

Combe B, Landewe R, Daien C, et al. (2016). 2016 update of the EULAR recommendations for the management of early arthritis. *Ann Rheum Dis* 76:948–59.

Rheumatoid arthritis

What is RA?

RA is a symmetrical polyarticular disease that affects ~0.8–1% of the population. The chronic systemic inflammation attacks the synovial tissues of moveable joints causing pannus formation, cartilage and bone degradation to joints, and systemic effects to other tissues (Figs. 4.1–4.3). Initial

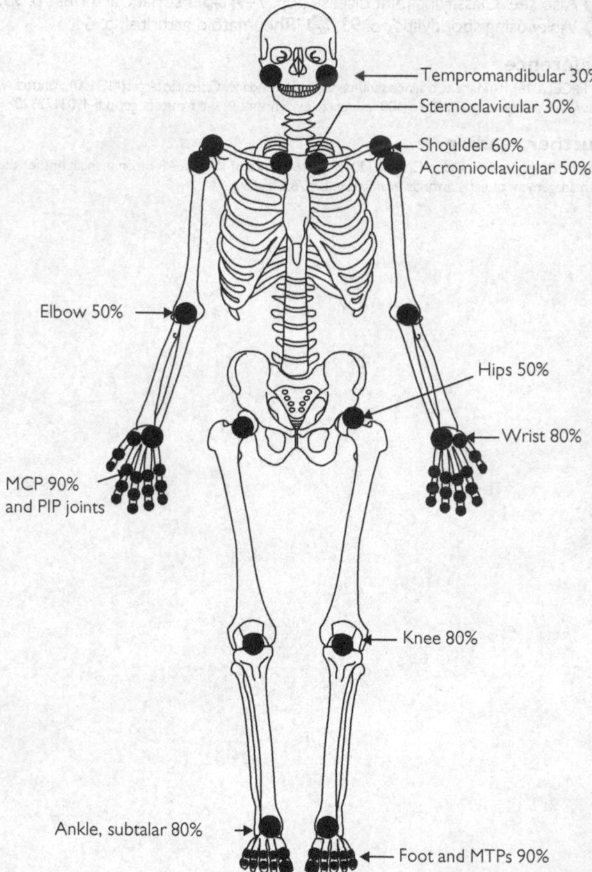

Fig. 4.1 Joints and tissues affected in RA and the percentage of those most commonly affected.

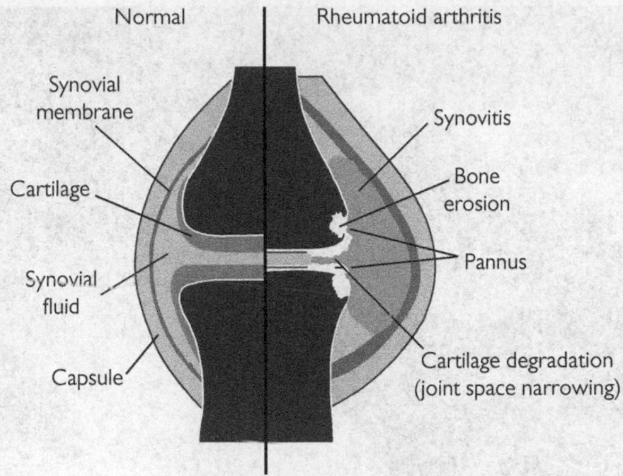

Fig. 4.2 The pathology of RA.

presentation of the disease may vary. RA has the potential to reduce life expectancy and result in progressive joint destruction and ultimately changes in function.

- The actual mechanism of triggering RA is unknown.
- A genetic predisposition to developing RA (human leucocyte antigen (HLA) DR class II molecules) has been identified, yet only 17% of both identical twins develop RA. Genetic and/or environmental factors may be associated with susceptibility.
- RA is a progressive and destructive disease with poor long-term outcomes.

➲ Also see 'Rheumatoid arthritis: clinical features', p. 68.

Who does it affect?

- RA can present at almost any age although the peak age of onset is between 35 and 50 years.
- RA affects 3♀:1♂.

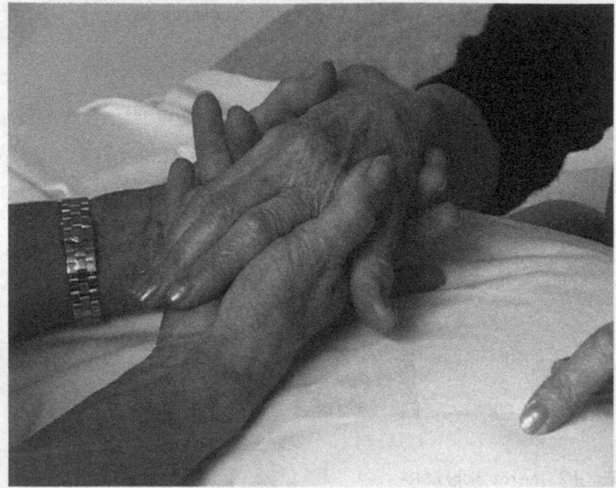

Fig. 4.3 The squeeze test—MCP or MTP joints. Positive squeeze test = if tender/painful on squeezing across MTP or MCP joints.

How is it diagnosed?

In early disease, the joints involved and symptoms may fail to adequately fulfil rigid criteria for established disease. The European League against Rheumatism (EULAR) advocates prompt referral for early arthritis based upon a high index of suspicion for IJD. The squeeze test is a simple pragmatic tool used to elicit synovitis in the commonly affected metacarpophalangeal (MCP) joints of the hands or MTP joints of the feet (Fig. 4.2). More detailed diagnostic criteria to support clinical examination findings have been devised (➲ see 'Rheumatoid arthritis: clinical features', p. 68).

However:

- RA can be difficult to diagnose, particularly in the early phases of the disease. May have a rapid or insidious onset.
- Commonly starts with joint pain (usually in the MCPs of the hands or MTPs of the feet). A high index of suspicion of an inflammatory joint disease should warrant prompt and early referral for diagnosis.
- A high positive titre for RF serology is a poor diagnostic tool, particularly in the absence of clinical signs. RA can be diagnosed in the absence of RF.
  - The use of anti-CCP serology test has shown to have a higher specificity and sensitivity than RF serology. Increasingly, anti-CCP is used to predict those with erosive disease, guiding optimum treatment pathways. Anti-CCP is present in serum of patients with RA years before signs and symptoms develop.

Further reading

Combe B, Landewe R, Daien C, et al. (2016). 2016 update of the EULAR recommendations for the management of early arthritis. *Ann Rheum Dis* 76:948–59.

NICE (2018). Rheumatoid arthritis in adults: diagnosis and management: evidence C: treat to target (NG100). https://www.nice.org.uk/guidance/ng100/evidence/evidence-review-c-treattotarget-pdf-4903172320

Oliver S (2007). Best practice in the treatment of patients with rheumatoid arthritis. *Nurs Stand*, 21:47–56.

Rheumatoid arthritis: clinical features

Predominant features that can be seen in RA

- Joint pain.
- Joint swelling.
- EMS—this is a predominant feature in the morning although with very active disease stiffness can continue for a significant period of the day.
- Fatigue and lethargy.
- Individuals may also experience low-grade fever and weight loss.
- Anaemia of chronic disease.
- See Box 4.2 and Fig. 4.4.

In addition, there are changes to joints and surrounding tissues

- Pannus formation of synovial tissues.
- Erosion of bone and joint space narrowing.
- Damage to tendon sheaths and cartilage.
- Deterioration in joint function and general functional ability.

Extra-articular manifestations of RA

Systemic organ involvement and extra-articular features including:

- Rheumatoid lung and interstitial lung disease.
- Vasculitis, anaemia of chronic disease.
- Ocular involvement—episcleritis, scleritis.
- Weight loss.
- Subcutaneous nodules; exocrine, salivary, and lachrymal glands involvement.
- Cardiovascular disease—pericarditis, myocarditis.

Box 4.2 Features of established rheumatoid arthritis

Signs

- Presence of EMS >30 min.
- Symmetrical polyarticular joint pain and swelling. Joints involved could be any of the synovial joints but classically might be:
    - Small joints and/or knuckles of the hand.
    - Wrists, elbows, and shoulders.
    - Knees, ankles, and small joints of the feet.
- Subcutaneous nodules.
- Genetic predisposition, e.g. family history of RA.
- Clinical evidence of synovitis or erosions—using X-ray, US, or MRI.
- Raised inflammatory indices, e.g. CRP or ESR.
- Anaemia of chronic disease.

Symptoms

- Joint changes—reduction in joint function, mobility, and ROM.
- Fatigue and joint pain.
- Sleep disturbances.
- Changes in mood and self-esteem.
- Short-term symptom relief achieved from NSAIDs or steroids.

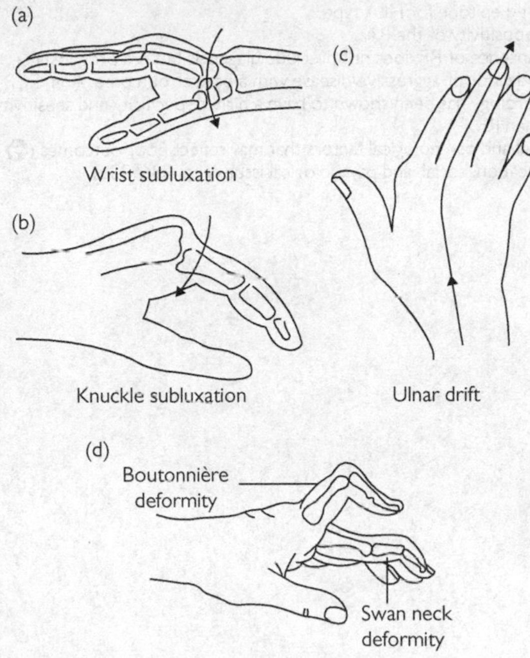

Fig. 4.4 Examples of changes in function. (a) Wrist subluxation; (b) knuckle subluxation; (c) ulnar drift; (d) Boutonnière and swan neck.

- Haematological—Felty's syndrome, lymphomas.
- Lymphadenopathy.
- Sjögren's syndrome.
- ↓ life expectancy and ↑ risk of malignancies.

Prognostic indicators of poorer disease outcomes

- Delayed access to treatment:
  - Longer disease duration at presentation—'window of opportunity'.
  - X-ray evidence of joint damage or erosions at presentation.
  - Poor functional status at presentation.
  - Inflammation of the MCP joints lasting >12 weeks.
  - Evidence of active and sustained synovitis using US or MRI.
- Raised acute phase response (CRP, ESR).

- Shared epitope for HLA type.
- Seropositivity of the RA:
  - Absence of RF does not preclude diagnosis but is a prognostic indicator of aggressive disease with a poorer outcome. Anti-CCP serology has been shown to have a higher specificity and sensitivity than RF.
- Social and psychological factors that may reflect poor outcomes (➔ see 'Education, social, and psychological issues', pp. 336–339).

Rheumatoid arthritis: assessment

RA is a long-term condition (LTC) characterized by pain, lethargy, and changes in functional ability. RA is a multisystem disease requiring long-term treatment with disease-modifying drugs. The diagnostic issues are only the beginning of the management plan; there is still much to be done, from a nursing perspective. The natural course of the disease varies, and short-term changes need to be considered in the context of the overall assessments.

The clinical assessment will:

- Inform management and guide diagnosis.
- Identify specific prognostic indicators that will define treatment strategies.
- Focus on a patient-centred approach.

Management of early RA requires an assessment to support:

- Time for the individual to discuss their anxieties and needs in the context of a holistic assessment, e.g. adjusting to diagnosis, expectations and beliefs, social support, psychological aspects, other co-morbidities, work-related issues, and relationships.
- Information, support, and advice about RA; pharmacological and non-pharmacological options; and risks and benefits of treatment and monitoring.
- A disease activity score (DAS28)—swollen and tender joints (Fig. 4.5).
- An assessment of pain (using a visual analogue scale (VAS)) and symptom control.
- Review all investigations:
  - Blood tests including haematology, biochemistry, inflammatory markers (CRP, ESE), and urinalysis.
  - Radiological investigations including chest, hand, and feet X-rays, US, or MRI results.
  - Assess current functional ability and need for prompt referral to other members of the multidisciplinary team (MDT)—occupational therapy, physiotherapy, and podiatry.
  - Fertility, sexuality, and relevant relationship issues.
- Immunological status, e.g. vaccinations, recent contact with infectious diseases, previous tuberculosis (TB), etc.
- ➲ Also see Chapter 14, 'Pregnancy and fertility issues', p. 415; ➲ Chapter 16, 'Pharmacological management', p. 445.

The window of opportunity

Radiographic joint damage, loss of function, and reduction of BMD are evident very early on in IJDs (up to 40% of early RA patients have erosive disease at presentation). Treating within the 'window' aims to:

- Focuses on prompt treatment.
- Improve long-term outcomes by ensuring early aggressive disease control based upon a 'treat to target' approach.
- Reduce the risks related to mortality and morbidity.

EULAR core data

PAIN

No pain ________________________________ **Pain as bad as it could be**

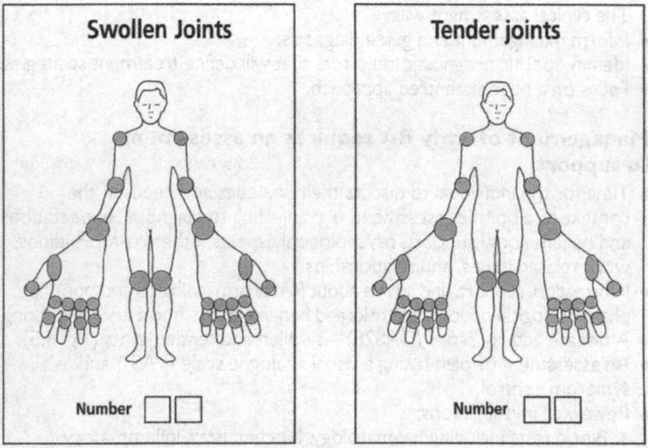

Swollen Joints	**Tender joints**
Number ☐☐	**Number** ☐☐

ESR ☐☐☐ **mm/hr** **C-reactive protein** ☐☐☐ **g/l**

PATIENT'S GLOBAL ASSESSMENT OF DISEASE ACTIVITY

Not active at all ________________________________ **Extremely active**

ASSESSOR'S GLOBAL ASSESSMENT OF DISEASE ACTIVITY

(1-5): ☐ 1 = asymptomatic; 2 = mild; 3 = moderate; 4 = severe; 5 = very severe.

Fig. 4.5 DAS28. Note: the assessor's global assessment of disease activity and pain VAS are not used to calculate the core DAS28 data.

Reproduced with kind permission from Scott DL, van Riel PL, van der Heijde D, et al. (1993). *Assessing disease activity in rheumatoid arthritis: the EULAR handbook of standard methods*. Pharmacia: Sweden.

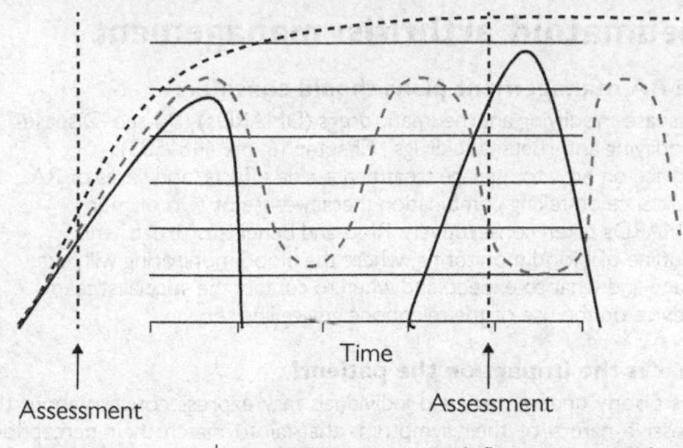

Fig. 4.6 Natural course of disease may vary from person to person, depending upon a range of factors. During their lifetime and in-between visits to hospital they may experience exacerbations of their disease and changes in their functional ability. These changes may be driven by a 'flare' of the disease or in some cases other factors that influence pain and functional ability such as anxiety and depression or changes due to the individual's social or work life.

Clinical distinctions need to be made between the wide spectrums of musculoskeletal disorders in order to:

- Make a firm diagnosis of the disease and optimum treatment.
- Identify the conditions that rapidly deteriorate and may result in life-threatening multisystem disorders.
- Identify acute, mild, self-limiting conditions.

Further reading

Smolen JS, Breedveld FC, Burmester GR, et al. (2016). Treating rheumatoid arthritis to target: 2014 update of the recommendations of an international task force. *Ann Rheum Dis* 75:3–15

Rheumatoid arthritis: management

The RA management plans should consider:

- Disease-modifying antirheumatic drugs (DMARDs) (➲ see 'Disease-modifying anti-rheumatic drugs', Chapter 16, pp. 445–503).
- Advice on how to manage treatments, side effects, and flares of RA.
- Guidance on taking combination therapy—use of two or more DMARDs taken consecutively. Risks and benefits of treatment.
- Outline of blood monitoring, where the blood monitoring will take place and what to expect, and when to contact the specialist team.
- Advice on the use of the telephone advice line service.

What is the impact on the patient?

RA is poorly understood, and individuals may express concern about the aggressive nature of their symptoms that fail to match their perceptions of what they perceived to be 'arthritis'. They may fear that they must have something 'more serious' such as cancer. RA can have a significant impact on the individual's lifestyle, including the need for long-term healthcare and medications, changes to quality of life, functional ability, and long-term health outcomes. The variable nature of the condition also adds to the stress of adjusting to the disease and the consequences of the disease (Fig. 4.6).

➲ Also see 'Education, social, and psychological issues', pp. 336–339; ➲ Chapter 22, 'Patient's perspective', Chapter 22, p. 621.

Social and psychological impact of RA

- Perceptions related to 'chronic disease status' and role in society.
- Changes to self-esteem and perceived level of control of life events and ability to manage the problems (self-efficacy).
- Loss of mobility, changes in functional ability and body image.
- The unpredictable nature of exacerbations (sometimes called 'flares') of the disease.

Nurse-led follow-up and review of RA

- A review of holistic needs.
- Documented evidence (outlined previously) should be compared and regular disease assessment (including DAS28) and patient-reported outcomes such as functional ability and symptom control (pain VAS).
- Review of treatment regimen, side effect profile, blood monitoring, and X-rays.
- Prompt access for advice and treatment/support for exacerbations of the disease—changes of DMARD regimen according to clinical pathway criteria.
- Referrals to multiprofessional team if required.
- Access to telephone advice line support.

➲ Also see Chapter 12, 'Ward-based care and referral to the multidisciplinary team', p. 385.

Rheumatoid arthritis: treatment

The key principles of treatment are:

- Control of symptoms.
- Preservation of functional ability.
- Effective control of the disease.
- Empower the individual to manage their condition and understand their treatment.

Control of symptoms

Pain, fatigue, and stiffness are common features of RA. Achieving effective disease control is imperative, but the drugs used to control the disease can take up to 3 months to work and additional medications may also be required to relieve pain. Pain relief options include pharmacological and non-pharmacological options:

- Simple or compound analgesia.
- NSAIDs—topical/oral/rectal.
- Corticosteroids—long-term maintenance therapy remains controversial but short-term relief is advocated, e.g. IA injection of joint with active synovitis:
  - Intramuscular (IM) injections.
  - IA.
  - IV.
  - Oral.

Non-pharmacological symptom relief

- Pacing/energy conservation/rest and relaxation/education and support.
- Joint protection.
- Application of cold packs/hot packs.
- Complementary therapies.

Disease control

DMARDs include conventional oral DMARDs (cDMARDs), biologic therapies/DMARDs (bDMARDs), and targeted synthetic DMARDs (tsDMARDs).

- DMARDs may be given in combination or triple therapy, e.g. methotrexate (MTX), sulfasalazine, hydroxychloroquine (➔ see 'Pharmacological management', p. 446).
- Biologic therapies are often prescribed with a cDMARD, usually MTX:
  - Anti-tumour necrosis factor alpha (anti-TNFα) adalimumab, etanercept, infliximab, certolizumab pegol, golimumab.
  - Anti-interleukin 6 inhibitor (tocilizumab)
  - B-cell depletion therapies (rituximab).
  - Co-stimulatory modulators (abatacept).
- tsDMARDs:
  - Tofacitinib.
  - Baricitinib.
- Refer to http://www.nice.org.uk for the latest guidance on all drug therapies and http://www.bnf.org.uk for detailed information on drugs.

Empowerment

- Education and information on condition and treatment options.
- Informed decision-making using a patient-centred approach.
- Enhancing patient self-efficacy and perceptions of control—including family, partner, and work-related issues.
- Acknowledging pain and fatigue are significant features of the condition.
- Access to advice and support (telephone advice line) for exacerbation of the disease.

➔ Also see Chapter 16, 'Pharmacological management', pp. 445–503; ➔ Chapter 18, 'Intra-articular, subcutaneous, and intravenous drugs', p. 537; ➔ 'Telephone advice', Chapter 11, p. 360; ➔ 'Self-management', Chapter 10, pp. 343–344; ➔ Chapter 10, 'Holistic and patient-centred care', p. 329.

Rheumatoid arthritis: nursing care issues in management and when to refer

During the lifetime of an individual with RA they will come in contact with a wide range of healthcare professionals (HCPs) due to the condition itself or complications of the disease, or treatment side effects, and, in some circumstances, other co-morbidities.

Nurses caring for individuals with RA must

- Provide adequate pain control.
- Maintain concordance with appropriate drug therapies that provide disease control.
- Monitor potential adverse events related to the treatment or the disease.
- Enable functional ability and independence wherever possible.
- To maintain dignity in all ADLs—including use of aids and devices to enable dressing, eating, and hygiene:
  - Take into account ward or other routines that may affect those with RA participating effectively—e.g. EMS affecting the ability to mobilize promptly in a ward environment.
  - Enable work-related activities and other social participation.
- To provide support and guidance on additional co-morbidities and needs in relation to that condition.

The specialist nurse: roles and management

Nurse specialists in rheumatology have developed significant expertise in the management of those with RA. These include:

- Providing information, education, and support about the diagnosis, treatment options, and managing symptoms.
- Undertaking a holistic assessment of social and psychological needs in relation to the diagnosis and ongoing management of the condition.
- Outlining risks and benefits of drug therapies and documenting informed consent.

Some nurses may undertake additional advanced roles that include:

- Drug monitoring clinics:
  - Reviewing blood, urine, and general health status to ensure safe continuation of treatment.
  - Assessing the effectiveness of disease control.
  - Adding a DMARD or titrating doses of DMARD therapies (as a nurse prescriber or protocol-driven care pathways).
- Nurse-led clinics:
  - Rapid access for flares/exacerbations of the condition.
  - Administering IA joint injections or IM steroids.
  - Manage a caseload.
  - Structured review process on follow-up appointments.
  - Undertake a structured DAS to guide treat to target decisions, and support regular assessments and reviews required to inform treatment decisions/criteria for new therapies.

- Running telephone advice line services:
  - Access to fast-track referrals via the advice line.
- Structured telephone follow-up consultations using telephone review.
- Nurse triage services reviewing early referral and treatment pathways.
- Act as a first point of contact to refer patients when required to the MDT (Box 4.3).

Box 4.3 When to refer to a nurse specialist or specialist team—occupational therapist (OT) physiotherapist (PT)

Referral should be considered for:

- Poor disease control—either frequent or sustained flares of RA with raised inflammatory markers and active synovitis.
- Poor symptom control including pain, stiffness, and fatigue.
- Inability to tolerate DMARD therapies either from toxicity or general intolerance.
- General trend in blood values that flag cause for concern (➲ see 'Drug monitoring', p. 473).
- Seek guidance on any potential adverse events related to cDMARD, bDMARD, or tsDMARDs—including infections, adverse trends in blood results, and new cardiac or respiratory symptoms.
- Guidance on immunization or challenges to immune status of patient particularly contact with infectious disease and conditions such as herpes zoster and chicken pox.
- Information or guidance on pregnancy or fertility issues while on/or being considered for DMARDs.
- Rapid changes in functional ability.
- Changes in general health status.
- Index of suspicion for infections, and respiratory, or cardiac complications.
- Skin integrity, rashes, and ulcers—seek advice.
- Poor psychological coping.

Referrals to OT and PT for:

- Those admitted to hospital—advice from OT or PT on postoperative recovery, mobilization and functional ability, exercises, and management will be beneficial to the patient.
- Access to aids and devices (including chair and bed raisers).
- Guidance on how to best handle patients postoperatively.
- Opportunity to undertake a review of functional issues and exercises including review of splints—where appropriate.
- Additional assessments required for those discharged and requiring further assessment/guidance before returning to work.
- ➲ See 'Specialist nurses and prescribing' Chapter 21, p. 613; ➲ 'Demonstrating the value of the nurse specialist', Chapter 23, p. 630.

Further reading

Bech B, Primdahl J, van Tubergen A, et al. (2019). Update of the EULAR recommendations for the role of the nurse in the management of chronic inflammatory arthritis. Ann Rheum Dis doi: 10.1136/annrheumdis-2019-215458. [Epub ahead of print]

Ndosi M, Johnson D, Young T, et al. (2015). Effects of needs-based patient education on self efficacy and health outcomes in people with rheumatoid arthritis: a multi-centre, single blind RCT. *Ann Rheum Dis* 75:1126–32.

Frequently asked questions: rheumatoid arthritis

I find the RA patients who come into the ward I work in difficult because they don't seem to want to get dressed or moving in the morning. I feel bad as it looks like we just have ignored them but they are very slow in moving around. Are there any tips to helping them in the morning?

The joint stiffness and pain makes movement difficult particularly after inactivity or first thing in the morning. Medication routines may also be altered by ward routines, especially if they are unable to self-medicate. Ensure the patient has been provided with effective analgesia (and possibly NSAIDs). If prescribed an NSAID they will need time for the therapeutic benefit before mobilizing (depending upon the drug, 30–45 min). Planning your work so they are left until last might help but also offering a hot bath or shower will ease their EMS, relieving the pain and stiffness and making mobility a little easier.

I see a lot of people with RA in my community but don't really have enough time to give them. What quick tips can you give me to focus on key issue?

The important quick points include:

- Observe their functional ability on entering and leaving the room; use of joint movements, guarding, or protecting joints due to active synovitis/ pain.
- How long does their EMS last (in minutes)? In general (in the context of all information) a reduction in EMS indicates less disease activity. Those who experience long periods of EMS may warrant closer questioning on how they are in general.
- Use a VAS scale for pain and global health—using a ruler to document the scores numerically to capture and track changes over time. The greater the score, the worse the pain and disease activity as perceived by the patient.
- Ask how many painful and swollen joints they have.
- An ↑ level of fatigue may indicate poor disease control.
- Review their blood results and inflammatory markers—an ↑ in inflammatory markers usually indicates ↑ disease activity. A trend towards lower haemoglobin may also indicate poor disease control— ! it could also indicate a GI bleed.
- Check they are concordant with their medications for DMARDs but also regular analgesia if they are experiencing a flare.
- If you are really challenged and can give minimal support, offer a patient organization website such as http://www.nras.org.uk.

When you have the information, you might want to discuss the case with the nurse specialist or review the patient notes and discuss with the specialist team or your local GP first. Telephone advice line services frequently provide guidance for community nurses or possibly a local community-based musculoskeletal team who you can discuss the patient with.

Juvenile idiopathic arthritis: classification and diagnostic criteria

JIA is the umbrella term to describe the differing types of arthritis in childhood. The term 'juvenile' refers to children under 16 years, idiopathic as cause unknown.

This classification was defined by the International League of Associations for Rheumatology (ILAR) in 1997, primarily for research purposes to demonstrate the diversity of JIA presentations and their subsequent management. JIA has formerly been known as Still's disease, juvenile chronic arthritis (JCA), and juvenile rheumatoid arthritis (JRA). It is worth noting the different nomenclatures when consulting international literature. In the US, all childhood arthritis is still defined as JRA while in the ILAR classification, JRA is one of the distinct subsets (one needs to consider this if consulting American literature). ➲ See 'Juvenile idiopathic arthritis: assessment' p. 84.

Clinical findings

Diagnosis is only considered once there has been a 6-week history of joint swelling. The subsets that come under this umbrella term (JIA) are outlined as follows:

1. Oligoarticular onset (oligo = few): 40–50% of all JIA

- Four or fewer joints affected in first 6 months of disease—typically affecting knees, ankles, and fingers, often asymmetrically.
- ♀:♂ ratio 4:1; peak incidence 2–4 years.
- Joint swelling often without pain, may have morning stiffness and/or fixed flexed joints.
- Associated with asymptomatic uveitis (inflammatory eye disease); the risk is higher if antinuclear antibodies are detected (ANA+).

The number of joints can remain constant during the period of follow-up. However, in some children more joints become involved in the first 6 months and if there are more than four joints involved, this is called 'extended oligoarticular JIA'.

2. Polyarticular onset (poly = many)

This is further subdivided into rheumatoid negative and rheumatoid positive (RF detected on two occasions, 3 months apart).

Polyarticular RF negative

- Five or more joints involved in first 6 months of disease—typically affecting small joints with symmetrical distribution.
- Can have minimal synovitis and flexor tendon involvement.
- May have constitutional features of lethargy and anaemia.

Polyarticular RF positive

- Similar to adult disease.
- Predominantly affects teenage ♀.
- Severe, aggressive, erosive disease affecting many joints.
- Group most likely to require joint replacement.

3. Systemic onset (sJIA)

sJIA (also previously called Still's disease) has similar manifestations to other autoinflammatory diseases with high levels of interleukin (IL)-1β and IL6. The 6-week history of joint swelling is not relevant to sJIA as joint manifestations often follow the systemic features.

- Affects ♂ and ♀ equally.
- 2-week history of spiking fevers >39°C. Typically late afternoon/early evening. Occurring rapidly and settling rapidly described. Quotidian describes the daily fluctuation of ups and downs of fever of a 24-hour period.
- Macular pale pink rash often appears with the fever pattern.
- Generalized lymphadenopathy, hepatomegaly and/or splenomegaly, serositis, and myalgia.
- May mimic malignancy and carries a risk of morbidity and mortality, although outcomes have improved significantly with better treatments. Amyloidosis used to be a cause of renal failure although now rarely seen.
- Macrophage activation syndrome (MAS) can occur as a result of overstimulated but ineffective immune response. This is also known as reactive haemophagocytic lymphohistiocytosis (reHLH).
- Joints affected—typically wrists, knees, hips, and ankles.

4. Psoriatic Arthritis (PsA)

- Dactylitis—'sausage-like' fingers or toes.
- DIP involvement.
- Nail pitting and/or onycholysis.
- Family history of psoriasis in first-degree relative.
- Associated with asymptomatic uveitis.
- Continues into adult life.
- Skin involvement with psoriatic lesions not always present but may evolve with time.

5. Enthesitis-related disease (previously defined as spondyloarthropathy)

- Predominantly affects ♂.
- Inflammation at the insertion of the tendons, ligaments, or fascia to the bone.
- Affecting feet and ankles with heel and foot pain.
- Responds poorly to anti-inflammatory drugs.
- Associated with family history of psoriasis and HLA-B27-related disease, AS, and inflammatory bowel disease.
- Can be Associated with acute anterior uveitis.
- Back and sacroiliac involvement rare in childhood, significant proportion of those affected will develop this in adulthood.

6. Unclassified
Any form of JIA which doesn't fit into the above-listed categories.

Arthritis in childhood has the additional complication that the skeleton is still developing and therefore joint deformity and poor growth can occur either as a result of disease activity, under-treatment, or excessive steroid usage. JIA, other than rheumatoid-positive polyarticular arthritis, is clinically distinct from arthritis in adults and will continue to be referred to as JIA in adulthood.

Further reading

Foster H, Brogan PA (2018). *Juvenile idiopathic arthritis*. In: *Paediatric Rheumatology*, 2nd edn, pp. 131–72. Oxford: Oxford University Press.

PMM online-Paediatric musculoskeletal matters online free educational resource (www.pmmonline.org)

Juvenile idiopathic arthritis: assessment

JIA is a diagnosis of exclusion based on a good clinical history and physical musculoskeletal examination. Blood tests are not diagnostic but may aid the diagnosis. It is important to exclude some differential diagnoses such as:

- Musculoskeletal non-inflammatory pain.
- Hypermobility.
- TB or other infections.
- Malignancy.

Assessment needs to cover physical, social, and psychological issues

- Precipitating factors, symptoms, speed of onset, and duration.
- Joint swelling—duration generally persistent lasting for weeks to months.
- Stiffness of joints—typically early morning or after being in one position for a period of time.
- Pain—areas, type, severity, and relieving factors.
- Growth—chart height and weight on appropriate growth chart.
- Nutrition—refer to dietician if necessary.
- Effects on ADLs. Use of functional assessment questionnaires such as the Childhood Health Assessment Questionnaire (CHAQ) allows objective comparisons of improvement/deterioration of condition over a period of time.
- School, play, and hobbies and sleep.

Physical examination

- Joint examination to identify active inflammation—joint tenderness, swelling, heat, and range of movement.
- Joint deformity, subluxation, and bone changes.
- The standardized tool for physical assessment is the Paediatric Gait Arms Legs and Spine Assessment (PGALS).
- Assessment of muscle bulk/strength.
- Dental hygiene and jaw opening (can be restricted with evidence of arrested jaw growth).
- In PsA assessment of skin, in particular groin area and scalp, nails, lipids. and BMI.
- Ophthalmic assessment forms part of the routine management of JIA up until the child is 11 years old.

There are 17 Tertiary Paediatric Rheumatology centres across the UK (two in Scotland, and two representing Ireland and Northern Ireland). The British Society of Paediatric and Adolescent Rheumatology (BSPAR) have set out 'standards of care' for JIA. In the UK, all children and young people, with rheumatological conditions, should have access to a paediatric and adolescent rheumatology service either, receiving their management at the tertiary centre or, managed as part of a formal paediatric rheumatology clinical network. All UK Paediatric Rheumatology Services are required to complete the 'quality dashboard'—and collect evidence of achieving certain standards. Examples of paediatric rheumatology standards include:

- Referral to first appointment within 4 weeks.
- Referral to ophthalmologist from JIA diagnosis—within 6 weeks.
- Joint injection undertaken within 6 weeks of assessed requirement.
- Counselling by paediatric rheumatology clinical nurse specialists (PRCNs) prior to starting immunosuppression therapy.

The provision of services varies across the UK. This chapter focuses on guidance from NHS England but references to other area with in the UK and internationally include:

- The American College of Rheumatology (ACR) (http://www.rheumatology.org):
    - Ringold S, Weiss PF, Beukelman T, et al. (2013). 2013 update of the update of the 2011 American College of Rheumatology recommendations for the treatment of juvenile idiopathic arthritis. *Arthritis Rheum* 65:2499–512.
- The European League Against Rheumatism (EULAR) (http://www.eular.org):
    - Bijlsma JWJ, Hachulla E (eds) (2015). *EULAR Textbook on Rheumatic Diseases*, 2nd edn. London: BMJ.
- Foster H, Brogan P (eds) (2018). *Paediatric Rheumatology*, 2nd edn. Oxford: Oxford University Press.

Juvenile idiopathic arthritis: management and treatment

There is no curative treatment for JIA, ∴ the aim of treatment is to achieve and maintain remission. This is achieved by ensuring each individual reaches their full potential as a result of:

- Knowledge of the condition and its management.
- Control of inflammation.
- Relief of pain—pharmacological and non-pharmacological.
- Preserving range of joint movement.
- Prevention of deformities and disability.
- Minimizing side effects and complications of disease and treatment.
- Promoting normal growth and development.

A comprehensive approach should:

- Be holistic, family centred, and well coordinated.
- Include a multiprofessional approach: consultant paediatric rheumatologist, paediatric rheumatology nurse specialist, physiotherapist, occupational therapist, psychologist, dietician, play specialist, pharmacist, social worker, and youth worker.
- Be multidisciplinary and, where possible, include utilization of combined clinics or referral to the following specialties:
    - Adult rheumatology.
    - Dermatology.
    - Endocrinology.
    - Gastroenterology.
    - Ophthalmology.
    - Orthodontics/maxillofacial.
    - Orthopaedics.
    - Podiatry.
- Include a vaccination history: prior to starting systemic treatment, assessment of varicella status and, depending on local policy, measles status. For varicella non-immune patients, consider varicella vaccination—please see the 'Green Book' for guidance.
- Include an assessment of TB status and hepatitis status prior to starting biologic therapies.

Treatment modalities

- NSAIDs—need to be given regularly for 3–4 weeks to relieve symptoms and reach maximum benefit.
- Steroids to expedite disease control by oral, IV, IM, or IA route. IA steroids to be administered under general or local anaesthetic (often with Entonox® (nitrous oxide and oxygen gas)) dependent on age and compliance of child and, in consideration of number and size of joints to be injected, with triamcinolone hexacetonide as the steroid of choice. These should be undertaken by paediatric rheumatologists, paediatric specialist nurses, or physiotherapists who have undertaken appropriate training. This enables a holistic assessment and an accurate appraisal of all joints that may need to be injected. Referral to an orthopaedic surgeon may result in only the joints requested being injected.

- Traditional disease-modifying antirheumatic drugs (tDMARDs) to effect remission. Methotrexate MTX is usually the drug of choice. In paediatric and adolescent care, standard practice is to use subcutaneous MTX over oral, see Royal College of Nursing (RCN) guidelines as outlined at the end of this topic.
- Biological therapies (bDMARDs) used in refractory JIA. In the UK these can only be prescribed by paediatric rheumatologists or paediatric rheumatology nurses who have a non-medical prescribing qualification with agreement from their Trust to prescribe such therapies. Further reading in respect of biologics is outlined at the end of this topic.
- Biosimilar therapies (tsDMARDS) are increasingly being used in JIA; further guidance is detailed at the end of this topic.
- Blueteq—online application process for using biologic therapies that are licensed and/or NICE approved.
- Individual Funding Requests (IFRs) are required to use unlicensed/NICE approved biologic therapies.
- Joint surgery, now rarely required due to modern therapies.

Further reading

Blueteq—case management system: http://www.blueteq.com

BSPAR. Guidelines for eye screening. http://www.bspar.org.uk

Children with Special Educational Needs and Disabilities (SEND). https://www.gov.uk/children-with-special-educational-needs/extra-SEN-help

Department of Health (DH) (2017). You're Welcome Pilot 2017: Refreshed Standards for Piloting—Quality criteria for making health services young people friendly. http://www.youngpeopleshealth.org.uk/yourewelcome/standards/

NHS England (2013). NHS Standard Contract Paediatric Medicine: Rheumatology. Particulars, Schedule 2—The Services, A—Service Specifications. https://www.england.nhs.uk/wp-content/uploads/2013/06/e03-paedi-medi-rheum.pdf

NHS England (2014). Paediatric Medicine: (Rheumatology) Quality Dashboard. https://www.england.nhs.uk/commissioning/wp-content/uploads/sites/12/2014/03/paediatric-rhematol.pdf

NHS England (2015). Clinical Commissioning Policy Statement: Biologic Therapies for the Treatment of Juvenile Idiopathic Arthritis (JIA). https://www.england.nhs.uk/wp-content/uploads/2018/08/Biologic-therapies-for-the-treatment-of-juvenile-idiopathic-arthritis.pdf

NHS England (2017). Commissioning Framework for Biological Medicines. http://www.england.nhs.uk

NHS Scotland. Scottish Paediatric and Adolescent Rheumatology Network (SPARN). http://www.sparn.scot.nhs.uk

NICE (2017). Implementing transition care locally using the 'Ready Steady Go' programme. https://www.nice.org.uk/sharedlearning/implementing-transition-care-locally-and-nationally-using-the-ready-steady-go-programme

Paediatric Musculoskeletal Matters: http://www.pmmonline.org

Paediatric Rheumatology European Association (PRES): http://www.pres.eu

Public Health England (2014). Immunisation Against Infectious Disease [The 'Green Book']. https://www.gov.uk/government/collections/immunisation-against-infectious-disease-the-green-book

Royal College of Nursing (2016). *Administering Subcutaneous Methotrexate for Inflammatory Arthritis*. London: RCN.

Royal College of Nursing (2017). *Assessing, Managing and Monitoring Biologic Therapies for Inflammatory Arthritis*, 4th edn. London: RCN.

Juvenile idiopathic arthritis: the role of the nurse in management

Nursing management—from a paediatric rheumatology clinical nurse specialist (PRCNS). PRCNSs are pivotal in the provision of care supporting the child and young person within the context of their family.

Meeting patients at or near to diagnosis and via nurse-led clinics offer

- Age-appropriate disease education/management for child, family, carers, and others involved in care.
- Extensive knowledge of treatment modalities and monitoring requirements, advocating patient-specific needs.
- Ongoing support and management in between clinic visits.
- Telephone clinics/email contact.
- Liaison as appropriate with the 1° care team, GP, community nurses, and education, social care, and voluntary agencies.
- Monitor compliance with treatment.
- Facilitate and coordinate admissions for inpatient or day care procedures—increasingly PRCNs are employing clinical support workers to assist with more administrative-based tasks.
- Prescription management liaising with pharmacy and homecare delivery companies.
- Psychosocial support for child and family/carers, especially help with needle aversion if present and use of distraction for injections/blood tests.
- Annual reviews to assess understanding and compliance. Preparation for transfer to adult services.
- Undertake extended roles as per local service need:
  - Joint injections.
  - Nurse prescribing.
  - Entonox®.
  - Phlebotomy.
  - Cannulation.
  - Pre-assessment prior to procedures.
- Liaising with nurses from other specialties.
- In some centres PRCNSs undertake home/school visits.
- Lead safeguarding referrals/plans.
- Development of patient literature and or resources.
- Facilitation of research—paediatric rheumatology has an extensive research portfolio with national and international collaborations.
- Commissioning, data collection, report writing, and service development.
- Family days, group education sessions, and activity weekends.
- Signposting to other resources, e.g. support groups:
  - Arthurs Place (http://www.arthursplace.co.uk).
  - BSPAR (http://www.rheumatology.org.uk).

- Childrens Chronic Arthritis Association (CCAA) (http://www.ccaa.org.uk).
- JIA@NRAS (National Rheumatoid Arthritis Society) (https://www.jia.org.uk/).
- JIA Matters support groups.
- Paediatric International Trials Organisation (PRINTO) (http://www.printo.it).
- Versus Arthritis (https://www.versusarthritis.org).
- Facilitation of effective transition to adult services.

Therapeutic interventions

- Physiotherapy and hydrotherapy—maintenance of normal function, posturing, pacing, and exercise.
- Occupational therapy—functional assessment, aids, adaptations, and splinting of joints as appropriate.
- Orthodontist—for mandibular surgery.
- Orthotics—for correction of foot positioning.
- Psychology.
- Play therapy.
- Youth work intervention.
- Teapot Trust Art Therapy (http://www.teapot-trust.org).

Further reading

PMM online-Paediatric musculoskeletal matters online free educational resource (www.pmmonline.org)

Ringold S, Weiss PF, Beukelman T, et al. (2013). 2013 update of the update of the 2011 American College of Rheumatology recommendations for the treatment of Juvenile idiopathic arthritis. *Arthritis Rheum* 65:2499–512.

Royal College of Nursing (2016). *Administering Subcutaneous Methotrexate for Inflammatory Arthritis*. London: RCN.

Royal College of Nursing (2017). *Assessing, Managing and Monitoring Biologic Therapies for Inflammatory Arthritis*, 4th edn. London: RCN.

Royal College of Physicians of Ireland, Health Service Executive (2017). A national model of care for paediatric healthcare services in Ireland. Chapter 43. Paediatric rheumatology. https://www.hse.ie/eng/services/publications/clinical-strategy-and-programmes/paediatric-rheumatology.pdf

Wyllie R, Camina N (2014). Competencies for paediatric rheumatology nurse specialists. BSPAR. http://www.bspar.org.uk

Juvenile idiopathic arthritis: social and psychological impact

A diagnosis of JIA impacts daily activities and functioning of both the affected child and the whole family. Families should be encouraged to maintain normal activities and routines but will have to adapt to:

- The child's reduced mobility, drug administration, assistance with ADLs, and additional exercise programmes.
- The need for parents to take time off work for frequent medical or therapy appointments which may compromise employment.
- Changes in behaviour—the child may deny they are in pain to avoid further treatment, be very moody after or during steroid therapy, or be non-adherent with medication.
- Changes in sleep patterns due to fatigue from disease and restlessness and discomfort due to pain, and slow starts due to EMS.
- The needs of siblings who may fear that they too will become ill with JIA or resent the attention given to their sibling.

The age of the child will also influence the impact of JIA. Help with ADLs is acceptable for a young child but inappropriate for a teenager.

Schooling

Most children can and do attend mainstream nurseries or schools, where they should be encouraged to participate in all aspects of school life. With parental/carers permission, key teaching staff and, if available, the school nurse should be made aware of the child's diagnosis, its management, and areas of concern. In particular, flexibility is required regarding the needs of the child as their condition can fluctuate from day to day, particularly during a flare of their illness.

- EMS may affect physical functioning, e.g. sitting on the floor in assembly, taking part in physical education (PE), or getting to school on time.
- If children experience pain, have difficulty in writing, or they need to move about to avoid becoming stiff, they can take additional rest breaks in exams. In severe cases, a scribe or laptop computer may be required. Schools require written evidence from the paediatric rheumatology team to facilitate this.
- Mainstream schools are required by law to appoint special educational needs coordinators (SENCOs). SENCOs ensure the child's educational needs are met by liaising with teaching staff, the multidisciplinary hospital team, and parents or carers.
- JIA, dependent on severity, can qualify as a special educational need (SEN). Schools apply for a formal assessment called a 'statement' to provide additional funding for non-teaching staff to assist with physical activities, e.g. getting changed after PE or carrying heavy equipment.
- Liaison with education welfare officers (EWOs)/inclusion staff where there are issues with attendance/school avoidance.

- Educational healthcare (EHC) plans are used to outline the pupil's specific needs, e.g. drug administration in school or being allowed to leave lessons 5 min early to avoid the rush in the corridor.
- OTs can undertake formal assessments of seating and hand writing and then provide specialist equipment.

Adolescence

Adolescence is a challenging time and JIA can impact significantly on the young person; the previously described assessment will help to explore the following issues:

- Communication with young people is key to their involvement in their care. One of the tools to assist this is the 'HEEADSSS' assessment:
  - Home.
  - Education.
  - Eating.
  - Activities.
  - Drugs and alcohol.
  - Sexual Health
  - Suicide/spirituality/sleep.
  - Social media/general safety.
- Reduced independence—physical limitations, dependence on others, and potentially overprotective parents.
- Awareness of being different—delayed puberty and/or poor growth.
- Limited fashion opportunities—swollen/atypical joints.
- Body piercing/tattoos—can be risky when taking immunosuppressant drugs due to potential infections and delayed healing of skin.
- Implications for risk-taking behaviours in relation to treatment, e.g. alcohol and MTX; pregnancy and MTX.
- Visible drug side effects, e.g. weight gain and cushingoid features.
- Lower expectations from parents and teachers—reduced career opportunities.
- Concerns about progression to university and accessing healthcare closer to education.
- Perceived disability, fear of pain, and reduced physical activity.
- Transition to adult rheumatology services:
  - All young people who need transfer to adult rheumatology services require a managed period of transition, e.g. the 'Ready Steady Go' programme in the absence of other locally organized transition packages.

Frequently asked questions: juvenile idiopathic arthritis

How many children have JIA?

1 in every 1000 children in the UK.

How long will the treatment last?

It varies according to subtype, and research is being undertaken to explore this. However, the current consensus is that immunosuppressive treatment should continue for a minimum of 2 years once symptom free, and possibly longer in uveitis-associated JIA. If relapse occurs, the treatment clock re-starts. It is impossible to predict the duration of the condition which is also influenced by subtype, compliance with treatment, and time to diagnosis.

Does it have a genetic element?

JIA is not 'genetic' although some forms (e.g. PsA and enthesitis-related arthritis) do have a familial link. Families with a strong history of auto-immune diseases may also be at greater risk.

Is there any special diet that would improve the symptoms?

Adequate amounts of calcium and vitamin D are recommended. However, restrictive diets are not recommended.

Further reading

PMM

Royal College of Nursing (2016). *Administering Subcutaneous Methotrexate for Inflammatory Arthritis.* 3rd edition London: RCN.

Royal College of Nursing (2017). *Biologic Therapies for Inflammatory Arthritis.* London: RCN. http://www.rcn.org.uk//professional-development/publications/pdf-005579

Spondyloarthritis

What is it?

Spondyloarthritis (SpA) is the umbrella term for a group of inflammatory rheumatic diseases that cause arthritis (Fig. 4.7). It differs from other arthritis as it involve the sites where the ligaments and tendons attach to the bones, called 'entheses'. It can be:

- Axial:
  - Radiographic axial spondyloarthritis (including AS) (AxSpA).
  - Non-radiographic axial spondyloarthritis.

Or:

- Peripheral:
  - Psoriatic arthritis (PsA).
  - Reactive arthritis (ReA).
  - Enteropathic spondyloarthritis.

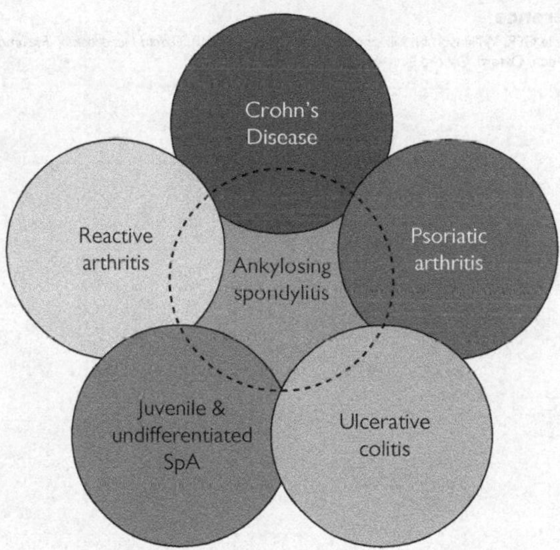

Fig. 4.7 Seronegative spondyloarthritis—disease overlap. The dotted line indicates the common link of all these conditions with HLA B27; the strongest association being with AxSpA. If there are no signs of associated spondyloarthropathy for Crohn's disease or psoriasis, then the HLA B27 association may not be present.

Common characteristics of spondyloarthritis

- Negative for RF.
- Peripheral inflammatory arthritis—usually asymmetrical and/or inflammatory back pain.
- Radiological/MRI evidence of sacroiliitis.
- Enthesopathic pain.
- Strong association with HLA B27—association not fully understood.

Who does it affect?

The prevalence varies among ethnic groups but is considered to be about 1% of the population in Europe. Spondyloarthritis affects ♀ and ♂, however in AxSpA it is usually at a ratio of ♀:♂ of 3:1 It can occur occasionally in childhood (adolescent ♀ presenting with a swollen knee).

How is it diagnosed?

Diagnostic criteria are outlined in detail in Clunie et al.[1] However, diagnostic criteria for spondyloarthritis remain a focus of research interest.

Reference

1. Clunie GPR, Wilkinson N, Nikiphorou E, et al. (eds) (2018). *Oxford Handbook of Rheumatology*, 3rd edn. Oxford: Oxford University Press.

Psoriatic arthritis: overview

What is PsA?

PsA is a chronic inflammatory joint disease that is strongly associated both with the skin disorder psoriasis and arthritis. The condition follows a variable and heterogeneous clinical course with some patients who experience very mild disease that responds well to treatment and others with erosive and destructive disease that is resistant to treatment resulting in poor long-term outcomes. A form of PsA called PsA mutilans causes severe destruction (Fig. 4.8). In a similar way to RA, PsA follows an erratic course with flare-ups and times of quiescence.

Relationship of skin and joints

- Simultaneous skin and joint involvement occur in about 15% of those with PsA.
- 60% have psoriasis before arthritis.
- Severe arthritis can have little or no skin involvement and visa versa.
- PsA has similarities to RA although there are some important differences which include:
  - PsA is classified as a spondyloarthropathy.
  - Affects ♀ and ♂ equally.
  - Diagnostic criteria differ (➲ see 'How is PsA diagnosed?', Chapter 4, p. 95).
- See Fig. 4.8.

Who does it affect?

- Prevalence of 0.1–2% of the population.
- 5–7% of psoriasis patients have PsA.
- 40% of those with extensive psoriasis have PsA.
- In specialist services, 40–60% of PsA have erosive and deforming arthritis.

How is PsA diagnosed?

PsA can be a difficult disease to diagnose due to the differing disease presentations with many clinical subgroups of PsA. New diagnostic disease classifications have been published.[1]

Key aspects of disease presentation and diagnosis include

- Seronegative for RF.
- Fewer joints involved and generally asymmetrical distribution.
- Axial manifestations of the disease are associated with HLA B27.
- Clinical features include a heterogeneous pattern of joint involvement.
- Imaging studies confirm the presence of enthesitis in PsA but not RA
- Entheses and soft tissues changes result in dactylitis (sausage-like digit) (Fig. 4.9c,d).
- Affects DIP joints.
- Nail involvement (Fig. 4.9a).

Axial disease

Shared features with AS:

- But less severe overall disease severity.
- Reduce association with positive serology for HLA B27 than AS.
- Fewer syndesmophytes, cervical involvement, and sacroiliitis.
- Better spinal mobility and sparing of apophyseal joints.

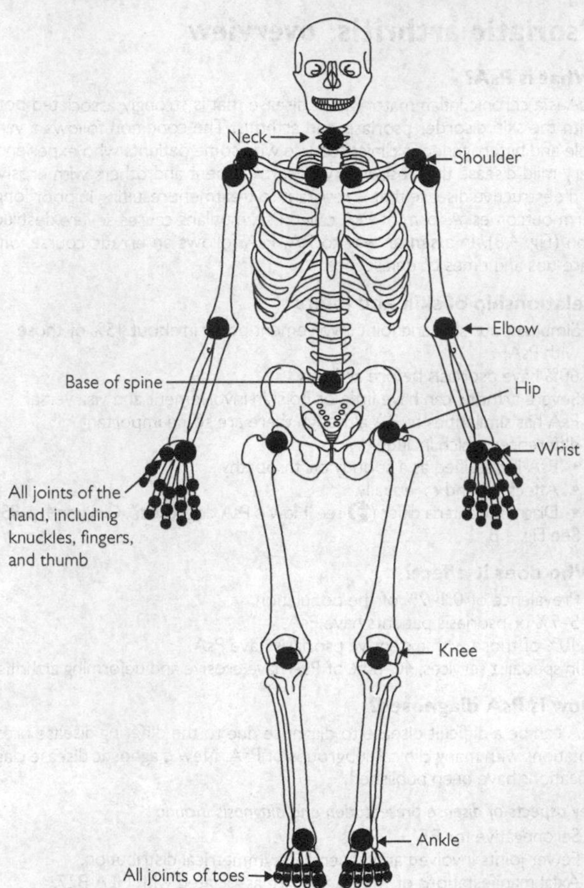

Fig. 4.8 Joints commonly affected by PsA.

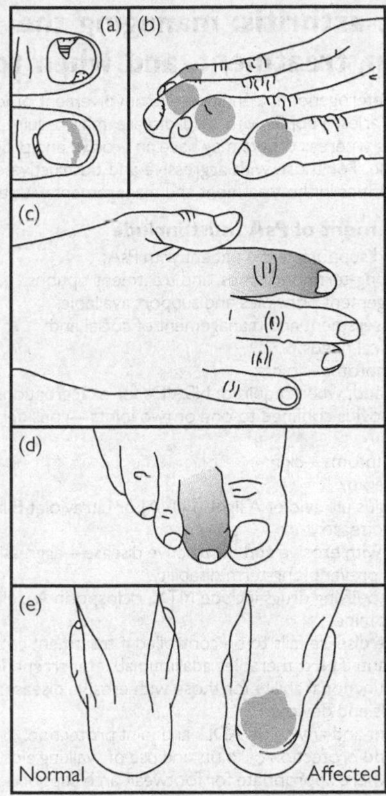

Fig. 4.9 Signs and symptoms of PsA.
Adapted with permission from the ARC.

Reference

1. Kavanaugh AF, Ritchlin C, GRAPPA Treatment Guideline Committee (2006). Systematic review of treatments for psoriatic arthritis: an evidenced based approach and basis for treatment guidelines. *J Rheumatol* 33:1417–21.

Psoriatic arthritis: managing the condition, treatment, and when to refer

PsA is a very heterogeneous condition with involvement of joints, and disease severity varies. People with mild disease may require treatment to treat symptoms whereas others may have an erosive and progressively destructive disease. For those with aggressive and destructive disease, there are many similarities in the treatment and management with that of RA.

The management of PsA must include

- Educating and supporting the patient with PsA:
  - Disease, long-term outcomes, and treatment options.
  - Self-management principles and support available.
  - Holistic assessment and management of social and psychological needs.
- Relieving symptoms—joints:
  - Analgesia and, when required, NSAIDs for exacerbations/flares.
  - Active synovitis confined to one or two joints—consider IA steroid injections.
- Relieving symptoms—skin:
  - Topical therapy.
  - Psoralen plus ultraviolet A light (PUVA) or ultraviolet B light (PUVB).
- Treating the disease:
  - For those with erosive and destructive disease—aggressive disease control to prevent long-term disability.
  - Disease-modifying drugs include MTX, ciclosporin A, sulfasalazine, and leflunomide.
  - Where the disease fails to be controlled if treatment criteria fulfilled—anti-TNFα therapies adalimumab, etanercept, infliximab.
- Maintaining functional ability for those with erosive disease:
  - Use of aids and devices.
  - Assessment and advice on ADLs and joint protection.
  - Exercise and protection of joints and use of walking aids.
  - Podiatry where appropriate for footwear, arch supports, etc.

Disease assessment

- Indices to measure joint, skin, and nail involvement (➔ see 'Indices to measure joint, skin and nail involvement', p. 101).
- Inflammatory markers—CRP and ESR.
- Pain and global health VASs.
- Functional ability.

When to refer

- Where the patient experiences numerous flares/exacerbations of the disease.
- Where there are toxicities or poor concordance issues with disease-modifying therapies.
- When symptoms are poorly controlled and require reassessment.

- For specialist support on functional changes may benefit from OT, PT, or podiatrist.
- For some patients, specific psychological needs may require referral to a psychologist (uniquely issues related to PsA and skin involvement).

What is the impact on the patient?

➲ See 'Nursing issues' Chapter 10, p. 330 and ➲ 'Patient-centred care', Chapter 10, p. 332.

Psoriasis

Psoriasis is a non-contagious skin condition. It is a systemic autoimmune disease. There is a link with psoriasis and arthritis in the seronegative spondyloarthropathies. PsA is a condition with inflammatory joint disease involvement and evidence of psoriasis (➔ see 'Psoriatic arthritis', Chapter 4, p. 95).

Epidemiology and incidence

- Psoriasis is a common inflammatory skin disease which affects 1–3% of the world's population.
- ♂ and ♀ are equally affected.
- Peak age of onset is between 20 and 35 years and then 50–60 years of age.
- 75% of all cases occur for the first time before the age of 40.
- Evidence varies but figures suggest 10–14% develop psoriatic arthritis.

The prevalence varies between races with the highest recorded numbers in the white populations of Scandinavia and Northern Europe and the lowest prevalence in Native American Indians and the Japanese population.

Causes

There is growing evidence that psoriasis is:

- Primarily a T-cell-driven disease where the usual process of skin replacement is accelerated.
- In 30% of cases there is a family history of psoriasis.
- Genetics play a role in about 40% of patients.
- Environmental triggers include infection (streptococcal infection accounts for 60% of guttate psoriasis), drugs (e.g. lithium, systemic steroids, and antimalarial), and physical and psychological stress.

History and examination

Important factors to consider in the history are:

- Persistent scaling in the ears and/or longstanding dandruff.
- Anal or vulval itching.
- Joint problems and concomitant or previously diagnosed autoimmune disease.

Clinical features

The regions commonly involved are the scalp, elbows, knees, sacrum, and the dorsal aspect of the hands, especially over the knuckles and the nails. All psoriasis lesions show varying degrees of three cardinal characteristics:

- Scaling.
- Thickening (induration).
- Inflammation (redness) and are highly symmetrical in most cases.

Types of psoriasis

Psoriasis is a very diverse skin disease which appears in a variety of forms; each form has its own distinct characteristics. It is usual for people to have one type at a time; however, it can occasionally change from one type to another.

There are five main types of psoriasis:

- *Plaque psoriasis*: the most prevalent form of the disease. About 80% of patients have this form of psoriasis. Features typically found on elbows, knees, scalp, and lower back are characterized by raised, inflamed, red lesions covered by a silvery, white scale.
- *Guttate psoriasis* ('guttate' from the Latin word meaning drop): typically starts in childhood or adolescence. Lesions usually appear on the trunk and limbs. They are thinner than in plaque psoriasis and resemble small, red, individual spots on the skin. Guttate psoriasis frequently appears following an upper respiratory tract or a streptococcal infection.
- *Flexural or inverse psoriasis*: found in skin folds (e.g. armpits, groin, under the breasts, and around the genitalia or buttocks). Flexural psoriasis appears as smooth and shiny and is particularly subject to irritation from rubbing and sweating from the skin folds.
- *Pustular psoriasis:* primarily seen in adults and is characterized by white pustules surrounded by red skin. Commonly seen on the palms of the hands and soles of the feet (called palmar plantar pustular psoriasis). Pustules are sterile and not contagious. Cycles of widespread pustular psoriasis covering most of the body can occur with reddening, followed by pustules, and then scaling.
- *Erythrodermic psoriasis*: the most common form of inflammatory psoriasis affecting most of the body surface. Can occur in association with widespread pustular psoriasis. Characterized by periodic, widespread, fiery redness of the skin with associated itching and pain. Protein and fluid loss can occur, leading to disrupted temperature regulation and severe illness such as infection, pneumonia, and heart failure. In severe cases, hospitalization may be required.

Trigger factors resulting in an episode of psoriasis

- Drugs—e.g. anti-malarial, NSAIDs, and some antibiotics.
- Ultraviolet exposure—sunshine is usually beneficial but can cause a flare of disease
- Trauma—e.g. scratching or piercings of area or surgery.
- Hormonal changes.
- Infections—streptococcal infection, HIV, and AIDS are associated with more severe psoriasis.
- Psychological stress.
- Smoking and alcohol.

Resource

Psoriasis Area and Severity Index (PASI) and Dermatology Life Quality Index (DLQI): ℛ https://www.pasitraining.com.

Further reading

NICE (2018). Psoriasis. ℛ https://cks.nice.org.uk/psoriasis#!backgroundsub

Axial spondyloarthritis

AxSpA is a relatively new term that encompasses both AS and non-radiographic axial spondylitis (nr-AxSpA). AS is classified when there is X-ray evidence of sacroiliitis and nr-axSpA and patients have early axial disease without X-ray changes, but with MRI evidence of active inflammation. Over a 10-year period, more than half of those with nr-AxSpA will progress to AS with radiographic evidence of sacroiliitis. AxSpA is a painful, progressive form of inflammatory arthritis that affects mainly the sacroiliac joints and spine. Extra-articular manifestations of the disease include enthesitis, uveitis, psoriasis, and inflammatory bowel disease.

Prevalence is thought to be 0.05–0.23% and it is three times more common in men than women and predominately in the <45 years age group.

Clinical features

The inflammation in AxSpA causes the bone to erode. When the inflammation subsides, the bone begins to repair itself but also replaces the previously inflamed elastic tissue of the tendons and ligaments with bone. The bones can slowly fuse and cause restriction of movement. In the spine, the outer annular fibres are replaced by bone and the vertebrae become fused, forming a long, bony column known as 'bamboo spine'. AxSpA is characterized by exacerbation and remission of disease activity; it is widely under-recognized, underdiagnosed, and undertreated. See Figs. 4.10 and 4.11.

Typical symptoms of AS

- Gradual onset of back pain over a period of weeks or months.
- Fatigue.
- EMS and pain that wears off during the day with exercise.
- Back pain that is worse after rest but better with exercise.
- Pain in the sacroiliac or gluteal region.
- Enthesopathy (bone erosion): Achilles tendonitis, plantar fasciitis, costochondral, and costovertebral abnormalities.
- Weight loss.
- Fever.
- Uveitis (iritis).
- Inflammatory bowel disease.
- Psoriasis.

Diagnostic criteria

- AS is not easily diagnosed; although there is no specific blood test, the gene encoding HLA B27 is associated with the disease and is positive in many patients. However, it is not a reliable guide to prognosis. Most patients are RF negative. Other blood tests that may indicate AxSpA include CRP—a marker of inflammation, and ESR—which can be elevated during active inflammation.

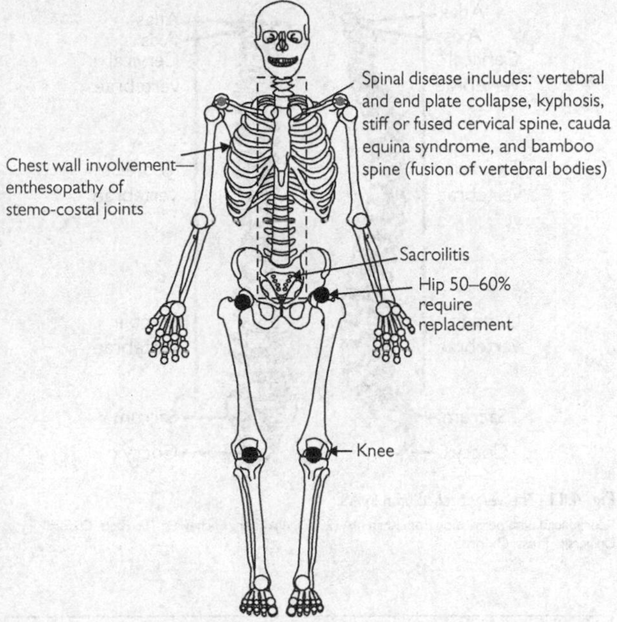

Fig. 4.10 Joints commonly affected in AS. Note: peripheral involvement (knees and hips)—can occur particularly in lower limbs in 20–30% (more severe disease).

- Diagnosis is based mainly on clinical features according to Assessment of SpondyloArthritis international Society (ASAS) criteria, which include MRI to detect active inflammation and establish an early diagnosis (Fig. 4.12).[1,2]
- AS is not solely a disease of the musculoskeletal system, it can manifest in other organs including the eyes, bowel, skin, lungs, and cardiovascular system.

Late clinical features

- Fusion of spine leading to restriction of movement—'bamboo spine'.
- Restriction in the range or movement of the hips and shoulders.
- 50% peripheral joint disease.
- 25% eye involvement, e.g. iritis.
- Flexion contractures of hips and knees.
- Reduction in chest expansion—can also appear early in disease.
- Heart valve involvement/aortic incompetence.
- Cauda equina syndrome.
- Amyloidosis.
- Osteoporosis.
- Classification is shown in Fig. 4.12.

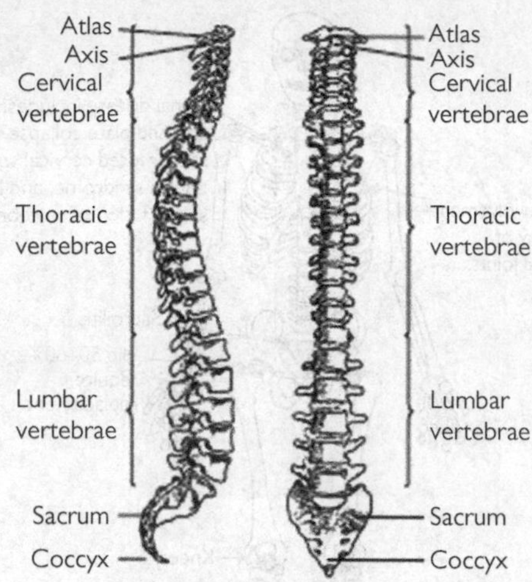

Fig. 4.11 The vertebral column in AS.

Reproduced with permission from Khan MA (2002). *Ankylosing Spondylitis: The Facts*. Oxford University Press, Oxford.

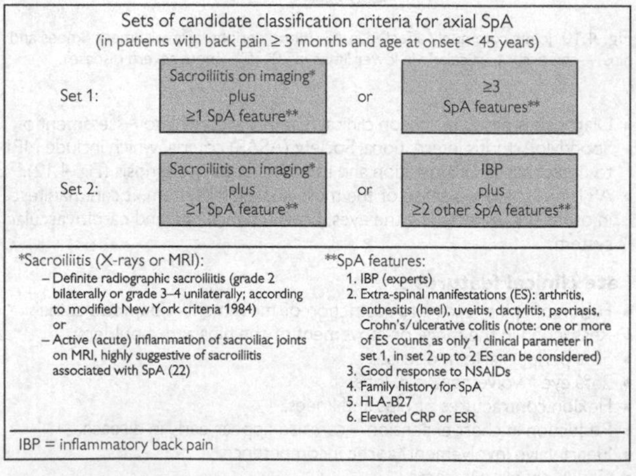

Fig. 4.12 ASAS classification of AxSpA.

Reproduced with permission from Rudwaleit M et al Ann Rheum Dis 2009. 68:777–783.

References

1. Rudwaleit M, Sieper J. (2012). Referral strategies for early diagnosis of axial spondyloarthritis. *Nat Rev Rheumatology* 8:262–8.
2. Rudwaleit M, van der Heijde D, Landewé R, et al. (2009). The development of Assessment of Spondyloarthritis international society classification criteria for axial spondyloarthritis (part II): validation and final selection. *Ann Rheum Dis* 68(6):777–783.

Further reading

Clunie GPR, Wilkinson N, Nikiphorou E, et al. (eds) (2018). *Oxford Handbook of Rheumatology*, 3rd edn. Oxford: Oxford University Press.

NICE (2017). Spondyloarthritis in over 16s: diagnosis and management (NG65). ℛ https://www.nice.org.uk/guidance/NG65

Axial spondyloarthritis: assessment

The most commonly used assessment tools are self-administered questionnaires—these are validated and used throughout the UK in determining treatment therapy.

- Bath Ankylosing Spondylitis Disease Activity Index (BASDAI).[1] Made up of six questions relating to the patient's self-reported disease activity.
- Bath Ankylosing Spondylitis Metrology Index (BASMI).[2] This is a way of measuring spinal and hip movement.
- Bath Ankylosing Spondylitis Functional Index (BASFI).[3] Made up of ten questions relating to the patient's self-reported functional ability.
- Bath Ankylosing Spondylitis Global (BAS-G) score.[4] Made up of two questions relating to the patient's self-reported global health.

Management

- Symptomatic relief of pain and stiffness.
- Disease control.
- Baseline assessments and review of changes in disease.

The nurse's role

- Patient education:
  - Information on the disease, treatment options, and pain relief.
  - Support patient empowerment/patient-centred care.
  - Self-management principles.
- Exercise.
- Physiotherapy.
- Hydrotherapy.
- Lifestyle modification—smoking cessation, work-related issues.
- Support Groups—National Ankylosing Spondylitis Society.[5]

Medications

- NSAIDs are a core treatment for pain relief but they do not alter the underlying mechanism of AxSpA.
- DMARDs—limited evidence for peripheral disease
- Biologic therapy including anti-TNFα and IL17.[6]

➲ Also see 'Biologics', Chapter 16, p. 485; ➲ 'Assessment tools: clinical indicators and disease-specific tools', Chapter 20 pp. 605–608; and ➲ Chapter 9, p 307.

References

1. Garret S, Jenkinson T, Kennedy LG, et al. (1994). A new approach to defining disease status in Ankylosing Spondylitis; The Bath Ankylosing Spondylitis Disease Activity Index (BASDAI). *J Rheumatol* 21:2286–91.
2. Jenkinson TR, Mallorie PA, Whitelock HC, et al. (1994). Defining spinal mobility in Ankylosing Spondylitis (AS): The Bath AS Metrology Index. *J Rheumatol* 21:1694–8.
3. Calin A, Garrett S, Whitelock H, et al. (1994). A new approach to defining functional ability in Ankylosing Spondylitis: the development of the Bath Ankylosing Spondylitis Functional Index (BASFI). *J Rheumatol* 21:2281–5.
4. Jones SD, Steiner A, Garrett SL, et al. (1996). The Bath Ankylosing Spondylitis Patient Global Score (BAS-G). *Br J Rheumatol* 35:66–71.
5. National Ankylosing Spondylitis Society. http://www.nass.co.uk
6. Hamilton L, Barkham N, Bhalla A, et al. (2016). BSR and BHPR guideline for the treatment of axial spondyloarthritis (including ankylosing spondylitis) with biologics. *Rheumatology (Oxford)* 56:313–16.

Frequently asked questions: seronegative spondyloarthritis

AxSpAaffects a lot of young ♀ of working age—does the condition mean they should give up work?

Many people give up work because of negative messages from their healthcare professionals. For the majority of patients they should be encouraged to stay at work as long as their employer is informed about their diagnosis and can be supportive while assessment and treatments are made. Teams play a really important role in helping patients stay at work—discuss work issues and put the condition, and how they should be once treatment is instigated, in context. The one difficult group can be those who work in heavy manual jobs although the continued physical activity reduces the stiffness that people with more sedentary roles may experience. Encourage them to see the OT and discuss their condition with their employers.

How effective are the treatments for AxSpA?

The disease itself can vary with some patients having mild disease that will benefit from lifestyle changes, regular exercise regimens, and the occasional use of NSAIDs. However, DMARDs are not recommended for AxSpA, although there is some evidence that sulfasalazine may be beneficial in peripheral joints. It is important to assess patients regularly so that they get the most effective treatment options as early as possible. The bDMARDs demonstrate significant treatment effects but not all patients will achieve the rigorous eligibility criteria for treatment (see NICE guideline[1] for treatment criteria with anti-TNFα therapies).

Who assesses and treats those patients who have skin involvement in PsA?

Patients may go to a dermatologist in the first instance (particularly if their first problems were related to the skin). However, in some places patients are seen in a clinic with dermatology and rheumatology expertise. There are some excellent models of nurses working across both specialties to ensure the patient has both issues (skin and joints) effectively assessed and treated. Scoring of joints, skin, and nail involvement does require training.

Reference

1. NICE (2017). Spondyloarthritis in over 16s: diagnosis and management (NG65). ☞ https://www.nice.org.uk/guidance/NG65

Reactive arthritis and enteropathic arthritis: overview

Reactive arthritis (ReA)

Clinical features and joints involved

ReA is a form of peripheral spondyloarthritis (Fig. 4.13). ReA is a term used to describe any infection that triggers a form of inflammatory arthritis. ReA usually develops following an infection within the previous month of presenting symptoms, which may be mild and unnoticed at the time.

ReA is most commonly triggered by GI or sexually acquired infections, though multiple other infections can trigger ReA.

The course of ReA is very variable. Most patients will have symptoms which settle within 12 months, though around 25% of patients will develop a chronic arthritis. Features include:

- Strong association with genetic HLA-B27 antigen-positive individuals.
- Predominately young (20–40-year-olds) onset, ♂ ≈ ♀.
- Asymmetrical oligoarthritis (usually weight-bearing lower limbs).
- Skin and mucous membrane lesions (mucosal psoriasis, urethritis, balanitis circinata, cervicitis, keratoderma blennorrhagica—rash on soles and palms of hands).
- Eye inflammation (uveitis, conjunctivitis).
- Lower back pain (unilateral sacroiliitis) or abdominal discomfort.
- Dactylitis, enthesopathy, tendonitis, tenosynovitis, and muscle pain.
- EMS.

ReA can present in many ways and mimics many other forms of arthritis. A good clinical history is essential to exclude other diagnoses and identify any potential infective event. See Box 4.4 and Table 4.1.

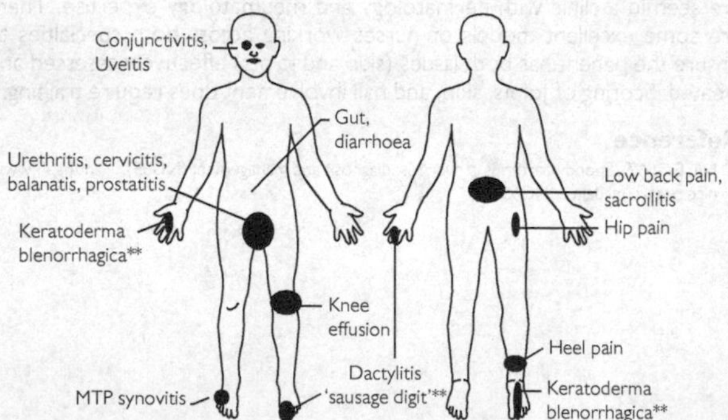

Fig. 4.13 Signs and symptoms of ReA. ** Less common but may be associated with long-term prognosis.

Box 4.4 Reactive arthritis investigations

- Aspiration of swollen joints for culture to exclude septic arthritis, gout, and HIV-associated arthritis. Microscopic analysis to exclude evidence of crystals (gout) if indicated.
  - ❗ Septic arthritis is a medical emergency and requires prompt medical treatment.
- Cultures for urine, blood, and stools as appropriate: check urethral discharge for chlamydial and gonococcal infection.
- Inflammatory markers may be raised (ESR, CRP).
- Consider RF and CCP antibodies.

Table 4.1 Reactive arthritis presentations

Common	Rare
REA incidence ~30–40 per 100,000 adults/ year	Radiological signs in early disease
20–40-year-olds	Small children and the elderly
65–96% positive to HLA-B27 antigen	Severe destructive disease
Pain on palpation of tendon insertion sites and difficulty in walking	Muscle wasting and severe disability
Ocular involvement including unilateral or bilateral conjunctivitis (sterile), acute uveitis	Glomerulonephritis and immunoglobulin (Ig)-A nephropathy
Enthesitis, especially heel pain (Achilles), metatarsalgia (plantar fasciitis), or 'sausage digits' (dactylitis)	Cardiac involvement

Enteropathic arthritis (EA)

The condition is not fully understood but has a number of similarities with spondyloarthropathies and ReA. ♂ ≈ ♀. Any age can be affected. EA tends to cause a large joint oligoarthritis, though it can affect any joint or the joints of the spine or pelvis.

Signs and symptoms

- Similar to ReA (sacroiliitis, mono- or asymmetrical arthritis).
- Enthesitis may be present (sites: elbow, foot, knee).
- Gradual onset.
- Skin lesions (e.g. erythema nodosum).

In EA there are three cardinal features:

- Joint pain and related symptoms follow an onset of bowel disease.
- Arthritis present in 20% of ulcerative colitis and Crohn's disease.

In the short term, there is a relationship between 'flares' of the arthritis and exacerbations of bowel disease.

Reactive arthritis and enteropathic arthritis: management and treatment

Managing the condition and treatment

Patients benefit from psychological and social support from the point of diagnosis through to treatment to minimize the impact of disease.

- Education and guidance on treatment, condition, and symptom control is essential and should be reinforced by written information.
- Consider social and psychological impact (➔ see 'Nursing issues', pp. 330–354; ➔ 'Patient-centred care', Chapter 10, p. 332).
- If sexually transmitted disease, counselling and contact tracing must be undertaken.
- Health promotion and disease prevention advice to avoid future infections.
- IA joint injection for swollen joints—consider referral to OT or PT.
- Antibiotics if an infective organism is identified (see local antibiotic policies for guidance on drug of choice and Table 4.2).
- Acute arthritis may be managed by NSAIDs, IA or systemic glucocorticoids.
- Suspected uveitis should be referred urgently to an ophthalmologist.

Prognosis

- Persistent synovitis may require DMARD therapy.
- Complete remission for the majority by 6–12 months. Almost all have complete remission at 2 years (70%). Poorer prognosis for those who have persistent symptoms and joint damage.

Treatment for EA

- Education and guidance on EA and the underlying bowel condition.
- Consider social and psychological impact (➔ see 'Nursing issues', Chapter 10, pp. 333–354; ➔ 'Patient-centred care', Chapter 10, p. 330).
- IA or oral steroids for swollen joints.
- Caution with NSAIDs which may precipitate a flare of the bowel disease.
  - For those failing to respond, DMARDs may be used (sulfasalazine (SAS), MTX).
  - Biologic therapy can be considered in patients who do not respond to DMARDs.

Table 4.2 Microorganisms implicated in reactive arthritis

Involvement	Microorganisms	Susceptibility	Comment
Gastrointestinal	*Campylobacter jejuni* *Clostridium difficile* *Escherichia coli* *Giardia lamblia* *Salmonella* *Yersinia*	HLA-B27 antigen positive	May complain of abdominal pain many months after initial attack
Genitourinary	*Neisseria gonorrhoea* *Chlamydia trachomatis* *Ureaplasma urealyticum*	HLA-B27 antigen positive	Mild dysuria or mucopurulent discharge may be present
Oral			Lesions—painless, shiny patches—occurring on palate, tongue, uvula, and tonsillar region

Polymyalgia rheumatica

Introduction

Polymyalgia rheumatica (PMR) is a common condition in the elderly population. It is a clinical syndrome of pain affecting the pelvic and shoulder girdle, EMS, and an elevated acute phase response. Onset may be sudden with clear diagnostic features (Box 4.5). An insidious onset with more systemic features may also present. PMR has an estimated prevalence of about 1% and is rare in those <50 years old. The ♀:♂ ratio is 2:1. Around 10% of patients with PMR will develop giant cell (temporal) arteritis (GCA)—this should always be excluded.

Social and psychological impact

Patients can feel anxious and fearful as the onset of disability and symptoms is sudden. General health education and instruction on protecting joints and muscles can help overcome anxiety. Relaxation and education—indicating steady, gradual, graded exercise—can also assist recovery.

Nursing care issues in management

Management of PMR, once diagnosed, is usually undertaken in 1° care. There are specific issues that will need to be considered and documented:

- A nurse specialist should undertake a patient-centred holistic assessment and provide education (verbal and written) about the condition, medications, and managing symptoms.

Box 4.5 Diagnosis of polymyalgia rheumatica

Classical presentation

- Age >50 years, duration >2 weeks.
- Bilateral shoulder or pelvic girdle aching, or both.
- Morning stiffness duration of >45 min.

Evidence of an acute phase response

Core exclusion criteria:

- Active infection.
- Active cancer.
- Active GCA.[1]

Investigations

- ESR.
- CRP.
- FBC.
- LFT.

Differential investigations

- Consider RF/CCP if joint pain.
- Immunoglobulins, protein electrophoresis, and Bence Jones urine test to exclude myeloma.
- Creatine kinase to exclude myositis.
- Thyroid function test to exclude hypothyroidism.
- Chest X-ray to screen for malignancy.

- The patient's functional ability and ADLs are affected (particularly in early phases and during exacerbations).
- Reported difficulties include rising from a chair, getting out of bed, and difficulties with washing and dressing.
- Physiotherapy or occupational therapy referral may be required to support management of ADLs (exercise and use of aids and devices).
- Practical advice on relief of pain and stiffness include the use of warm showers and gentle exercise.
- Nurses in all care settings should advise patients about 'flares' of PMR, which may be related to reducing prednisolone. If there is a relapse of symptoms—particularly aching and stiffness in the shoulder and hip girdles—monitor CRP, review prednisolone dose, and seek specialist help where necessary.

Review

Review the patient after starting initial treatment (Box 4.6). Recheck inflammatory markers every 2–6 weeks after changes in treatment to assess response. Fracture risk assessment should be undertaken.

Response to treatment

Relapse is most common in the first 18 months of treatment but may recur when steroids are stopped. Steroids should be very slowly tapered down to reduce the risk of relapse. Pain is a predominant feature and will provide a good indicator of reductions in disease activity.

► Although not indicated as core treatment, an analgesic or NSAID may be prescribed in the short term for pain relief while weaning off prednisolone (refer to the *BNF* for cautions and contraindications).

Box 4.6 Treatment of polymyalgia rheumatica

- Low-dose prednisolone—commence on 15 mg once daily.[1]
- Dose reduction should be tailored to individual patients; BSR guidelines suggest: daily prednisolone 15 mg for 3 weeks; then 12.5 mg for 3 weeks; then 10 mg for 4–6 weeks; then reduction by 1 mg every 4–8 weeks or alternate-day reductions (e.g. 10/7.5 mg alternate days, etc.).
- For those that fail to achieve dose reductions, this may take longer and require a steroid-sparing agent (e.g. MTX).
- Analgesia may aid pain relief while reducing prednisolone.
- Monitor CRP, though clinical assessment is more important than blood tests results.
- Fracture risk assessment should be undertaken on commencing treatment.

Response to treatment

- 70% global response usually achieved within 1 week—a less complete response suggests an incorrect diagnosis.
- Return to normal values in acute phase responses.
- If response not demonstrated—stop treatment and review diagnosis.

Reference

1. Dasgupta B, Borg FA, Hassan N, et al. (2010). BSR and BHPR guidelines for the management of polymyalgia rheumatica. *Rheumatology* 49:186–90.

Frequently asked questions: polymyalgia rheumatica

What if the CRP remains elevated after starting prednisolone?

Diagnosis should be reviewed.

What if the patient with PMR is unable to stop prednisolone after 2 years?

Is the initial diagnosis correct? Other causes of pain such as OA should be considered.

Occasionally patients can require longer courses of treatment.

What if you suspect an underlying malignancy?

Refer to a consultant/physician for an urgent opinion.

What if a patient is unable to tolerate oral bisphosphonate therapy?

Consider parenteral bisphosphonates.

Further reading

Dasgupta B, Borg FA, Hassan N, et al. (2010). BSR and BHPR guidelines for the management of polymyalgia rheumatica. *Rheumatology* 49:186–90.

Hennell SL, Busteed S, George E (2007). Evidence-based management for polymyalgia rheumatica for rheumatology practitioners, nurses and physiotherapists. *Musculoskeletal Care* 5:65–71.

Giant cell arteritis

There is an association between PMR and GCA; 10% of patients with PMR will develop GCA. The majority of patients with GCA will have PMR symptoms.

GCA is inflammation of the larger blood vessels commonly affecting the extra cranial branches of the carotid artery. When monitoring PMR, ensure screening for GCA:

▶ Screening for GCA when monitoring PMR should include:

- Symptoms of unilateral headache or any visual symptoms.
- Scalp tenderness and jaw claudication.

▶ Seek urgent specialist opinion if GCA suspected.

Management of PMR and GCA

GCA will require more aggressive steroid treatment (➲ see Box 4.6, p. 113) including gradually reducing the dose when symptoms are effectively managed.[1]

▶ If new visual disturbances are reported, seek ophthalmology opinion.

➲ See also: Chapter 5, pp. 127–184, 'Connective tissue diseases', pp. 127–184.

Reference

1. Dasgupta B, Borg FA, Hassan N, et al. (2010). BSR and BHPR guidelines for the management of giant cell arteritis. *Rheumatology* 49:1594–7.

Crystal arthropathies

Crystal arthropathies describe a group of inflammatory joint disorders that develop as a result of micro crystal formation in the joints or in periarticular tissues. Other organs vulnerable to crystal deposition include excretory organs (e.g. liver, kidneys). For incidence and features see Table 4.3.

Crystal arthropathies are an important differential diagnosis for conditions such as inflammatory and septic arthritis where acute extremely painful joint pains are a presenting symptom; gout is the most common inflammatory arthritis. This section will provide an overview of crystal arthropathies with a specific focus on gout. For further more detailed information on crystal arthropathies refer to the British Society for Rheumatology (BSR) guidelines.[1]

Types of crystal arthropathies

Three major crystal arthropathies develop as a result of crystal deposits and these include:

- Monosodium urate monohydrate (MSM) ≈ gout.
- Calcium pyrophosphate deposition (CPPD) ≈ pseudogout.
- Calcium hydroxyapatite ≈ acute calcific periarthritis.

Crystal arthropathies can cause:

- Arthritis.
- Tenosynovitis.
- Bursitis.
- Cellulitis.
- Tophaceous deposits (usually late disease—gout only).
- Renal disease.

Presenting features and joints affected

- Symptomatic condition results in an 'acute' attack of arthritis.
- Joints become hot, swollen, and extremely tender to touch.
- The affected joint(s) may appear red and have a shiny appearance.

❶ Also signs of septic arthritis (a medical emergency).

Distribution of joints

The distribution of joints and tissues affected varies according to the type of crystal arthropathy:

- Gout: usually affects peripheral joints (big toe 50–70%; foot 50%; knee 30%; wrists 10%; elbows 10%; fingers 25%).
- CPPD: knees, wrists, hips, symphysis pubis, shoulders.
- Hydroxyapatite: central joints usually shoulders, rarely hips, spine, and knees.

Table 4.3 Incidence and features of crystal arthropathies

Condition	Gout	Pseudogout
Age of onset	Mean age of onset: • >40 years ♂ • >50 years ♀; rare before menopause	Rare in those <60 years of age
♂:♀ ratio	4 ♂:1 ♀	1 ♂:1 ♀
Mechanism	High levels of serum uric acid (SUA) develop as a result of overproduction or failure to adequately secrete SUA	Calcium pyrophosphate crystals (CPPC) released and shed into joint capsule causing inflammatory response (acute episode of pseudogout) CPPC can also deposit in tendons resulting in calcific tendonitis
Common precipitating factors	↑ SUA predisposing factor to developing may be combined with: • Menopausal status in ♀ • Impairment of renal function • Hypertension • Co-morbidities that comprise the metabolic syndrome • Diuretic use	There may be: • No obvious precipitating cause • Injury to joint • Generalized illness (especially if associated with ↑ temperature)
Co-morbidities	• Hypertension • Hyperglycaemia • Hyperlipidaemia	Strong associations with: • Hyperparathyroidism • Haemochromatosis • Hypomagnesaemia • Wilson disease
Differential diagnosis	• Septic arthritis • RA • PsA • ReA • Exacerbation of OA	• Several subcategories of CPPD • Septic arthritis and other inflammatory joint diseases (as for gout)

Reference

1. Hui M, Carr A, Cameron S, et al. (2017). The BSR guidelines for the management of gout. *Rheumatology* 56:e1–e20.

Gout and pseudogout

Gout and pseudogout are the two most common forms of crystal disease. For joints they affect, see Fig. 4.14.

Gout

Gout is a condition where urate crystals occur in joints, connective tissues, and urinary tract. Gout is associated with co-morbid conditions including renal impairment and cardiovascular disease. The incidence and prevalence is rising. In the UK, ~250,000 people every year consult their GP with a diagnosis of gout (➲ see Table 4.3, p. 117). Overall prevalence in the UK in 2012 was 2.5%.[1]

The predominant cause of gout is hyperuricaemia (SUA concentration >7 mg/dL). Uric acid is the end-product of protein metabolism and is usually excreted by:

- Kidneys (two-thirds).
- GI tract (one-third).

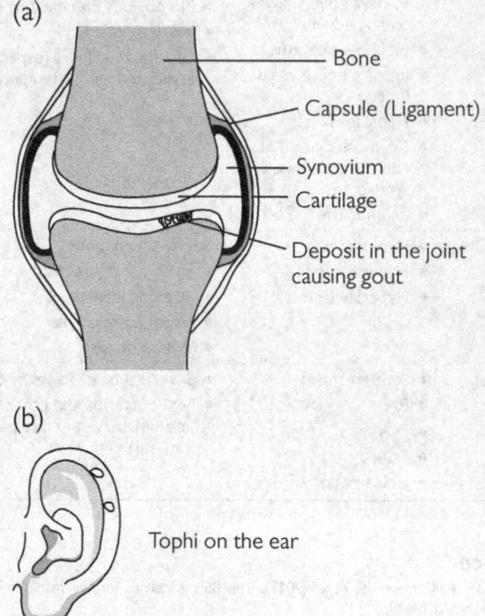

Fig. 4.14 Joints affected in gout and pseudogout. Urate may collect under the skin forming small white pimples ('tophi') but these are not usually painful.

Precipitating factors for gout

The risk of developing gout ↑ as SUA rises. Hyperuricaemia + precipitating factor (e.g. a patient starting diuretics or cytotoxic therapy) = gout (➲ see Table 4.3, p. 117). Gout can be described as either:

- 1°: no known cause or inherited metabolic disorder.
- 2°: to conditions that result in ↑ SUA.
  - High SUA can be attributed to either overproduction or underexcretion of uric acid and in some cases a mixture of both.
  - >90% cases are due to reduced clearance of SUA.[2]

The presentations of gout include:

- Acute attacks: sudden presentation of disabling pain (usually during the night), red, shiny skin, tender joint (usually big toe 50–70%, or lower limbs). Untreated can last days or weeks.
- Recurrent gout: can result in joint damage and residual disability.
- Chronic tophaceous gout: following recurrent attacks tophi are formed from accumulation of uric acid crystal and inflammatory cells forming under the skin and in periarticular tissues (the ear, bursae, and tendon sheaths).
  - Also seen in elderly patients (usually ♀) on diuretics.

Pseudogout

Pseudogout develops following the shedding of calcium pyrophosphate crystals from articular cartilage and is strongly associated with chondrocalcinosis (calcium crystals in hyaline cartilage, e.g. menisci). There are many similarities to gout as well as differences (➲ see Table 4.3, p. 117). The presentation of pseudogout is similar to that outlined in an acute attack of gout; however, the long-term course of the condition is usually more benign than gout. Symptoms can develop over a period of 24 hours and the clinical picture can sometimes mimic OA. Precipitating factors include:

- Injury to joint.
- Generalized illness (especially with associated fever).
- Surgery.

References

1. Kuo CF, Grainge MJ, Mallen C, et al. (2015). Rising burden of gout in the UK but continuing suboptimal management: a nationwide population study. *Ann Rheum Dis* 74:661–7.
2. Mount HK, Reginato AM (2005). Pathogenesis of gout. *Ann Intern Med* 143:499–516.

Crystal arthropathies: investigations and treatments

The diagnosis of a crystal arthropathy relies upon a thorough clinical history and good musculoskeletal examination (➲ see Chapter 8, 'Assessing the patient', p. 289).

❶ Septic arthritis is an important differential diagnosis (urgent medical treatment required).

Investigations for gout and pseudogout

Joint aspiration and microscopy

Microscopy of the synovial fluid analysis aids identification of the crystals implicated in the joint pain.

Microscopy should examine for:

- Urate crystals (gout)—negatively birefringent (murky, pus-like appearance).
- Calcium pyrophosphate—positive birefringent (may be bloodstained).
- Hydroxyapatite—stain with alizarin red.

Failure to identify crystals does not exclude the diagnosis.

❶ Culture of synovial fluid is important to exclude/confirm septic arthritis.

Blood tests

- Full blood count (FBC)—leucocytosis.
- Uric acid (may be normal during an acute attack but does not preclude gout). May be useful for monitoring treatment.
- Acute phase response—a normal CRP suggests an alternative diagnosis.
- U&E and creatinine. Further investigations may be required if abnormal results.
- Bloods to consider contributing factors, e.g. alcohol (raised gamma-glutamyl transferase or liver function tests (LFTs)), glycated haemoglobin (HbA1c) (diabetes), and lipids (hyperlipidaemia).

Radiological investigations—not always required

- X-rays can exclude trauma, fracture, or infections.
- In pseudogout, may identify additional factors such as OA.
- Soft tissue swelling, periarticular osteoporosis, and erosion may be evident in gout.
- ➲ See also Chapter 17, 'Blood tests and investigations' pp. 505–535.

Treatment

- Advise lifestyle modification; diet, alcohol, and obesity.
- Consider stopping causative drugs, e.g. diuretics.
- Removal of crystals by aspiration (especially in large joints) and IA steroid injection.
- Immediate relief of symptoms (analgesia, NSAIDs, colchicine, corticosteroids, rest, ice, elevation).
- Exclude/manage exacerbating factors related to 1° or 2° causes of gout.

- Urate-lowering therapy (ULT) should be discussed and offered to all patients who have a diagnosis of gout. ULT should particularly be advised in patients with the following: recurring attacks (two or more attacks in 12 months); tophi; chronic gouty arthritis; joint damage; renal impairment (estimated glomerular filtration rate <60 mL/min); a history of urolithiasis; diuretic therapy use; and 1° gout starting at a young age.
- Nursing care including education, symptom relief.

See Box 4.7.

❗ Important: septic arthritis is a differential diagnosis for acute onset of very painful joints.

Box 4.7 Treatment for calcium pyrophosphate deposition

- CPPD management similar to gout at initial presentation.
- Rest, information about the condition, management, and pain control.
- Paracetamol + codeine or NSAID for pain (although a very painful condition—review benefit); consider IA steroids.
- Colchicine—only recommended for recurrent attacks (rare).
- Exercises to reduce muscle wasting/weakness should be advocated when attack has resolved.
- Diet—no specific dietary factors.

Crystal arthropathies: nursing care issues in management

The commonest crystal arthropathy is gout followed by pseudogout. Gout is an extremely painful condition and requires prompt management to relieve the pain and distress and aid recovery. Individuals who are affected by these conditions initially require very similar nursing support and management, particularly in relation to:

- Pain-relieving strategies.
- Functional limitations.
- Monitoring of the condition and results of investigations.
- Lifestyle modification.

Severity of attacks and resolution will vary from mild (1–2 days) to severe (1 to several weeks).

Aims of management

Treatment and rapid relief of symptoms

See Table 4.4.

- Relief from the immediate attack of gout, with a focus on pain-relief strategies.
- Analgesia.
- Rest, ice packs, and pressure-relieving devices (e.g. bed cradle).
- Functional limitations.
- Reassurance/education and advice.

Self-management principles

- Education on condition and the causes of gout and hyperuricaemia
- Advice on resolution of attacks and managing future attacks.
- Managing medications.
- Lifestyle advice and issues related to concordance:
  - Moderation of alcohol consumption.
  - Dietary modification to achieve gradual reduction in body weight and subsequent maintenance.
  - Avoid sugar-sweetened soft drinks containing fructose.
  - Avoiding high-purine foods.
  - Weight loss if appropriate. Avoid crash diets (gout).
  - Encourage fluid intake of ~2 L per day.
  - Sensible moderate exercise—avoid intense physical exercise.

Prevention of future attacks (gout)

See Table 4.5.

Management must focus on treating the 1° or 2° causes related to the overproduction or underexcretion of SUA resulting in ↑ SUA.

- Urostatic—inhibit production: allopurinol and febuxostat.
- Urosuric—promote renal excretion of urate (sulfinpyrazone):
  - Urosuric drugs are less commonly used.
- Identification of contributing factors—related to co-morbidities etc.
- Guidance on managing a future attack—prompt NSAIDs.

Table 4.4 Prophylactic treatment for gout (also refer to the *BNF* and full summaries of product characteristics (SPCs))

Treatment • Do not commence treatment during acute attack • Commence treatment: 1–2 weeks after resolution of acute episode	Uricostatic drugs: • Febuxostat • Allopurinol	Uricosuric drugs (less commonly prescribed) • Sulfinpyrazone • Benzbromarone (unlicensed in UK prescribing named patient basis). Can ↑ LFTs
Mode and onset of action	• Requires metabolism by liver (prodrug) • Half-life ~24 hours (depending on renal function)	• Reduces renal reabsorption of SUA
Treatment regimen ► Allopurinol and febuxostat should be co-prescribed with low-dose NSAID or colchicine (0.5 mg twice daily) as risk of precipitating acute attacks (co-prescribe for ~12 months)	• Aim for SUA <300 mcg/L • Start with allopurinol 50–100 mg with 50–100 mg/day increments every few weeks adjusted for SUA target and renal function (max. dose 900 mg/day)	• Aim for SUA <300 mcg/L • Prescribe for underexcretors of SUA • 200–800 mg/day normal renal function • 50–200 mg/day mild/moderate renal insufficiency • Note: ineffective generally in patients with mild renal insufficiency
Side effects	• Hypersensitivity reactions (rare) • Hepatic toxicity/GI symptoms, central nervous system • Be aware of drug interactions	• Avoid in renal insufficiency;/disease or blood disorders/porphyria/risk of urinary stones • Do not co-prescribe with aspirin/salicylates • GI symptoms (common) • Blood disorders (rare
Monitoring Note: patient concordance is generally poor (50%), indicating a greater need for education	Monitor SUA levels every 3 months in the first year: then annual SUA, creatinine clearance, and patient knowledge/lifestyle	• Ensure adequate fluid intake (2–3 L daily) • Monitor SUA levels every 3 months in the first year: then annual SUA, creatinine clearance, and patient knowledge/lifestyle

Table 4.5 Treatment during an acute attack (refer to the SPCs and *BNF*)

Pain control	Nursing care	Analgesia	Corticosteroids	NSAIDs/COX-2	Colchicine (gout only)
Consider contraindications and cautions: GI/ cardiovascular (CV)/renal/ hepatic/elderly	Identify precipitating factors (e.g. diuretics) and refer to clinician Rest, ice, elevation Relief of pressure on affected joint(s)/evaluate functional limitations Consider MDT referral if appropriate	Avoid aspirin-based analgesia (low dose for CV risk can continue) Opiates can be used as adjunct to core treatment. NSAIDs/COX-2s/ colchicine	*IA injections per joint* Consider if confined to 1 joint: or contraindicated other therapies/refractory to treatment Aspirate: culture and microscopy. *IM injections* See for IA injections	Review risk factors: NSAIDs/COX-2s: contraindicated: consider steroids or colchicine	Narrow therapeutic window (efficacy vs toxicity/side effects) Used while initiating prophylactic treatment with allopurinol—for at least 6 weeks (if tolerated)
Onset of action	Review pain scores/ assessments and review nursing support/treatment required	Consider risk factors, tolerance, and pain relief needs Select: compound analgesia or opiate with dosing regimens to add to therapeutic benefit of NSAIDs	Rapid onset of benefit	Select NSAID/COX-2 Full licensed dose, short half-life, rapid onset NSAID: indometacin 50 mg three times daily. Consider: diclofenac, ibuprofen, naproxen, etoricoxib	Alternative for those contraindicated NSAIDs/COX-2s. Side effect profile inhibits use

Pain control	Nursing care	Analgesia	Corticosteroids	NSAIDs/COX-2	Colchicine (gout only)
Treatment regimens	Regular analgesia Monitor benefit Monitor bloods Observations: fluid intake, pyrexia, skin integrity Education and advice on medications, lifestyle (when appropriate time). Use resources for dietary advice (https://www.versusarthritis.org/)	Assess risk factors and consider: Compound analgesia: Co-codamol at different dose ranges 1–2-, 4–6-hourly Co-dydramol 10/500 1–2 tabs 4–6-hourly: Or select: opioid Tramadol hydrochloride 50–100 mg 4-hourly	IA injection to affected joint: triamcinolone acetonide (40–80 mg) IA or IM methylprednisolone acetate (80–120 mg)	Limit treatment to 6 weeks max. Traditional NSAID + PPI COX-2: if GI but no CV risk ± PPI Select NSAID/COX-2 in relation to patient individual risk factors	Start: 500 mcg twice daily (max. 6 mg per course of treatment) Do not repeat within 3/7 days
Benefits	Essential to aid recovery/ functional ability and encourage positive coping styles	Adjunct to NSAIDs	IA: aspirate can also be diagnostic Relieves swelling promptly	Highly effective for pain relief	Valuable for heart failure patients or those on warfarin
Risks	Psychological distress Pain, fatigue, and loss of appetite	Constipation Nausea Encourage fluid intake	! Consider: septic arthritis IA: small risk of infection on injecting Steroid-related side effects:	Side effect profile of NSAIDs/COX-2s Should be lowest optimal dose for shortest duration	Side effect profile: narrow therapeutic window IV colchicine: **not recommended**

Also see Chapter 9, 'Symptom control'.

Frequently asked questions: crystal arthropathies

Is gout hereditary?

A genetic predisposition means some people will have a higher chance of developing gout, e.g. people who have a familial hyperuricaemia due to an inability to secrete uric acid (~30% of ♂). However, otherwise gout itself is not hereditary.

What is the long-term risk related to having gout?

The long-term damage to joints (such as a chronic arthritis) tends to happen only if there are repeated attacks of gout over a sustained period—ULT reduces this risk.

Gout is associated with chronic disability and impaired quality of life. Gout is also associated with co-morbidities such as obesity, diabetes mellitus, chronic kidney disease, hypertension, cardiovascular disease, depression, and an ↑ in mortality.[1]

How many people have more than one attack of gout?

The first attack usually occurs between 40 and 60 years of age and some people may never experience another attack. Around 50% of patients will suffer a further attack; the risk ↑ depending on the number of risk factors a patient has. Attacks are more frequent in those who receive no ULT. Patients should be warned that starting ULT may precipitate another attack and that the treatment will need to be long term.

Reference

1. Kuo CF, Grainge MJ, Mallen C, et al. (2015). Rising burden of gout in the UK but continuing sub-optimal management: a nationwide population study. *Ann Rheum Dis* 74:661–7.

Chapter 5

Connective tissue diseases

Systemic lupus erythematosus

Introduction

Lupus (SLE) is an autoimmune disease of unknown aetiology. This is a complex autoimmune disease that is multifactorial in nature and currently has no known cure. It is the commonest of the connective tissue diseases (CTDs) and follows a pattern of unpredictable activity with quieter phases of the condition.

Genetic, hormonal, and infective causes have all been cited as playing an important part in the development of lupus in any one individual. Lupus is 10–20 times more commonly seen in ♀ than in ♂, and frequently presents in young ♀ of child-bearing age. Although lupus is reported worldwide, certain ethnic groups have a higher incidence (Afro-Caribbean, Chinese) which reflects in epidemiological figures.

Widespread inflammation leads to symptoms ranging from simple joint aches and pains, with fatigue and skin rashes, to life-threatening multisystem organ failure. Organs that can be targeted are the kidneys, the heart, the lungs, and the central nervous system (CNS). Less commonly, the inflammatory component of lupus also has the potential to damage other organs including the:

- Pancreas.
- GI system.
- Circulatory system.

Classification criteria

Criteria for the classification of SLE were published in 1982,[1] and revised in 1997 (Box 5.1).[2] These classification criteria, devised by the ACR, are of value for clinical trials but play a small part in the clinical diagnostic process. In routine daily practice, a full clinical examination, presenting symptoms, and blood results together enable the clinician to confirm diagnosis.

Prognosis

Lupus still carries a significant risk of mortality and long-term morbidity despite advances in treatment. Renal lupus remains one of the major causes of death in lupus; however, more recently, cardiovascular events are increasingly being recognized as playing an important role in improving long-term outcomes.

➲ Also see 'Diagnosing lupus: the importance of blood and urine tests', p. 129; ➲ 'Pregnancy in Sjögren's syndrome', p. 147.

References

1. Tan EM, Cohen AS, Fries JF, et al. (1982). The 1982 revised criteria for the classification of systemic lupus erythematosus. *Arthritis Rheum* 25:1271–7.
2. Hochberg MC (1997). Updating the American College of Rheumatology revised criteria for the classification of systemic lupus erythematosus. *Arthritis Rheum* 40:1725.

Diagnosing lupus: the importance of blood and urine tests

Lupus is diagnosed through clinical history and systemic examination. Confirmation of the diagnosis is through positive autoantibody tests. Blood abnormalities are common in lupus, including anaemia, leucopenia, thrombocytopenia, and other clotting disorders. Iron deficiency and immune-mediated anaemia are also common.

Red blood cells (RBCs)

Up to 40% of lupus patients will become anaemic at some point during the course of their disease. There are numerous causes related to the anaemia including iron deficiency, GI bleeding, or medications (steroids and NSAIDs). Anaemia of chronic disease can lead to antibody formation, which target the RBCs leading to a normochromic-normocytic anaemia.

Thrombocytopenia (low platelets) occurs in 25–35% and can respond to low-dose steroids. Coombs-positive haemolytic anaemia occurs in 10% of lupus patients. In cases of haemolytic anaemia/thrombocytopenia, high-dose steroids with immunosuppression (azathioprine (AZA), mycophenolate mofetil (MMF)) are required. Liaison with haematology is essential in those with platelet counts regularly <100 × 10^9/L.

White blood cells (WBCs)

Low levels of WBCs are common and can lead to a greater risk of infection. Leucopenia is found in 15–20% and is common in active lupus.

Autoantibodies

Specific autoantibody testing is a valuable diagnostic tool in lupus. The commonly presenting autoantibodies are as follows:

- Antinuclear antibody (ANA): over 90% of those with lupus have a positive ANA, above a titre of 1/40. This is not specific for lupus and needs to be considered with other more specific tests. ANAs can also be present in other autoimmune rheumatic conditions and chronic infections.
- Anti-Sm: Sm is a ribonucleoprotein found in the cell nucleus. Highly specific for lupus, present in about 30% of those with lupus.
- Anti-dsDNA: an immunoglobulin that is highly specific for lupus that can fluctuate with disease activity and therefore serial testing is a useful monitoring tool. Associated with a higher risk of lupus nephritis.
- Extractable nuclear antigen (ENA) anti-Ro and anti-La: these immunoglobulins are commonly found together and are specific against RNA proteins. Anti-Ro is found in 30% of lupus and 70% of those with 1° Sjögren's syndrome (SS). Anti-La found in 15% with lupus and 60% of 1° SS. Anti-Ro is associated with photosensitivity and both are associated with neonatal lupus.
- Antiphospholipid antibodies should always be checked in lupus, with or without any history of thromboembolic disease. These include antibodies directed against cardiolipin and β2 glycoprotein 1. To confirm a positive result, the tests should be repeated 6–12 weeks apart.

Box 5.1 Revised criteria of the ACR for the classification of SLE

4 out of these 11 criteria must be present for a diagnosis of SLE:

1. Malar rash.
2. Discoid rash.
3. Photosensitivity.
4. Oral ulcers.
5. Arthritis.
6. Serositis: pleuritis or pericarditis.
7. Renal disorder: proteinuria >0.5 g/24 hours at 3+ persistently or cellular casts.
8. Neurological disorder: seizures or psychosis (excluding other causes such as drugs).
9. Haematological disorder:
   - Haemolytic anaemia *or*
   - Leucopenia or $<4.0 \times 10^9$/L on two or more occasions *or*
   - Lymphopenia or $<1.5 \times 10^9$/L on two or more occasions *or*
   - Thrombocytopenia $<100 \times 10^9$/L.
10. Immunological disorders: raised dsDNA antibody binding or anti-Sm antibody or positive antiphospholipid antibodies (abnormal serum level IgG/IgM anticardiolipin antibodies and a positive lupus anticoagulant) or a false-positive serological test for syphilis known to be positive of at least 6 months and confirmed by *Treponema pallidum* immobilization or fluorescent treponemal antibody absorption test.
11. ANA in raised titre.

Source: data from Tan EM, Cohen AS, Fries JF, et al. (1982). The 1982 revised criteria for the classification of systemic lupus erythematosus. *Arthritis and Rheumatism*, 25(11), 1271–7.

- In addition, the lupus anticoagulant should be checked in all lupus patients (activated partial thromboplastin time (APTT), dilute Russell's viper venom time (dRVVT), and kaolin clotting time (KCT)).

Other tests

- *Complement proteins (C3 and C4)*: help to mediate inflammation. Levels of C3 and C4 may be low in active lupus especially lupus nephritis.
- *Inflammatory markers*: general measure of inflammation such as PV and ESR are useful in lupus, although CRP can be normal. A raised CRP in lupus may indicate infection.
- *U&Es, creatinine, LFTs, and creatine kinase*: routine blood testing must always include U&Es and LFTs. Protein/creatinine ratio is important in suspected renal involvement.
- *Vitamin D_3 and thyroid function tests.*
- *Urine testing*: essential at every clinic visit, the routine dipstick alerts the nurse to early signs of kidney disease. Protein and haematuria should be investigated further by looking for red cell casts. Protein excretion

should be quantified by urine protein/creatinine ratio. If leucocytes or nitrites are present, then the urine should be cultured for infection.

►► Immediate action must be taken in anyone with lupus who shows signs of early renal disease. This should include referral to a renal physician for potential kidney biopsy to determine the extent and type of inflammation and/or damage.

► *Any rise in blood pressure may be an associated sign of renal complications.*

❗ A flare of lupus is often seen as a rising titre of dsDNA antibodies and PV/ESR, falling complements and lymphocytes, accompanied by systemic symptoms (➔ see 'Nursing care of lupus patients', p. 140).

Lupus: antiphospholipid syndrome, fertility/pregnancy, and hormone replacement therapy issues

Lupus: antiphospholipid syndrome (APS)

APS can be either 1° or 2° to lupus. This classically presents as blood clotting (thrombosis) and, in ♀, a tendency to miscarriage. This can be both arterial and venous clotting leading to a wide range of symptoms. It is also described as 'sticky blood' which can be worse during pregnancy when blood viscosity is naturally thicker. This can lead to a higher risk of pre-eclampsia and premature birth.

Classically APS can cause:

- Thrombosis—venous (DVT), arteries (cerebrovascular accident, hypertension) and brain (memory loss, seizures, migraine).
- Recurrent miscarriages.
- Livedo reticularis—blotchy skin rash.
- Thrombocytopenia.

Treatments for APS depend on the history of clotting but can include low-dose aspirin, warfarin, and during pregnancy, low-molecular-weight heparin. Close supervision is required to enable a healthy fetus to survive. In those ♀ with lupus and APS, who carry the Ro/La antibodies, prepregnancy counselling and close nurse specialist support is vital.

Lupus: contraception, pregnancy, and HRT

Lupus is known to be exacerbated by hormones and can lead to flares when the menstrual cycle is due and often postpartum. Oestrogen is known to flare lupus, so contraception and HRT should always be progesterone-only where possible.

Steroid management during pregnancy can be life-saving. At the same time it must be recognized that pregnant ♀ with lupus—especially those on steroids—are more likely to develop hypertension, diabetes, hyperglycaemia, and renal complications. Pregnancy itself may also cause the disease to flare. However, many ♀ with lupus have normal pregnancies and these should be encouraged in ♀ when their disease is quiescent.

Pregnancy carries some risks, especially in those ♀ with the anti-Ro/La antibodies and 2° APS. Babies from mothers who carry the anti-Ro/La antibodies can be born with a transient neonatal lupus (➔ see 'Pregnancy in Sjögren's syndrome', p. 147). Mothers carrying Ro/La are at risk of fetal heart block and should be referred for fetal echocardiography at a centre experienced in the management of this complication. It affects 1:20 women with Ro/La.

The risk of miscarriage is high for those with positive anticardiolipin antibodies and positive lupus anticoagulant. Figures suggest up to a 30% risk of miscarriage with the first pregnancy, and with a history of at least two spontaneous miscarriages, up to 70% during the following pregnancy. 50% of miscarriages occur in the second and third trimesters. Aspirin and low-molecular-weight heparin should replace warfarin and be continued throughout pregnancy and the postpartum period.

Where possible, all medications should be reduced to a minimum and drugs such as MTX and mycophenolate must be stopped in advance of conception as they are teratogenic. Medication reviews and prepregnancy counselling are a vital part of the nurse's role in giving information about these risks and ensuring where possible, that pregnancies are planned events. A consultant-led hospital birth should be booked and ♀ and their partners allowed time to discuss any issues at length.

➔ See 'Nursing issues', pp. 140 and 330; ➔ Patient-centred care, p. 332.

Further reading

Gordon C, Amissah-Arthur MB, Gayed M, et al. (2018). The British Society for Rheumatology guideline for the management of systemic lupus erythematosus in adults. *Rheumatology (Oxford)* 57:e1–45.

Lupus: musculoskeletal system and the skin

Up to 90% of lupus patients describe musculoskeletal symptoms of flitting symmetrical joint and muscle aches and pains. There is usually little erosive damage to joints but tenosynovitis is common. Subluxation of some joints can occur, which is typically seen as a reversible deformity, though it can be severe and disabling as in the case of Jaccoud's arthropathy.

Investigations of musculoskeletal symptoms

- Plain X-ray to exclude erosive arthritis suggestive of RA.
- MRI or US can reveal characteristic signs of soft tissue changes and bony alterations although this investigation is not indicated routinely.

Management of musculoskeletal symptoms

- Symptoms can be improved by simple NSAIDs or hydroxychloroquine, an antimalarial.
- DMARDs such as MTX may be required in rare cases of lupus overlap disease with some components of erosive disease.
- Surgical referral to orthopaedics may be necessary in severe cases of tenosynovitis.
- Patients who have lupus with musculoskeletal involvement can see the condition impact their work, home, and social life, ultimately affecting their quality of life.
- Arthralgia can cause a range of functional limitations affecting work and home life.
- Managing children and juggling work and home commitments can lead to high levels of fatigue and subsequent depression.
- Nursing management of musculoskeletal symptoms includes assessment of active disease and patient education relating to understanding the disease process and the importance of balancing exercise and rest.
- Self-management techniques as part of formal education programmes are beneficial, but require high levels of support and resources.[1]
- Referrals to occupational therapy for ADL assessment and physiotherapy for graded exercise programmes are essential to encourage the individual to optimize sometimes limited personal resources.

Lupus and the skin

Cutaneous involvement of lupus is very common, with the classic 'butterfly rash'. The butterfly rash is:

- Seen in about one-third of those diagnosed with lupus.
- Is a disc-shaped lesions seen across the face (sparing the nasal folds) and light exposed areas of the skin.
- In discoid lupus (skin only), these rashes can be scarring.
- Sun exposure can trigger systemic disease flares of lupus.
- Oral manifestations include:
    - Recurrent crops of mouth ulcers (a feature of active disease).
    - Dryness related to 2° SS, affecting the eyes, mouth, skin, and vagina.

Management of lupus skin problems

Again, hydroxychloroquine can be helpful, with mepacrine as an options for severe rashes. Collaborative working with a dermatologist is essential for those with severe rashes.

Nursing advice is important in order to help patients successfully manage skin flares of lupus. Nursing advice includes:

- Use of high-factor sun cream (above SPF50) UV-A and-B on a regular basis all year round.
- Sunsense and Uvistat both provide comprehensive ranges or other high-quality products that also include moisturizer and tint for the face.
- Simple advice such as avoiding the midday sun, using sun hats for protection, wearing sun-protective clothing, and choosing an appropriate holiday resort will help to prevent skin flares.
- Referral to the British Red Cross cosmetic camouflage service enables successful covering of scars.

➔ Also see 'Nursing care of lupus patients', p. 140.

Reference

1. Brown S, Somerset ME, McCabe CS, McHugh NJ (2004). The impact of group education on participants' management of their disease in lupus and scleroderma. *Musculoskeletal Care* 2:207–17.

Lupus: fatigue and psychological manifestations

Nurses play a vital role in enabling individuals to share their feelings and provide support during difficult phases of the condition and symptoms experienced.[1] Fatigue is one of the most frequently reported symptoms of lupus, and is the most challenging to treat. Fatigue can lead to:

- Frustration and anger. These symptoms can be compounded by the despair experienced in the protracted processes involved in achieving a diagnosis.
- A sense of helplessness fuelled by the fatigue and inability to undertake normal ADLs.
- Problems with personal relationships and in working life.
- Associated fibromyalgia can worsen fatigue.
- Depression is common, is complicated by fatigue, and requires careful management and support.

General management issues

- Psychological effects can worsen symptoms, and it is important for the nurse to be alert to any signs of potential psychological repercussions.
- In some cases the treatments such as hydroxychloroquine may help improve feelings of fatigue.
- For those requiring additional psychological support, initiation of antidepressive treatment and referral to psychology teams should be considered in severe cases.
- Contact with others patients with lupus may enable individuals to share common feelings. Local support groups and access to national support should be available and are often provided by national organizations such as Lupus UK.[2]

➲ Also see 'Nursing care of lupus patients', p. 140; ➲ 'Education, social, and psychological aspects of a new diagnosis', pp. 336–340.

References

1. Waldron N, Brown SJ, Hewlett S, et al. (2011). 'It's more scary not to know': a qualitative study exploring the information needs of patients with systemic lupus erythematosus at the time of diagnosis. *Musculoskeletal Care* 9:228–38.
2. Lupus UK: http://www.lupusuk.org.uk

Lupus: cardiopulmonary, renal, and central nervous system

Lupus and the cardiopulmonary system

All cardiac and pulmonary symptoms should be taken seriously and referred to a cardiologist and a pulmonary physician to undergo thorough investigations. These can include pulmonary function tests (PFTs) (including gas transfer), echocardiogram, high-resolution computed tomography (HRCT) of the chest, and right-heart catheterization where pulmonary hypertension is suspected. Cardiovascular disease is becoming the leading cause of death in lupus. Cardiac/cardiovascular abnormalities include:

- Pericarditis with a rub.
- Myocarditis (in up to 15%) with combinations of tachycardias and dysrhythmias, systolic murmurs, and endocarditis.
- Accelerated atherosclerosis, due to the chronic inflammatory nature of the disease and the use of steroids to control inflammation.
- Risk of myocardial infarction (MI). Screening for those at high risk is an important part of the clinic consultation.

Pulmonary abnormalities

Pulmonary involvement of lupus is often described as subclinical, with late presentation sometimes limiting treatment.

Pulmonary hypertension in lupus is rare, and is usually pulmonary arterial hypertension which is managed with targeted therapies such as endothelin receptor antagonists (bosentan, sitaxsentan). Immunosuppression may need to be reviewed in the light of evidence of a flare of lupus. PH can also be 2° to lung fibrosis or pulmonary emboli as a result of antiphospholipid antibodies.

- Pulmonary arterial hypertension.
- Pulmonary fibrosis.
- Pleurisy—the most common respiratory problem and pleuritic chest pain is a common feature.

Managing cardiopulmonary systems

- Cholesterol should be measured (aim for the cholesterol ratio to be <5), blood pressure aim for <125/75 mmHg, weight, BMI, and dietary intake should all be addressed.
- Blood glucose should be measured.
- Cessation of smoking is imperative to reduce the ↑ risk of cardiovascular events.

The role of the nurse is to enable the patient to make informed choices about their risks and treatment options in the context of the individual's lifestyle. Nurses should also be informed about detecting changes in cardiac and pulmonary function and alerting specialist teams.

Lupus and the kidneys

Renal involvement is one of the most life-threatening complications of lupus. Regular investigations at *every clinic visit* must include a blood test for renal function, urinalysis for protein, and blood pressure. Renal biopsy can be helpful in guiding treatment. Treatments include:

- High-dose steroids.
- Immunosuppression with cyclophosphamide and/or MMF/AZA.
- Diuretics and antihypertensives as needed.
- Or anti-B-cell ablation with the anti CD-20 monoclonal antibody, rituximab.

Lupus and the CNS

This is the most worrying complication for the individual with lupus. Symptoms can be vague and somewhat difficult to distinguish from other diseases. There is no one single diagnostic test. Symptoms can range from:

- Headaches and seizures.
- Mood swings.
- Depression/psychosis.
- Cranial or peripheral neuropathy.

If these symptoms occur, they can result in extreme fear and distress for the patient. Nurses play an important role by providing:

- Relevant information, anticipating concerns, and helping the individual and their family to develop coping skills, allowing time and attention to all involved. Support from and referral to local psychiatric services may be required.
- ► Nursing support in identifying early referral to specialist teams.
- This support is often achieved by providing a first point of access with a telephone advice lines. Vigilance in identifying fluid retention, weight gain, lethargy, hypertension (with proteinuria), raised creatinine, or other signs indicating renal failure or fluid and electrolyte imbalance can limit damage.
- ➲ Also see 'Nursing care of lupus patients', Chapter 5, p. 140.

Assessment tools to evaluate lupus activity

Evaluating lupus activity is divided into:

- Disease activity.
- Disease severity.

These measures are system based and calculate a score based upon evidence reviewed through clinic assessment over the last 6 months. The BILAG-2004 and the SLEDAI-2K or the SELENA-SLEDAI are recommended tools for assessing disease activity.

The SLICC/ACR Damage Index X is used to measure damage. Health status is usually measured using the SF-36 or LupusQoL.

➲ See Chapter 20, 'Assessment tools', pp. 595–612.

Prognosis

Lupus still carries a significant risk of mortality and long-term morbidity despite advances in treatment. Renal lupus remains one of the major causes of death in lupus; however, more recently cardiovascular events are increasingly presenting. Knowledge of the impact of premature atherosclerosis must be at the forefront of the nurse's mind when managing lupus patients, where prevention is the key. Early management and intervention of any atherosclerosis will improve long-term prognosis in those who survive the early years of the illness.

➲ See 'Nursing care of lupus patients', p. 140.

Nursing care of lupus patients

Nursing care management of lupus is aimed at enabling individuals to make informed choices through access to up-to-date information and support. From the patient perspective they have invariably been referred to numerous specialists over time, with a significant delay in receiving a diagnosis. This delay can vary from a number of months to many years of 'non-specific' symptoms, and can often depend on a chance referral to an enlightened specialist for correct diagnosis.

Treatments are aimed at managing acute periods of potentially life-threatening illness, minimizing the risk of flares when the disease is quiescent, and controlling day-to-day symptoms.

Some specialist rheumatology units have access to lupus nurse specialists who can offer:

- Specialist support through consultations and telephone advice lines.
- Education—vital to those newly diagnosed who need to recognize potentially serious symptoms and know how to gain early access to specialist treatment.[1] The key areas for nursing input in lupus are in providing education, support, information, and counselling in helping individuals to work towards accepting lupus as a chronic illness. The difficulty for nurses is balancing the right level of information without causing distress or worry to the lupus patient.
- Proactive support to the patient to prevent common problems related to the condition such as fatigue and depression. Diagnosis can depend on a chance referral to an enlightened specialist. Delay in diagnosis impacts the individual's ability to cope with their diagnosis, its treatment, and potential complications. Furthermore, lupus can also be misdiagnosed, and is known as a mimic of other diseases such as multiple sclerosis or syphilis.
- Knowledge of the impact of premature atherosclerosis must be at the forefront of the nurse's mind when managing lupus patients, where prevention is the key. Early management and intervention of any atherosclerosis will improve long-term prognosis in those who survive the early years of the illness.
- Nursing interventions include explanations of the significance of the blood and urine tests and giving education to ensure patients attend the surgery for regular tests when they are known to have systemic manifestations of lupus. Alerting specialist teams when developing symptoms such as ↑ fatigue and bruising/bleeding may enable early intervention.

Assessment of vaccination status

- Medication reviews and prepregnancy counselling is a vital part of the nurse's role in giving information about these risks and ensuring, where possible, that pregnancies are planned events.
- Monitoring for drug toxicities and blood, cervical, vulval, lung, and thyroid malignancies.

Key points

- Education about the disease process, early warning signs, recognizing and managing a flare, knowing when to contact the specialist team.
- Assisting in adjusting to physical and psychological changes, encouraging lifestyle and self-management skills.
- Empathy and support: enabling contact with specialist teams and self-help groups such as Lupus UK.[2]
- Availability by telephone for ongoing support between consultations.
- Body image problems: addressing worrying concerns such as rashes or scarring.
- Pregnancy advice and prepregnancy counselling.
- Setting realistic achievable goals in maintaining best level of health and optimize resources.
- Balancing the need for information, relevant to the individual and their lupus, without causing distress or worry.
- Monitoring for drug toxicities and malignancies.

References

1. Arthritis and Musculoskeletal Alliance (2007). Standards of care for people with connective tissue diseases. http://arma.uk.net/wp-content/uploads/pdfs/ctdweb.pdf
2. Lupus UK: http://www.lupusuk.com

Further reading

Gordon C, Amissah-Arthur MB, Gayed M, et al. (2018). The British Society for Rheumatology guideline for the management of systemic lupus erythematosus in adults. *Rheumatology (Oxford)* 57:e1–45.

Sjögren's syndrome: overview

Introduction

Sjögren's syndrome (SS) is a systemic autoimmune disease of unknown aetiology. It is a chronic condition that can have a significant impact on an individual's quality of life and working capacity and is characterized by lymphocyte infiltration of the exocrine glands leading to a dry mouth (xerostomia) and dry eyes (keratoconjunctivitis sicca). Inflammatory cells target both the salivary and lachrymal glands, resulting in atrophy of the glands and subsequent dryness of not only the eyes and the mouth, but in severe cases the vulva/vagina, pharynx, oesophagus, and skin. SS affects:

- Nine times more ♀ than ♂. Incidence figures vary, but it has been reported as affecting between 3% and 4% of the UK population.
- Tends to occur between the ages of 40 and 60 years (but can affect children and the elderly).
- One of the complex CTDs, SS has some genetic, environmental, and infective causes although there is currently no clear evidence to support any one cause. It has been associated with certain viruses, in particular the Epstein–Barr virus and retroviruses. There is no cure for SS, and treatments aim to reduce symptoms and preserve organ function.

Diagnosis

Box 5.2 outlines the revised international criteria for diagnosis of SS.[1] Diagnosis is also supported by excluding other diagnoses or medication-related symptoms (e.g. sarcoidosis can mimic the clinical picture of SS). SS can be either a 1° or 2° diagnosis:

- 1° SS is associated more with more systemic (extra-glandular) disease and carries with it a 40-fold relative risk of lymphoma (although the absolute risk is very small). 1° SS patients often report significant fatigue, fever, Raynaud's phenomenon, myalgias, and arthralgias.
- 2° SS is reported in 10–20% of those with lupus and RA.

Tests of reduced tear/salivary secretion can be useful, but not wholly diagnostic of SS, as keratoconjunctivitis sicca occurs in many different conditions. Extra-glandular features are seen in about one-third of SS patients. Most frequently seen extra-glandular features include:

- 60% with arthritis/arthralgias.
- 40% with Raynaud's phenomenon.
- 14% with lymphadenopathy.
- 14% with lung involvement.

The importance of blood tests

As SS is a syndrome (that can appear in many different forms), it can be difficult to diagnose and there are no specific simple diagnostic tests. Blood tests to aid diagnosis include:

- ANA—89% positive in SS.
- Anti-Ro/La antibodies on testing of ENA:
  - Anti-Ro (SSA) seen in 70%.

Box 5.2 Classification criteria for Sjögren's syndrome

Diagnosis of SS confirmed if four out of the following six criteria are met:

1. Ocular symptoms: a positive response to at least one of the following questions:
   - Have you had daily, persistent, troublesome dry eyes for >3 months?
   - Do you have a recurrent sensation of sand or gravel in the eyes?
   - Do you use tear substitutes more than three times a day?
2. Oral symptoms: a positive response to at least one of the following questions:
   - Have you had a daily feeling of a dry mouth for >3 months?
   - Have you had recurrently or persistently swollen salivary glands as an adult?
   - Do you frequently drink liquids to aid in swallowing dry food?
3. Ocular signs: positive Schirmer's test without anaesthesia <5 mm in 5 min or rose bengal score ≥4 according to van Bijsterveld's scoring system.
4. Histopathology: in minor salivary glands, focal lymphocytic sialadentitis with a focus score ≥1.
5. Salivary gland involvement: objective evidence defined by a positive result in at least one of the following:
   - Unstimulated whole salivary flow <1.5 mL/min.
   - Parotid gland sialography showing presence of diffuse sialectasias.
   - Salivary scintigraphy showing delayed uptake, reduced concentration, and/or delayed excretion of tracer.
6. Autoantibodies: presence in the serum of the following autoantibodies: antibodies to Ro (SSA) or La (SSB) antigens, or both.

Source: data from Vitali et al. (2002). Classification criteria for Sjögren's syndrome: a revised version of the European criteria proposed by the American-European Consensus Group. *Annals of the Rheumatic Diseases*, 61, 554–8.

- Anti-La (SSB) seen in 60%.
- Up to 60–90% of Europeans who are Ro/La positive also carry the HLA-DR3 association.

- Raised PV/CRP/ESR, acute phase response to inflammation.
- Always exclude other diagnoses. Clinicians should always test for hepatitis C, AIDS, pre-existing lymphoma, sarcoidosis, and graft-versus-host disease.

Reference

1. Vitali C, Bombardieri S, Jonsson R, et al. (2002). Classification criteria for Sjögren's syndrome: a revised version of the European criteria proposed by the American-European Consensus Group. *Ann Rheumat Dis* 61:554–8.

Sjögren's syndrome and the glands

Symptoms of glandular involvement can be very non-specific, making diagnosis difficult and sometimes protracted. Dry eyes are commonly the first presentation and the intensity of symptoms can worsen over time. Other conditions and medications can also be responsible for presenting symptoms and they should always be excluded as part of the screening process for SS.

Oral signs and symptoms

Lymphocytic infiltrate of the exocrine glands can result in significant symptoms. Enlargement of the parotids can be episodic or frequent and occurs in 50% of those with 1° SS, leading to chronic enlargement. The 1° symptom that causes most problems is dryness (xerostomia), leading to symptoms such as:

- Difficulty in swallowing food.
- Difficulty in holding a conversation, an inability to speak continuously.
- Experiencing disturbed sleep.
- Dental caries, periodontitis, and gingivitis.
- Oral thrush.
- Change in taste sensation.
- Pain and burning.

Treatment for oral symptoms using simple remedies, such as:

- Use of room humidifiers.
- Sips of water frequently, sucking ice cubes.
- Avoiding sugared drinks or highly sugared foods.
- Drink water regularly.
- Chewing xylitol containing sugar-free gum to stimulate salivary production.
- Brush teeth twice a day using a high-fluoride toothpaste.
- 3–6-monthly dental check-ups.
- Avoid alcohol-containing mouthwashes.
- Saliva sprays—Saliva Orthana® or Luborant® (contain fluoride) or Glandosane® (fluoride free).
- Biotene range including gels, gums, and toothpastes.
- Spoonful of natural sugar-free Greek yoghurt before bed.

Ocular signs and symptoms

This is the major glandular manifestation that can lead to significant eye infections and possible corneal and conjunctival damage. Symptoms described include:

- Gritty, burning sensation in the eye.
- Redness and itchiness in the eye.
- Photosensitivity.

Schirmer's test evaluates tear secretion and is measured through a filter strip of paper 30 mm long, that is placed on the lower eyelid. The result is positive if ≤5 mm is wet in 5 min. A further measure of tear secretion is the rose bengal test where a dye is applied to the ocular surface which is taken up by devitalized epithelial cells. Positive staining is consistent with SS.

Treatments for ocular symptoms include:

- Using a warm compress daily to stimulate meibomian gland secretion.
- Use a weak solution of bicarbonate to wipe eye lids daily with a cotton bud.
- Use of liposomal sprays.[1]
- Simple lubricants such as hypromellose drops (preservative free), with longer-acting agents such as Viscotears® single dose unit (SDU) or Celluvisc® SDU if necessary.
- Ointments such as Lacri-Lube® are helpful at night.
- If there is mucus stranding, then mucolytics are prescribed such as acetylcysteine 5–10% non-preserved eye drops.[1]
- Punctal occlusion should be considered in those with severe symptoms, with temporary performed first.
- For long-standing inflammation, referral to an ophthalmologist for consideration of ciclosporin 0.1% (Ikervis®) as recommended by NICE.[2]
- In severe cases, pilocarpine 5 mg once daily increasing to 5mg four times daily may be of benefit.[1]

Treatment for chronic enlargement of parotids can require:

- Use of US to assess the extent of inflammation and evidence of stones.[1]
- A short course of steroids can be used for acute inflammation after infection has been excluded.[1]
- Massaging the glands can help.

References

1. Price EJ, Rauz S, Tappuni AR, et al. (2017). The British Society for Rheumatology guideline for the management of adults with primary Sjögren's syndrome. *Rheumatology* 56:1643–7.
2. NICE (2015). Ciclosporin for treating dry eye disease that has not improved despite treatment with artificial tears. ℘ https://www.nice.org.uk/guidance/ta369

Sjögren's syndrome and extra-glandular manifestations: systemic disease

Systemic disease is seen in one-third of those with 1° SS. Most commonly presenting symptoms include fatigue, arthralgias, myalgias, and low-grade fevers. Raynaud's phenomenon is also present in up to about 35% and this symptom can predate sicca symptoms by many years. Digital fingertip ulceration is not a feature. Treatments depend on severity of systemic damage, with immunosuppression often required using high-dose steroids, DMARDs, and newer agents such as rituximab and other B-cell targeted therapies currently producing promising results.

Musculoskeletal symptoms

In 1° SS patients, 70% report arthralgias, with 25% of those developing arthritis. In those with Raynaud's, they are more likely to develop a non-erosive arthritis. Arthralgias and fatigue respond well to hydroxychloroquine, and in those who have erosive disease, other DMARDs such as MTX would be appropriate. The use of steroids would be reserved for those with significant flare of musculoskeletal symptoms, including chronic recurrent glandular enlargement.

Skin

The skin can be very dry leading to symptoms of stinging, itching, and patchy alopecia. Hypersensitivity vasculitis can also develop. The dryness can also affect the vulva and vagina, and can lead to major complications in sexual relationships. Treatments of dry skin include use of non-lanolin-based products for washing (such as aqueous cream), tissue nourishment with moisturizers—either ointments or creams—and avoiding highly scented products. Vaginal dryness can impact a sexual relationship and most women with SS will be using simple lubricants regularly. Hormonal moisturizers or oestrogen creams and HRT are sometimes needed when symptoms are severe.

Pulmonary and renal involvement

Interstitial lung disease with dryness of the trachea can lead to a dry cough and airways obstruction due to dryness in the pleura; 25% will develop pulmonary abnormalities. Steroids are effective in reducing inflammation and can be used effectively with DMARDs such as AZA.

Renal disease is found in about 10% of those with 1° SS. Glomerulonephritis is uncommon, but would need to be treated with steroids and DMARDs such as AZA, MMF, or cyclophosphamide if present.

Neurological complications and neuropathies

Neurological complications present in many different ways, from diffuse sensorimotor neuropathy to a multiple sclerosis-like illness. Diffuse sensory motor neuropathy occurs in up to 20%; sensory symptoms predominate. Mononeuritis multiplex is seen in 1–3% of these with SS and often presents as a lateral popliteal nerve palsy. This is associated with vasculitis and responds well to high-dose steroids and DMARDs such as cyclophosphamide.

Lymphoma

There is a 40-fold higher relative risk of developing lymphoma in SS. Persistent parotid gland enlargement, lymphadenopathy, splenomegaly, and glomerulonephritis are all associated with a higher risk of developing lymphoma. SS patients must be screened when first diagnosed, at frequent intervals when there is any suspicion. Nurses must be available to counsel patients about this diagnosis and offer support and information on an individual basis as needed. Patients should be advised to report any parotid gland swelling.

Pregnancy

♀ with SS who carry the Ro and/or La antibodies will need to be counselled for pregnancy-related complications. Antibodies pass through the placental barrier during pregnancy:

- Can lead to a transient neonatal lupus rash in the newborn (~5%).
- A lower risk of congenital heart block is <2% of first pregnancies.
- Risk ↑ in subsequent pregnancies to about 12%.

♀ should also be screened for antiphospholipid antibodies. Birth plans need to be hospital based, with an obstetric-led birth and frequent scans. Pregnancies need to be planned during an inactive phase of the underlying SS.

➔ Also see 'Disease-modifying antirheumatic drugs', Chapter 16, pp. 445–452; ➔ 'Rituximab', Chapter 16, p. 496.

Sjögren's syndrome: fatigue and psychological manifestations

Fatigue affects the majority of those diagnosed with SS and can be extreme, causing incapacitation, influencing daily activities, and work, social, and personal relationships. Hydroxychloroquine can help in some, with mastery of self-management techniques influencing an individual's ability to cope with this frustrating chronic illness. Symptoms are difficult to treat in SS and can result in physical changes that can affect a personal relationship. These difficult symptoms are often little recognized and result in depression, isolation, and anger.

Support for symptoms of fatigue

- Counselling and psychology services should be accessed early to prevent any further distress, encouraging the individual with SS to develop positive strategies to manage their symptoms.
- Referral to occupational therapy and physiotherapy is essential and a MDT approach benefits the patient immensely.
- Pacing and planning advice, balanced with assessment of individual needs and the introduction of a graded exercise programme, can enable an individual to find purpose and direction.
- Patients can benefit from sleep management, relaxation techniques and cognitive behavioural therapy (CBT).
- Access to nurse specialist support is essential both in the consultation settings and between appointments through the telephone advice line.

Evaluation tools

Two validated tools have been developed for use in the assessment of 1° SS. The EULAR Sjögren's syndrome disease activity index (ESSDAI) and the EULAR SS Patient Reported Index (ESSPRI).[1,2]

References

1. Seror R, Ravaud P, Bowman SJ, et al. (2010). EULAR Sjögren's syndrome disease activity index: development of a consensus systemic disease activity index for primary Sjögren's syndrome. *Ann Rheum Dis* 69:1103–9.
2. Seror R, Theander E, Brun JG, et al. (2014). Validation of EULAR primary Sjogren's syndrome disease activity (ESSDAI) and patient indexes (ESSPRI). *Ann Rheumat Dis* 74:859–66.

Nursing care in Sjögren's syndrome

Nursing care management is aimed at enabling the patient with SS to participate in shared decision-making by having access to current evidence-based information in order to manage their symptoms effectively. In common with other CTDs, care is aimed at reducing organ failure and maintaining periods of remission from disease flare.

Patients need to know how to access specialist resources and when to call for help. SS is commonly seen in rheumatology units, often as a 2° diagnosis, and for many the symptoms are overlooked in favour of the underlying 1° conditions. It is these frustrating sicca symptoms that can lead to poor sleep patterns, exhaustion, severe fatigue, and, ultimately, significant depression when not addressed and treated appropriately. ♀ are the predominate group affected and as such, these symptoms can impact on home, work, and relationships. Relationships suffer due to physical sicca changes and fatigue, and this affects the patient's ability to have a comfortable physical relationship. There is no one treatment that is beneficial all round to treat these difficult symptoms.

Nurses provide a key role to SS patients through education and support, information, and counselling. Some specialist rheumatology units have access to a nurse specialist who can offer:

- Education: most important in times of a new diagnosis, when the disease is flaring, when complex treatment regimens are being initiated, and in helping an individual to come to terms with the psychological effects of living with a chronic illness. Education about SS is balanced on individual need, but individuals need to understand that SS is a multisystem autoimmune disease, where symptoms are manageable with early intervention to prevent systemic failure.
- Information: importance of blood results and autoantibody status is crucial in the young ♀ with SS, where pregnancy must be discussed and should be a planned event where possible.
- Support: nurses are able to refer patients to self-help groups such as the British Sjögren's Syndrome Association (BSSA), which are vital to enable patients to have the opportunity to meet others with similar symptoms and problems.[1]
- Counselling: this should be available for those requiring support and in times of distress. In particular, for ♀ with personal sexual problems to enable them to manage a reasonable physical relationship with their partner (➔ see 'Sexuality', Chapter 14, p. 423).
- Symptom management: sicca symptoms are challenging to live with and nurses can support patients, offering simple measures that can have effective results. Patients should be encouraged to develop a close relationship with their dentist and hygienist in maintaining good oral health.
- Advocate: nurses become the advocate of the SS patient, giving them appropriate information to help them to manage their disease more effectively and encouraging them to make lifestyle choices that will have a positive impact on their health and well-being. Self-management should be encouraged to enable individuals to gain control and lead fulfilling lives.

Nursing care of the patient with SS: key points

- Simple management of sicca symptoms.
- Pacing and planning, with exercise to help with fatigue symptoms.
- Sleep management, relaxation techniques, and CBT.
- Pregnancy advice and prepregnancy counselling.
- Support via telephone advice line in between clinic appointments.
- Providing clear information about risks of lymphoma and systemic disease in 1° SS.
- Empathy and support: contact with specialist teams and groups such as the BSSA.
- Balancing the need for information, relevant to the individual and their SS, without causing distress and worry.

➔ Also see 'Diagnosis', p. 153; ➔ 'Outcome measures', Chapter 20, pp. 595–612.

Reference

1. British Sjögren's Syndrome Association: http://www.bssa.uk.net

Further reading

Price EJ, Rauz S, Tappuni AR, et al. (2017). The British Society for Rheumatology guideline for the management of adults with primary Sjögren's syndrome. *Rheumatology* 56:1643–7.

Seror R, Ravaud P, Bowman SJ, et al. (2010). EULAR Sjögren's syndrome disease activity index: development of a consensus systemic disease activity index for primary Sjögren's syndrome. *Ann Rheum Dis* 69:1103–9.

Vitali C, Bombardieri S, Jonsson R, et al. (2002). Classification criteria for Sjogren's syndrome: a revised version of the European criteria proposed by the American-European Consensus Group. *Ann Rheumat Dis* 61:554–8.

Scleroderma: overview

Scleroderma is an uncommon autoimmune CTD. The word comes from two Greek words: 'sclero' meaning hard and 'derma' meaning skin. Scleroderma occurs when immune dysfunction leads to damage of the small blood vessels and production of excess collagen. This in turn causes fibrosis of the skin and its underlying structures, and in the systemic form affects the internal organs.

Scleroderma spectrum of disorders

Although the term scleroderma is often used as if it were a single disease, it is a generic or umbrella term for a family of diseases (Box 5.3). The two forms of systemic scleroderma—limited scleroderma and diffuse scleroderma—together make up 90% of all cases of scleroderma.

Epidemiology

- Occurs worldwide but more frequently in North America and Australia compared to Europe and Japan.
- Systemic scleroderma prevalence is estimated to be between 3 and 24 per 100,000 population.
- Systemic scleroderma is consistently more frequent in ♀ with a mean sex ratio of around 3:1. Can develop at any age although typically presents between the ages of 30 and 60 years.
- Systemic scleroderma is almost unseen in children <12 years and the very elderly.

Cause

The cause of scleroderma is unknown. Scleroderma is characterized by extensive fibrosis and damage to the blood vessels. Although the disease is driven by activation of an autoimmune mechanism, the triggers for this process are not clear. It is likely that several factors combine to cause scleroderma which may include:

- Genetic predisposition.

Box 5.3 The scleroderma spectrum of disorders

- Raynaud's phenomenon:
  - 1° Raynaud's phenomenon.
  - Autoimmune Raynaud's phenomenon.
- Systemic:
  - Limited cutaneous systemic sclerosis.
  - Diffuse cutaneous systemic sclerosis.
  - Scleroderma sine scleroderma.
- Localized:
  - Morphoea plaque—single or disseminated
  - Generalized morphoea.
  - Linear scleroderma.
  - En coup de sabre.

- Hormonal changes, e.g. pregnancy, childbirth, and menopause.
- External trigger, e.g. exposure to infection or chemicals.

Prognosis

Prognosis varies depending on the type and severity of the disease. A patient with localized (i.e. not systemic) scleroderma is unlikely to have their life expectancy shortened. Systemic scleroderma has a poorer prognosis; however, again it varies depending on the extent and type of organ involvement. The overall 5-year survival rate for systemic scleroderma is in excess of 80%.

➔ Also see 'Scleroderma: clinical features and investigations', pp. 153–155.

Further reading

Poudel DR, George M, Dhital R, et al. (2018). Mortality, length of stay and cost of hospitalization among patients with systemic sclerosis: results from the National Inpatient Sample. *Rheumatology* 57:1611–22.

Khanna D, Tashkin DP, Denton CP, et al. (2019). Ongoing clinical trials and treatment options for patients with systemic sclerosis-associated interstitial lung disease. *Rheumatology* 58:567–79.

Scleroderma: clinical features and investigations

Clinical features

Also see Table 5.1.

- Raynaud's phenomenon: circulatory disorder causing colour changes to the digits and often the first presenting feature of scleroderma.
- Skin: tight, thick skin, sclerodactyly (thickening of fingers), inflammation and itching, digital pitting, telangiectasia, hyper/hypopigmentation, calcinosis, microstomia, digital ulcers.
- Musculoskeletal system: fibrosis, arthritis, myositis, joint contractures, synovitis, tendon friction rubs, compression neuropathies, e.g. carpel tunnel syndrome.
- GI system: reflux oesophagitis, dysmotility, gastric antral vascular ectasia, which may cause bleeding into the GI tract, bacterial overgrowth, diarrhoea and constipation, incontinence, nutritional failure.
- Sicca symptoms (dry eyes, dry mouth).
- Viscera: pulmonary fibrosis pulmonary arterial hypertension, myocarditis, pericardial effusion, renal disease.
- Other: fatigue, sexual problems, changes to appearance and body image issues.

❗ Any patient showing signs of renal crisis—sudden rise in blood pressure, headaches, vomiting, nose bleeds, blurred vision, breathing difficulties, or seizures—should be reviewed immediately by a doctor.

Investigations and diagnosis

Scleroderma is often quite difficult to diagnose as symptoms vary in prevalence and severity in each individual. In the majority of cases, Raynaud's phenomenon or skin tightening and swelling are the initial presenting features. A wide range of clinical tests are used in scleroderma for initial diagnosis as well as ongoing review of the disease to assess the extent of organ involvement and the efficacy of some treatments.

► Early diagnosis is critical to allow implementation of treatment and to reduce complications and level of potential disability.

Autoantibodies

Specific autoantibody testing is a valuable diagnostic tool in scleroderma and can indicate potential organ involvement. The autoantibodies most commonly found in scleroderma are:

- ANAs: a positive ANA test can be a non-specific indicator of immune system dysfunction and is found in almost all people with scleroderma. Two patterns of ANAs are associated with scleroderma:
  - Anti-topoisomerase (also called anti-Scl-70): this antibody is specific for scleroderma and indicates that a patient may be at risk of developing interstitial lung disease.
  - Anti-centromere antibody (ACA): this antibody is specific for the limited subset of scleroderma and is associated with the development of pulmonary arterial hypertension.

Table 5.1 The American College of Rheumatology/European League Against Rheumatism criteria for the classification of systemic sclerosis

Item	Sub-item(s)	Weight/score
Skin thickening of the fingers of both hands extending proximal to the metacarpophalangeal joints (*sufficient criterion*)	–	9
Skin thickening of the fingers (*only count the higher score*)	Puffy fingers	2
	Sclerodactyly of the fingers (distal to the metacarpophalangeal joints but proximal to the proximal interphalangeal joints)	4
Fingertip lesions (*only count the higher score*)	Digital tip ulcers	2
	Fingertip pitting scars	3
Telangiectasia	–	2
Abnormal nailfold capillaries	–	2
Pulmonary arterial hypertension and/or interstitial lung disease (*maximum score is 2*)	Pulmonary arterial hypertension	2
	Interstitial lung disease	2
Raynaud's phenomenon	–	3
SSc-related autoantibodies (anticentromere, anti-topoisomerase I [anti-Scl-70], anti-RNA polymerase III) (*maximum score is 3*)	Anticentromere	3
	Anti-topoisomerase I	
	Anti-RNA polymerase III	

These criteria are applicable to any patient considered for inclusion in a systemic sclerosis study. The criteria are not applicable to patients with skin thickening sparing the fingers or to patients who have a scleroderma-like disorder that better explains their manifestations (e.g. nephrogenic sclerosing fibrosis, generalized morphoea, eosinophilic fasciitis, scleroderma diabeticorum, scleromyxoedema, erythromyalgia, porphyria, lichen sclerosis, graft-versus-host disease, diabetic cheiroarthropathy).

†The total score is determined by adding the maximum weight (score) in each category. Patients with a total score of ≥9 are classified as having definite systemic sclerosis. SSc, systemic sclerosis. Reprinted from van den Hoogen, Khanna, Fransen et al. (2013). 2013 classification criteria for systemic sclerosis: an American college of rheumatology/European league against rheumatism collaborative initiative *Ann Rheumat Dis* 2013; 72: 1747–1755 with permission from the BMJ Publishing Group.

Tests used in diagnosis and investigation of scleroderma

- Blood tests: FBC, ESR/CRP, biochemistry and muscle enzymes, autoantibody screen, thyroid function.
- Urine: urinalysis, microscopy, glomerular filtration rate.
- Lungs: chest X-ray, PFTs, HRCT.
- Heart: ECG, echocardiogram (particularly pulmonary arterial pressure and left ventricular ejection fraction), cardiac catheter.

Others: capillary microscopy, infrared thermography, joint X-rays, laser Doppler, investigations of small and large bowel, electromyography, and nerve conduction studies.

Scleroderma: treatment and follow-up care

There is no cure for scleroderma; however, treatments are available which aim to slow down disease progression.

Immunosuppressants

The choice of immunosuppressant used depends on the extent of skin, joint, or organ involvement. Immunosuppressants in most common use are:

- MMF.
- MTX.
- Hydroxychloroquine.
- Cyclophosphamide, used less frequently now than in the past.
- Biologics are an emerging treatment option and currently an area of research.

Most immunosuppressant drugs require regular monitoring of kidney and liver function and FBC. Low-dose corticosteroids are used sparingly in lung involvement or acute inflammation as they are thought to precipitate a renal crisis.

➲ Also see Chapter 16, 'Pharmacological management', pp. 445–503.

Symptom-specific medications

- PPIs (e.g. omeprazole, lansoprazole) to treat reflux oesophagitis due to sclerosis of the gastro-oesophageal junction.
- Prokinetics (e.g. metoclopramide, domperidone) used when sclerosis of the GI system results in reduced peristalsis and stomach emptying.
  - Domperidone now used with caution due to links with QT prolongation.
- H2-receptor antagonists (e.g. ranitidine) to mediate gastric secretion.
- Rotational antibiotics (e.g. ciprofloxacin, metronidazole) to treat bacterial overgrowth in the small bowel.
- Vasodilators (e.g. diltiazem, losartan) to ↑ blood flow to the extremities thereby treating and preventing digital ulcers and improve symptoms of Raynaud's phenomenon.
- Phosphodiesterase type 5 (PDE5) inhibitors (e.g. sildenafil) given for persistent digital ulceration.
- Prostacyclin IV (e.g. iloprost) to dilate blood vessels and aid circulation to help heal digital ulceration and improve symptoms of Raynaud's phenomenon.
- Endothelin receptor antagonist (bosentan) to reduce incidence of new digital ulceration formation (specialist centre prescribing only).
- Antibiotics (e.g. flucloxacillin) to treat infected digital ulcers.
- Antihistamines (e.g. chlorphenamine/hydroxyzine) helpful in reducing itching in the early stages of diffuse scleroderma when skin can be very inflamed.

Follow-up care

Patients with suspected scleroderma should be referred to a specialist centre as soon as possible with initial diagnosis and treatment implementation taking place under the guidance of the specialist team.

Much follow-up care can take place at the patient's local hospital with less frequent visits to the specialist team. Follow-up care, which will continue for life, may include:

- Regular follow-up appointments with the rheumatologist and team.
- Annual echocardiogram, lung function tests, and pulmonary function tests.
- Blood tests/monitoring while on immunosuppressant therapy.
- Psychosocial support.
- Referrals to appropriate specialists if further organ involvement develops, e.g. GI, dermatology, cardiology, respiratory.

Further reading

Moots RJ (2010). Manifestations of systemic sclerosis necessitate a holistic approach to patient care: a case report. *Musculoskeletal Care J* 8:164–7.

Nursing issues in management of patients with scleroderma

As scleroderma is a complex and unpredictable condition, nurses have a key role in helping patients to manage their condition (Table 5.2).

Nursing care is aimed at offering a holistic and individualized approach to each patient. The key issues in nursing management are:

- Enabling patients to make informed choices by providing ongoing information, advice, and support.
- Providing a continuing programme of education to empower patients to take responsibility for their own health and become active participants in their care.
- Teaching self-management strategies to help the patient recognize and manage common symptoms early in order to avoid complications of the disease and its treatment.
- Enabling patients to understand the diagnosis, prognosis, and chronic nature of the condition.
- Liases to ensure appropriate MDT involvement, e.g. PT, OT, social worker, podiatrist, counsellor, and palliative care team.

❗ *Patients should be taught to recognize the symptoms of, and seek immediate medical attention for:*

- Infected digital ulcers.
- Hypertension/renal crisis.
- Digital gangrene.

Patients with scleroderma may have an assessment of the skin thickening on their body. This gives an indication of the severity of the skin involvement; however, most importantly, serial assessments at each visit allow evaluation of whether skin thickening is deteriorating further or responding to treatment. The extent of skin involvement may, although not always, be an indicator of disease severity.

The assessment tool used is the modified Rodnan Skin Score Tool (Fig. 5.1). The body is broken down into 17 smaller areas and each area is pinched to assess skin tightening and thickening and given a score between 0 (no skin involvement) and 3 (hidebound skin). The total is then calculated (for a detailed outline of scoring see Khanna et al.[1]).

Reference

1. Khanna D, Furst DE, Clements PJ, et al. (2017). Standardization of the modified Rodnan skin score for use in clinical trials of systemic sclerosis. *J Scleroderma Relat Disord* 2:11–8.

Table 5.2 Nursing care plan

Patient problem	Nursing management	Expected outcome
Raynaud's phenomenon	Advice about keeping warm Stop smoking Natural remedies Hand warmers Counselling on starting drug treatment if conservative therapy ineffective	Reduction in frequency and severity of attacks
Digital ulcers	Recognize infection Dry dressing Antibiotics if required Regular assessment advised	Expedite healing of ulcers, reduce likelihood of further recurrence
Calcinosis	Paraffin wax baths	Exit of calcinotic lumps through skin
Tight dry skin	Paraffin wax baths, massage, moisturizers	Moisturize skin to improve tightness
Joint problems	Exercises, refer to physio/OT, heat and ice, waxing	Relieve pain and stiffness, ↑ flexibility, mobility
Foot problems	Refer to podiatrist	↓ pain and ↑ mobility
Breathlessness	Coping strategies	↑ ability to manage ADLs independently Signpost to appropriate help if required
Itchy skin	Moisturizers, anti-itch creams, antihistamines	↓ pruritus to improve quality of life
Telangiectasia	Camouflage make up, refer for laser treatment	Camouflage or remove telangiectasia reducing psychosocial burden
GI problems	Practical coping strategies, dietary advice, refer to dietician	Reduction in severity of symptoms improving nutritional intake and quality of life
Dry eyes	Practical measures, over-the-counter eye drops Ophthalmology assessment if required	Relieve dry eyes

Continued

Table 5.2 (*Contd.*)

Patient problem	Nursing management	Expected outcome
Oral problems	Advice about good mouth care, over-the-counter remedies for dry mouth and ulcers, mouth exercises. Referral to specialist at dental hospital if required Stress importance of regular dentist and hygienist visits	Reduce need for future dental intervention
Emotional problems	Provide support, refer to counsellor, social worker, ensure awareness of national patient groups and helplines	Patient to feel supported in managing condition
Fatigue	Coping strategies. OT referral	↑ ability to manage ADLs
Sexual problems	Identify problem—refer to gynaecologist, urologist, or counsellor as appropriate	Maintain sexual activity at desired level

Frequently asked questions: scleroderma

What causes scleroderma?

The exact cause of scleroderma is unknown; however, it is thought to be a combination of abnormal immune activity, genes, hormones, and an environmental trigger (e.g. viral infection, exposure to chemicals).

Can complementary therapies help in scleroderma?

Complementary therapies can be beneficial, particularly in helping to manage Raynaud's phenomenon and digital ulcers. As always, they should be used to complement medical treatment and only used with the knowledge of the specialist.

Will scleroderma reduce life expectancy?

In some cases, life expectancy may be reduced due to scleroderma; however, this depends on the type and extent of organ involvement.

Can patients be seen at their local hospital rather than travelling to the specialist so frequently?

Most patients with scleroderma can be seen at their local hospital for follow-up appointments with only yearly visits to a specialist; however, it is advisable to be seen by a specialist for initial diagnosis and ongoing treatment advice.

How do you prevent/treat digital ulcers?

Treatment for digital ulcers is by vasodilation thereby improving blood supply to the affected areas. Calcium channel blockers (e.g. diltiazem) and angiotensin-II receptor antagonists (e.g. losartan) are the most commonly used medications. A maintenance dose can be used permanently, or during cold weather, and the dose ↑ if an ulcer does occur.

What is iloprost?

Iloprost is a prostacyclin analogue which is given intravenously over several days in order to induce vasodilation to treat or prevent digital ulcers. It is used as an unlicensed indication and given according to local guidelines.

Will my scleroderma ever get better?

There is no cure for scleroderma. Many people find that skin and musculoskeletal symptoms are worst for the first 2 years and then slowly improve. However, a person will remain at risk of developing organ involvement throughout the rest of their lives.

Can anything be done about changing facial features?

Changes in appearance are common in scleroderma and may be significant. There is little that can be done; however, a consultation with a plastic surgeon familiar with scleroderma may be helpful.

Modified Rodnan Skin Score (MRSS) Document

Subject ID: ______________________

Date of Examinaion: ________________

	Right				Left			
Fingers	0☐	1☐	2☐	3☐	0☐	1☐	2☐	3☐
Hands	0☐	1☐	2☐	3☐	0☐	1☐	2☐	3☐
Forearms	0☐	1☐	2☐	3☐	0☐	1☐	2☐	3☐
Upper Arms	0☐	1☐	2☐	3☐	0☐	1☐	2☐	3☐
Face			0☐	1☐	2☐	3☐		
Anterior Chest			0☐	1☐	2☐	3☐		
Abdomen			0☐	1☐	2☐	3☐		
Thighs	0☐	1☐	2☐	3☐	0☐	1☐	2☐	3☐
Legs	0☐	1☐	2☐	3☐	0☐	1☐	2☐	3☐
Feet	0☐	1☐	2☐	3☐	0☐	1☐	2☐	3☐
Column Totals								
Total:								

Key: *0 – No Thickening* *1 – Mild Thickening* *2 – Moderate Thickening* *3 – Severe Thickening*

Notes:

Examiner:

Printed Name: ______________________

Signature: ______________________ Date: ____________

Fig. 5.1 Modified Rodnan skin score (mRSS). Assessed in 17 different areas. Case report form to capture mRSS.

Reprinted from Khanna D et al. (2017) Standardization of the modified Rodnan skin score for use in clinical trials of systemic sclerosis. *Journal of Scleroderma and Related Disorders* 2(1):11–18 with permission from SAGE.

Where can patients get ongoing information and advice between doctors' appointments?

There are patient groups for patients with scleroderma which can provide valuable information, advice, and support. Most specialist centres for scleroderma also have nurse-led telephone helplines for the use of patients and other healthcare professionals.

Do patients need to take medication for life?

Immunosuppressant therapy is taken until the disease is under control, usually for a period of several years. Management of ongoing complications such as reflux or Raynaud's phenomenon or organ involvement is likely to require ongoing treatment.

How can patients alleviate skin itching?

Skin itching can be severe in the early stages of diffuse scleroderma and is caused by the inflammatory response. Keeping skin well moisturized is very important and anti-itch creams (available over the counter) can be beneficial. Antihistamine tablets can help and in very severe cases a small dose of corticosteroid may be prescribed.

Will physiotherapy help?

Physiotherapy is valuable in scleroderma and regular exercises will significantly improve range of movement both in the joints of the fingers and hand and in larger joints, especially if started early and done regularly.

In the childhood forms of localized scleroderma, physiotherapy has a very important role to play in treatment and referral should be prompt to prevent problems with growth and development. Hand waxing is also very helpful in helping to maintain and improve skin condition and joint suppleness.

Why do I need to keep having the same tests done?

It is important to have regular organ tests to ensure that any deterioration in function is detected early in order to implement or switch treatment if it may be required.

Is it right that treatments prescribed are usually used for cancer patients?

Immunosuppressant medications used in scleroderma are the same as those sometimes used for cancer. They are given in lower doses in scleroderma and often produce only minimal side effects.

Does scleroderma affect pregnancy?

Scleroderma has a varied effect on pregnancy. It is not advisable to get pregnant while the disease is active or while on immunosuppressant medications; however, once the disease is under control, pregnancy (under close medical supervision) is likely to be safe both for mother and child although it is possible a flare may occur due to pregnancy. Sometimes pregnancy seems to trigger scleroderma in a ♀ who had previously been healthy.

Further reading

Denton CP, Hughes M, Gak N, et al. (2016). BSR and BHPR guideline for the treatment of systemic sclerosis. *Rheumatology (Oxford)* 55:1906–10.

NHS England (2015). Clinical Commissioning Policy: Sildenafil and Bosentan for the Treatment of Digital Ulceration in Systemic Sclerosis. https://www.england.nhs.uk/commissioning/wp-content/uploads/sites/12/2015/10/a13pb-sildenafil-bosentan-oct15.pdf

Steen VD, Medsger TA Jr (1997). The value of the Health Assessment Questionnaire and special patient-generated scales to demonstrate change in systemic sclerosis patients over time. *Arthritis Rheum* 40:1984–91.

Van den Hoogen F, Khanna D, Fransen J, et al. (2013). 2013 classification criteria for systemic sclerosis: an American college of rheumatology/European league against rheumatism collaborative initiative. *Ann Rheumat Dis* 72:1747–55.

ANCA-associated vasculitis

The antineutrophil cytoplasmic antibody (ANCA)-associated vasculitides (AAV)—granulomatosis with polyangiitis (GPA, formerly known as Wegener's granulomatosis), eosinophilic granulomatosis with polyangiitis (EGPA, formerly known as Churg–Strauss syndrome), and microscopic polyangiitis (MPA)—are a group of rare, potentially life-threatening conditions, characterized by inflammation and necrosis of blood vessel walls.

It is often difficult to diagnose these conditions as early presentation is often non-specific and may mimic other diseases.

- Non-specific features.
- Malaise.
- Fever.
- Weight loss.
- Arthralgia.
- Arthritis.
- Headache.

These features are common to many other diseases but especially infection and malignancy. Specific clinical features, such as a vasculitic rash which is often purpuric, needs to be differentiated from other causes of purpura such as thrombocytopenia and cutaneous vasculitis, this can also be a feature of infectious disease such as bacterial endocarditis. Necrotic lesions in the skin due to vasculitis are also seen in thrombotic disorders such as APS and the whole spectrum of systemic upset, purpura, and sometimes skin infarcts can be seen in the rare but important condition atrial myxoma.

Vasculitis should be considered with presentation of unexplained multisystem disease, pyrexia of unknown origin, rash, and renal involvement. ANCA-associated vasculitis affects small to medium-sized blood vessels. The annual incidence is 20 per million adults per year, with a median age of onset of 65 years in the UK.

Diagnosis

Often made when all other causes are excluded, i.e. infection and malignancy. It is the combination of presenting symptoms and clinical features, the pattern of organ involvement, and the results of blood tests, urinalysis, and X-rays, coupled with ANCA status and tissue biopsy results that leads to a diagnosis of 1° systemic vasculitis (PSV). The three most common types—GPA, EGPA, MPA—will be presented.

The nurse's role in the management of AAV

The treatment of AAV is usually overseen by a consultant with a special interest in vasculitis who leads the MDT. A holistic patient-centred approach to care must be considered in the context of the nurse's role. Key aspects of the role of the nurse:

- Provide psychosocial support and education.
- Patient education about their disease, treatments, possible side effects, and the monitoring process is vital.

- It is the responsibility of the nurse in caring for the patient with AAV to administer IV cyclophosphamide. Cyclophosphamide is a cytotoxic agent used to treat cancer and a number of other conditions. It can be administered either orally daily or as an IV pulse regimen.

➲ Also see 'Pretreatment assessment of cyclophosphamide', pp. 174–175.

Further reading

Mooney J, Poland F, Spalding N, et al. (2013). 'In one ear and out the other – it's a lot to take in': A qualitative study exploring the informational needs of patients with ANCA Associated Vasculitis. *Musculoskeletal Care* 11:51–9.

Mooney J, Spalding N, Poland F, et al. (2014). The informational needs of patients with ANCA-associated vasculitis—development of an informational needs questionnaire. *Rheumatology (Oxford)* 53:1414–21.

Ntatsaki E, Carruthers D, Chakravarty K, et al. (2014). BSR and BHPR guidelines for the management of adults with ANCA associated vasculitis. *Rheumatology (Oxford)* 53:2306–9.

Robson JC, Dawson J, Cronholm PF, et al. (2018). Health-related quality of life in ANCA-associated vasculitis and item generation for a disease-specific patient-reported outcome measure. *Patient Relat Outcome Meas* 9:17–34.

Yates M, Watts RA, Bajema IM, et al. (2016). EULAR/ERA-EDTA recommendations for the management of ANCA-associated vasculitis. *Ann Rheum Dis* 75:1583–94.

Yates M, Watts R (2017). ANCA-associated vasculitis. *Clin Med* 17:60–4.

Granulomatosis with polyangiitis

GPA is a rare, potentially life-threatening disease that classically affects the upper and lower airways and kidneys but can affect other systems (Table 5.3). It is more common in Caucasians than other ethnic groups, peak age of onset is 60 years, with equal sex distribution. It is a small to medium-sized vessel vasculitis characterized by inflammation, and necrosis of these vessels and frequently accompanied by granuloma formation, particularly in the upper airway. The antibody associated with GPA is ANCA which usually stains with cytoplasmic staining (c-ANCA) with specificity against proteinase 3 (PR3).

Common presentations

- Bleeding from the nose.
- Deafness.
- Haemoptysis.
- Haematuria.
- Proteinurea.

Table 5.3 Clinical features of granulomatosis with polyangiitis

Systemic	ENT	Lung
Fever	Sinusitis	Cough
Night sweats	Nasal crusting	Haemoptysis
Malaise	Oral ulcers	Pleuritis
Arthralgia	Subglottic stenosis	Nodules—chest X-ray
Weight loss	Epistaxis	Fixed infiltrates (>1 month)
	Hearing loss	
	Late clinical presentation	
	Saddle nose deformity	
Kidney	**Skin**	**Eye**
Haematuria	Rash	Epi/scleritis
Proteinurea	Purpura	Proptosis
↑ creatinine		
Nerve		
The commonest is a mild peripheral neuropathy/ but mononeuritis multiplex is the most classical form of vasculitis (commoner in EGPA, than in GPA or MPA)		

Investigations

Blood tests, urinalysis, X-rays, and tissue biopsies are all used to aid diagnosis, exclude differential diagnosis, assess organ involvement, and disease severity.

Blood tests

- FBC may reveal anaemia (low Hb), raised platelets, and a raised WBC count (as the consequence of any chronic inflammatory response).
- A mild eosinophilia is common in allergies and other inflammatory diseases, but a very high eosinophil count is particularly characteristic of EGPA ($>1.5 \times 10^9$/L). But mild eosinophilia is also not uncommon in GPA.
- U&Es and creatinine useful in assessment of kidney function/impairment. ESR and CRP raised in inflammation and ANCA status.

Urinalysis

Dipstick urinalysis for haematuria and proteinurea is essential for detection of renal involvement. Send midstream specimen of urine for culture and sensitivity. Quantify protein excretion with protein/creatinine ratio.

► Red cell casts indicate renal involvement; this is one of the most serious outcomes in AAV.

►► It is important to recognize this as early as possible, so that appropriate treatment can be given.

Biopsies

Tissue biopsies from various organs can be helpful in reaching a diagnosis, the most common sites are:

- Skin.
- Kidney.
- Nose.
- Lung.

Typical appearances are those of necrotizing vasculitis in the skin, focal segmental necrotizing glomerulonephritis in the kidney (indicating small vessel vasculitis), and tissue from the upper airways reveals non-specific changes and granuloma is sometimes seen but this is rare. Needle biopsies of the lung also often reveal non-specific changes but an open biopsy will often show granuloma in GPA.

X-rays

Chest X-ray may show lung inflammation, nodules, or cavitating nodules that are associated with GPA. Sinus X-rays often show evidence of inflammation/infection with fluid levels but chronic disease causes bone destruction which also may be seen on CT or MRI.

Key nursing issues

It is vital that routine temperature, pulse, and respiration, blood pressure, and urinalysis are carried out and any abnormalities discussed with medical staff. A rise in creatinine, haematuria, and proteinurea should be discussed with medical staff. Skin rashes should be observed and monitored. Yearly cardiovascular disease assessment.

Eosinophilic granulomatosis with polyangiitis

EGPA consists of asthma, eosinophilia, fever, and accompanying vasculitis of various organ systems. It is associated with antibodies to ANCAs, usually perinuclear ANCA (p-ANCA), with specificity against myeloperoxidase (MPO) seen in ~5% of cases.

Clinical features

- Asthma.
- Nasal polyps.
- Allergic rhinitis.
- Eosinophilia.
- Sinusitis.
- Rashes.
- Palpable purpura.
- Haematuria/proteinurea.
- Hypertension.
- Malaise.
- Loss of appetite.
- Weight loss.
- Mononeuritis multiplex.
- Neuropathy.

Classic pulmonary feature is of a flitting pulmonary shadowing on chest X-ray (which is similar to eosinophilic pneumonia). Pulmonary haemorrhage is much more commonly seen in MPA.

Asthma is one of the essential features of EGPA. Asthma symptoms may begin long before the onset of vasculitis—e.g. many years before any other symptoms arise, and long before the diagnosis of EGPA is made. Other early symptoms/signs include nasal polyps and allergic rhinitis.

Peripheral nerve involvement includes pain, numbness, or tingling in extremities (neuropathy/mononeuritis multiplex).

Investigations

- FBC.
- U&Es.
- CRP/ESR.
- ANCA.
- Chest X-ray.
- Eosinophilia is characteristic of EGPA ($>1.5 \times 10^9$/L).
- Biopsy results show a necrotizing granulomatosis and eosinophilic vasculitis.

Key nursing issues

It is common for the heart to be affected, so any chest pain, shortness of breath (SOB), hypertension, dependent oedema, or an abnormal pulse rate or rhythm should be reported to medical staff. Yearly cardiovascular disease assessment.

Microscopic polyangiitis

MPA is a small-vessel vasculitis which occasionally can affect medium-sized and/or large vessels, involving the skin, lungs, digestive system, and kidneys. Renal involvement is common. It is associated with antibodies to ANCAs usually p-ANCA with specificity against MPO.

Clinical features

- Tiredness.
- Fever.
- Malaise.
- Flu-like symptoms.
- Myalgia.
- Weight loss.
- Haematuria.
- Proteinurea.
- Breathlessness.
- Skin rash.
- Haemoptysis.
- Pulmonary haemorrhage.
- Cough.
- Peripheral neuropathy.
- GI bleeding.
- Abdominal pain.

Inflammation of the kidney (glomerulonephritis) is a common presentation, symptoms/signs include tiredness, haematuria/proteinurea, and elevated creatinine. The speed of renal involvement is unpredictable, ranging from slow to rapid progression necessitating a need for close monitoring of creatinine levels.

Investigations

See Table 5.4.

- Chest X-ray may show evidence of haemorrhage with widespread shadowing; this contrasts with GPA, which shows fixed infiltrates or granulomas with fluid levels, and EGPA, where there are transient shadows more suggestive of pneumonia.
- Skin biopsy shows leucocytoclastic vasculitis.
- Bronchoscopy may confirm pulmonary haemorrhage.
- Lung biopsy may also show a small-vessel vasculitis.
- Renal biopsy:
  - In all ANCA-associated vasculitis, the changes are identical with the characteristic change being a pauci-immune focal segmental necrotizing glomerulonephritis.

The characteristic feature differentiating MPA from other autoimmune kidney conditions is the relative absence of immunoglobulin and complement deposition in the kidney (pauci-immune).

Key nursing issues

- It is vital that routine urinalysis is performed. Any haematuria/proteinurea and/or elevated creatinine must be discussed with medical staff. Yearly cardiovascular disease assessment.
- Any SOB and haemoptysis should be reported to medical staff.

Table 5.4 Blood and immunology investigations

Test	Result	Indication	Disease
FBC	Hb (anaemia)	Chronic disease/pulmonary haemorrhage	EGPA, GPA, MPA
	Platelets >400 × 10^9/L	Inflammatory response (note: seen with active disease)	EGPA, GPA, MPA
	WBC >11.0 × 10^9/L	Infection (note: also seen as an effect of steroids)	All
	WBC <4.0 × 10^9/L	Drug induced: cyclophosphamide, MTX, AZA	All
	Neutrophils <2.0 × 10^9/L	Drug induced: cyclophosphamide, MTX, AZA	Withhold all cytotoxic drugs (cyclophosphamide), recheck bloods, screen for infection
	Eosinophils >0.4 × 10^9/L	Allergy, inflammation	EGPA (>1.5 ×10^9/L) Smaller ↑ in GPA
	ESR >15 mm/hour	Non-specific indicator of inflammation	All
	CRP >10 mg/L	Inflammation/infection	All
U&Es[a]	Creatinine <150 µmol	Mild kidney inflammation/ early disease	MPA, GPA, EGPA
	Creatinine >150 but <500 µmol	Generalized/kidney failure	MPA, GPA, EGPA
	Creatinine >500 µmol	Severe kidney failure/ life-threatening	MPA, GPA, EGPA
ANCA	Negative	Does not exclude vasculitis	All
	Positive c-ANCA	PR3 specificity	Strongly associated with GPA
	Positive p-ANCA	MPO specificity	Associated with MPA, EGPA

[a] Renal involvement: renal function can change rapidly and results need to be interpreted carefully in respect of previous values. Any abnormality of urinalysis, even with apparently normal creatinine can indicate glomerulonephritis—always discuss renal function tests with the medical team in these circumstances.

Treatment for ANCA-associated vasculitis

Treatment should commence as early as possible to avoid irreversible organ damage. Assessment of the target organs involved and the severity of the disease is vital, as this determines the immunosuppressive regimen. The severity of the disease can be categorized into three groups and the EULAR guidelines for management of AAV should be followed.[1]

►► Treatment should not be delayed when waiting for biopsy confirmation in those with organ/life-threatening disease (Fig. 5.2).

Treatment is divided into induction and maintenance. The aim of induction treatment is to gain control of active disease—the majority of patients require cyclophosphamide; increasingly, rituximab is being used as an alternative.

Cyclophosphamide (always given together with corticosteroids)

- Administered orally or intravenously.
- Oral dose is 2 mg/kg daily; maximum dosage 200 mg daily.
- Given for 3–6 months.
- IV dosage is 15 mg/kg; maximum dosage 1500 mg.
- Given as 2–3-week pulses.
- Dosage should be adjusted for age and renal impairment.
- For those on an IV pulse regimen, 2-mercaptoethane sulfonate (mesna) should be considered as this may protect against bladder toxicity.
- Initial treatment is aimed at inducing remission, this can take 3–6 months.
- Then switch to maintenance therapy.

Maintenance therapy

Cyclophosphamide should be stopped and replaced with either AZA, MMF, or MTX plus prednisolone. Maintenance therapy should be for a minimum of 2 years, except for ANCA-positive GPA patients who should continue treatment for up to 5 years.[1]

Reference

1. Ntatsaki E, Carruthers D, Chakravarty K, et al. (2014). BSR and BHPR guidelines for the management of adults with ANCA associated vasculitis. rheumatology. *Rheumatology (Oxford)* 3:2306–9.

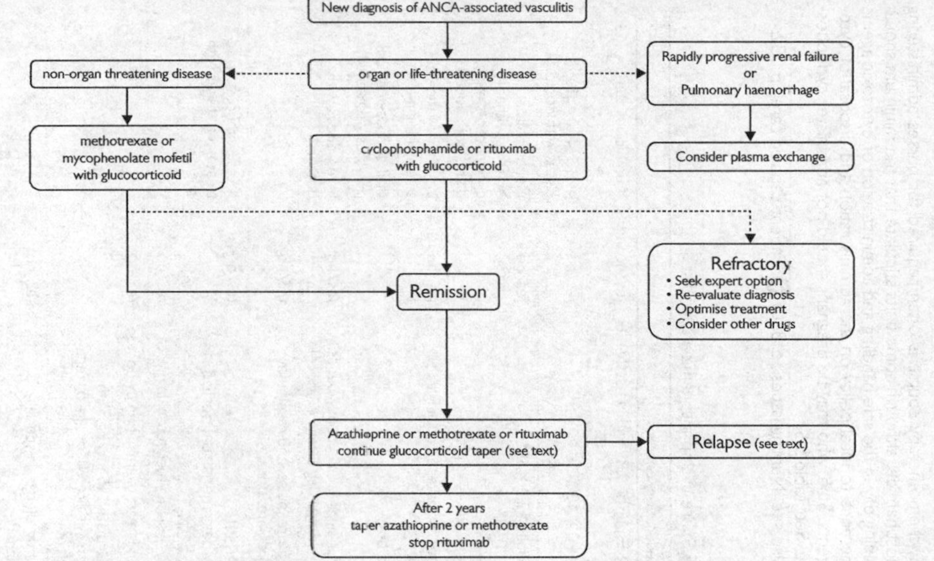

Fig. 5.2 Algorithm to describe the management of new ANCA-associated vasculitis.

Reprinted from Yates, Watts, Bajema et al. (2016). EULAR/ERA-EDTA recommendations for the management of ANCA-associated vasculitis *Ann Rheum Dis* 75:1583–1594 with permission from the BMJ Publishing Group.

Administration of intravenous cyclophosphamide

An N59 chemotherapy course is often required for nurses administering cyclophosphamide, although some units stipulate that the minimum should be a training day in the safe handling and administration of cytotoxic agents and adherence to local policy on the administration and disposal of cytotoxic agents. Staff who may be pregnant should not administer cyclophosphamide. See Table 5.5.

➲ Also see 'Nursing issues', p. 330; ➲ 'Patient-centred care', p. 332.

Table 5.5 Pre-cyclophosphamide checklist

Patient education/consent	Yes/no	
FBC, U&Es, LFTs, CRP within last 24–48 hours	Yes/no	If no bloods stat
WBC >4.0 × 10^9/L	Yes/no	WBC <4.0 × 10^9/L discus with doctor
Neutrophils >2.0 × 10^9/L	Yes/no	Neutrophils <2.0 × 10^9/L withhold cyclophosphamide, discus with doctor
Exposure to chickenpox/shingles	Yes/no	Yes check varicella status, inform doctor
Varicella titre		(If first dose and not previously screened)
Check for signs of infection: wounds, urinary catheter, leg ulcer, cough, cold	Yes/no	If yes, discus with doctor
Temperature, pulse, and respiration; blood pressure, urinalysis	Yes/no	
♀ pregnant Date of last menstrual period	Yes/no	If yes, withhold treatment, discus with doctor
Infertility—discus sperm banking	Yes/no	
Chest and heart examination by doctor	Yes/no	
Dose calculated 15 mg/kg, with reduction if indicated for age or renal impairment		
Check drug allergies, especially sulphonamides	Yes/no	
Mesna and antiemetic prescribed	Yes/no	
Septrin® prophylaxis prescribed	Yes/no	
Bone prophylaxis prescribed	Yes/no	
Future invasive procedure planned	Yes/no	

Further reading

Dougherty L, Lister S (eds) (2015). *The Royal Marsden Manual of Clinical Nursing Procedures*, 9th edn. Oxford: Wiley- Blackwell Publishing.

Nursing and Midwifery Council (2015). *The Code: Professional Standards of Practice and Behaviour for Nurses and Midwives*. London: Nursing and Midwifery Council.

Polyarteritis nodosa

Classic PAN is a non-granulomatosis vasculitis of medium-sized arteries. It is rare in the UK with a mean age of onset of 50 years with equal distribution between the sexes. It is ANCA negative, and rarely causes glomerulonephritis.

Clinical features

- Tiredness.
- Fever.
- Malaise.
- Weight loss.
- Loss of appetite.
- Hypertension.
- Testicular pain.
- Frank haematuria—indicates severe renal disease.
- Abdominal pain—mainly due to gut infarction with a very poor prognosis.
- Skin rash—the most common are skin ulceration/gangrene (due to infarction) and livedo reticularis (a reticular discolouration pattern generally seen peripherally). Diagnosis of livedo reticularis is confirmed by biopsy. In addition, occasionally angiography will show microaneurysms under the skin, which can rupture, causing haemorrhage, as well as infarction due to blockage of similar-sized blood vessels. Angiography more commonly is used to show these changes in the visceral circulation (coeliac axis and renal vessels).

Investigations

- FBC.
- U&Es.
- CRP/ESR.
- ANCA.
- Chest X-ray.
- Eosinophilia is characteristic of EGPA ($>1.5 \times 10^9$/L).
- Biopsy results show a necrotizing vasculitis.

Key nursing issues

- It is essential that blood pressure is monitored as hypertension is common.
- Any abdominal pain should be reported to medical staff (to rule out gut infarction).
- Haematuria should be discussed with medical staff.

Behçet's disease/syndrome

Introduction

Behçet's disease is characterized by oral and genital ulcers, eye inflammation, and arthritis. The dominant features of oral/genital ulceration are inflammatory in nature. Blood vessels are sometimes affected with frequent features such as:

- Phlebitis indicating inflammation of the veins.
- Arteritis and the development of aneurysms involving large arteries as well as small arteries.

Other non-vasculitic symptoms include:

- Arthritis.
- Neurological involvement, when there is an aseptic meningitis and ocular Behçet's disease when there is inflammation, rather than vasculitis within the eye.

Behçet's disease is uncommon in the UK but is much commoner in the Eastern Mediterranean region and the Middle East. Many of the large series of patients come from Turkey where Behçet's disease was first described. Other areas where Behçet's disease is seen frequently include Greece, South East Asia, and Japan. It is rare in children <16 years; the peak age of onset is 20–40 years with an equal distribution between ♂ and ♀.

Clinical features and presentation

See Box 5.4 and Table 5.6

❗ Eye manifestations can be serious and must be treated; complications are frequent and can cause blindness if untreated; commonest cause of blindness in Middle and Far East.

Classification criteria for Behçet's disease

Must have recurrent oral ulceration plus two of the following[1]:

- Recurrent genital ulceration.
- Eye manifestations.
- Skin lesions.
- Positive pathergy test.

Box 5.4 Common presentation of Behçet's disease

- Recurrent painful oral ulcers (almost 100% of patients).
- Genital ulcers (90%):
  - On the scrotum in ♂.
  - On the outer labia and cervix in ♀.
- Eye manifestations—uveitis (70%).

In severe disease:

- Young ♂ 20–25 years old.
- Eye involvement.
- CNS involvement (up to 10% in some series).
- Pulmonary artery aneurysm (associated with a high mortality rate).

Table 5.6 Clinical features of Behçet's disease

Mucosal surfaces	CNS	Eyes
Multiple episodes of oral ulcers	Headaches	Multiple episodes of uveitis
Multiple episodes of genital ulcers	Memory loss	Blurred vision
	Stroke	Retinal
		vasculitis
	Impaired balance	Hypopyon (pus in anterior chamber)
Skin	**Other**	**Vasculature**
Erythema nodosum	Fatigue	DVT
Papulopustular lesions	Arthritis	Haemoptysis
Acneiform or papulopustular rash	GI ulceration	Pulmonary artery aneurysm
	Epididymitis	Thrombophlebitis
	Aseptic meningitis	

The classification criteria[1] were developed for research purposes and in clinical practice diagnosis is made by presenting symptoms and clinical features and exclusion of other differential diagnosis such as:

- Herpes simplex virus.
- Sweet's syndrome.
- ReA.
- AS.
- Crohn's disease.
- Oral aphthous ulcer.

Reference

1. International Study Group for Behçet's Disease (1990). Criteria for diagnosis of Behçet disease. *Lancet* 335:1078–80.

Behçet's disease: investigations and treatment

As there are no specific diagnostic tests, diagnosis is made using:

- Clinical examination and an assessment of the degree of inflammation. Formal slit lamp examination of the eyes is necessary to assess ocular inflammation. Sexual health examination of genital ulcers to confirm the diagnosis.
- Blood tests such as FBC, ESR/CRP, U&Es, and LFTs.
- Pathergy testing has been used in Middle East, but has not been of use in the UK population, because the positivity rate is much lower.
    - A pathergy test involves using a sterile 20–22-gauge needle, to obliquely pierce the skin to a depth of 5 mm; a positive is determined if an erythematous papule develops at the test site after 2 days.
- Genetic tests for HLA-B51 can be helpful when positive but again is not a helpful diagnostic test usually in a Caucasian population.
- For recurrent oral or genital ulceration where diagnosis is in doubt:
    - Tissue biopsy is important if the diagnosis of recurrent oral or genital ulceration is in doubt.
    - Virology—to exclude other causes particularly of genital ulcers.

► The differential diagnosis includes inflammatory bowel disease which may need investigating separately, other causes of aphthous ulceration such as infection with herpes.

Treatment of Behçet's disease

Treatment is aimed at the dominant clinical problem, usually advised by the appropriate specialist, i.e. ophthalmologist, dermatologist, rheumatologist, or neurologist.

Eye manifestations

Evidence supports the treatment of severe eye disease with AZA and ciclosporin. Short courses of steroids maybe needed as an adjunct therapy (➲ see 'Pharmacological management: ciclosporin and azathioprine', p. 428). Interferon and TNF inhibitors are increasingly used.

Arthritis

Treat with NSAIDs and as any inflammatory arthritis.

Skin

- Treat ulcers with topical steroids.
- Systemically unwell patients will require treatment with steroids/immunosuppression.
- Oral and genital ulcers may require treatment with colchicine.

For a small minority of patients who fail to respond to the described treatment, there is an emerging role for TNF inhibitor blockade.

Thalidomide

This is an unlicensed drug in the UK, that can be used to treat serious oral and genital ulcers but should only be used in severe disease or when other treatment modalities have failed. It is very rarely used now.

Dosage: 50–100 mg daily, then reduce to 50 mg every 2 or 3 days once in remission. Thalidomide must only be prescribed by a consultant who is experienced in its use. Special assessment and monitoring of patients is required due to the two most serious side effects:
- Teratogenic effects.
- Peripheral neuropathy.

A prescription can only be issued for 28 days and repeat prescriptions only issued on each monthly visit after a negative blood pregnancy test (where appropriate).

Doctors and pharmacists must be registered in the thalidomide Pharmion Risk Management Programme (PRMP) to prescribe and dispense the drug. Patients must also register with the programme and comply with its requirements to receive the drug.

❗ Particular care is necessary in ♀ with child-bearing potential.

Also see 'Treatment with thalidomide and cyclophosphamide: the nurse's role', p.181.

Monitoring—requires hospital supervision
- Monthly follow-up:
  - Signs of peripheral neuropathy, pins and needles, stop drug immediately.
- 6-monthly nerve conduction tests or after each 10 g.
- Monthly pregnancy test.
- Routine blood tests, e.g. for leucopenia.

Must take contraceptive precautions for 3 months on stopping thalidomide.

Further reading
de Wazieres B, Gil H, Magy N, et al. (1999). Treatment of recurrent ulceration with low doses of thalidomide. Pilot study of 17 patients. *Rev Med Interne* 20:567–70.

McDonald DR, Lee C, Fowler RA, et al. (2007). Behçet's disease. *CMAJ* 176:1273–4.

Powell RJ, Gardner-Medwin JM (1994). Guidelines for the clinical use and dispensing of thalidomide. *Postgrad Med J* 70:901–4.

Saenz A, Ausejo M, Shea B, et al. (2000). Pharmacotherapy for Behçet's syndrome. *Cochrane Database Syst Rev* 2:CD001084.

Wu J, Huang DB, Pang KR, et al. (2005). Thalidomide: dermatological indications, mechanisms of action and side-effects. *Br J Dermatol* 153:254–73.

Treatment with thalidomide and cyclophosphamide: the nurse's role

Cyclophosphamide

Patients receiving cyclophosphamide must be screened and monitored closely to observe for potential side effects (e.g. bone marrow suppression, haemorrhagic cystitis, or ↑ risk of bladder cancer).

Administration of IV cyclophosphamide

An N59 chemotherapy course is usually required for nurses administering cyclophosphamide. In some organizations the minimum amount of training (e.g. safe handling and administration of cytotoxic agents) together with adherence to local policy on the administration and disposal of cytotoxic agents may be acceptable (Table 5.7). Staff who may be pregnant must not administer cyclophosphamide.

➲ Also see 'Post-cyclophosphamide treatment', p. 183; ➲ 'Nursing issues' pp. 330 and 336; ➲ 'Patient-centred care', p. 332.

Further reading

Dougherty L, Lister S (eds) (2015). *The Royal Marsden Manual of Clinical Nursing Procedures*, 9th edn. Oxford: Wiley-Blackwell Publishing.

Nursing and Midwifery Council (2015). *The Code: Professional Standards of Practice and Behaviour for Nurses and Midwives*. London: Nursing and Midwifery Council.

Table 5.7 Cyclophosphamide—pretreatment assessment checklist

Patient education/consent	Yes/no	
Chest and heart examination by doctor	Yes/no	
Temperature, pulse, and respiration; blood pressure, urinalysis	Yes/no	Report any abnormalities
Check drug allergies especially sulphonamides	Yes/no	
Exposure to chickenpox/shingles	Yes/no	If yes, check varicella status: discuss with doctor
Varicella titre		If 1st dose and not previously screened
Check for signs of infection: wounds, urinary catheter, leg ulcer, cough, cold	Yes/no	If present, discuss with doctor
FBC, U&Es, LFT's, CRP within last 24–48 hours	Yes/no	If no, bloods stat
WBC >4.0 × 10^9/L	Yes/no	WBC <4.0 × 10^9/L discuss with doctor
Neutrophils >2.0 × 10^9/L	Yes/no	Neutrophils <2.0 × 10^9/L withhold treatment—discuss with doctor
♀ pregnant Date of last menstrual period	Yes/no	If pregnant or uncertainty regarding pregnancy, withhold treatment and discuss with doctor
Infertility—discuss sperm banking	Yes/no	
Dose calculated 15 mg/kg, ↓ dose if indicated for age or renal impairment		
Mesna and antiemetic prescribed	Yes/no	
Septrin® prophylaxis prescribed	Yes/no	
Bone prophylaxis prescribed	Yes/no	
Future invasive procedure planned	Yes/no	

Post-cyclophosphamide treatment

- Patients must drink at least 3 L of fluid to reduce bladder toxicity.
- Empty bladder frequently.
- Ensure patient knows when to have follow-up bloods and when to take mesna and co-trimoxazole.
- Avoid live vaccines for 3 months after stopping immunosuppressive treatment.

Follow-up care

These diseases can relapse at any time and require regular follow-up to assess the extent of organ involvement, progression of the disease, and toxicity of treatment especially infection.

Assessment and monitoring

- Regular bloods.
- FBC and differential count.
- U&Es.
- ESR/CRP.
- ANCA status.
- Urinalysis: dipstick for haematuria and proteinurea. Red cell casts indicative of significant kidney inflammation. Cyclophosphamide can cause haemorrhagic cystitis and ↑ risk of bladder cancer (>30-fold). Routine blood monitoring of AZA/MTX.
- The Birmingham Vasculitis Activity Score (BVAS) can be used to assess disease activity and severity of disease and the Vasculitis Damage Index (VDI) can be used to monitor long-term outcome.

► It is important to note that ANCA titre is not always associated with disease activity; however, a positive ANCA should alert the clinician to assess the patient more frequently due to a possible imminent relapse.

►► Early detection of relapse and prompt treatment is essential, minor relapse (no threat to vital organs) is treated with an ↑ in prednisolone and a major relapse (threated vital organs) is treated with cyclophosphamide.

Further reading

Bacon PA, Luqmani RA, Moots RJ, et al. (1994). Birmingham Vasculitis Activity Score (BVAS) in systemic vasculitis. *QJM* 87:671–8.

Frequently asked questions: vasculitis

What is vasculitis?

Inflammation of blood vessels.

What causes AAV?

We still do not know. An environmental agent interacting with a genetically predisposed host.

What is the prognosis?

PSV: early mortality is 10%, thereafter prognosis for GPA/EGPA is good with a 5-year survival rate of 80%. For MPA there is a worse prognosis because of renal involvement; mortality is 50% at 5 years.

What is the risk of bladder cancer from cyclophosphamide?

Up to 30-fold higher but highest with long-term cyclophosphamide, probably much less with short-term intermittent (<6 months).

Should patients with AAV be given the influenza and pneumococcal vaccine?

Yes.

Can EGPA be diagnosed without a biopsy?

Yes, it is preferable to have biopsy evidence, however this is not always possible but the diagnosis can be made from clinical signs and symptoms, blood tests, and ANCA serology.

How many patients with EGPA have asthma?

95%.

Cyclophosphamide can be given orally or as an IV pulse, is there a difference?

No, there is no difference in time to remission but using the IV route allows for a reduction in total dose of cyclophosphamide administered.

Can patients who are ANCA positive become ANCA negative?

Yes, many will become ANCA negative during treatment.

What advice should we give patients?

Aim for a blood pressure of 120/80 mmHg; do not smoke; eat a healthy balanced diet; and control body weight.

Is Behçet's disease a sexually transmitted disease?

No, there are no links to sexually transmitted diseases.

Can patients receive vaccinations?

Yes, unless they are immunosuppressed, when they should avoid live vaccines.

Chapter 6

Chronic non-inflammatory pain

Chronic musculoskeletal pain

Over 80% of the population will consult a GP for musculoskeletal pain in their lifetime. Widespread pain, fibromyalgia, and regional pain have a similar occurrence and shared risk factors which suggest they are all part of the same spectrum of chronic pain. Chronic musculoskeletal pain has several key attributes:

- Pain persists over time.
- Pain affects physical, psychological, and social function.
- Often there is no identifiable pathological cause for the pain.
- The individual is not able to carry out their normal activities.

Consequently, the aim of management is not the abolition of pain but to help individuals optimize their function and learn how to cope with the pain.

Defining pain

The most widely used definition of pain is from the International Association for the Society of Pain which regards pain as 'an unpleasant sensory and emotional experience associated with actual or potential tissue damage or described in terms of such damage'.[1] It is worth remembering that pain is a very individual experience and it is important to understand the impact of pain from the perspective of the individual.

The difference between chronic and acute pain

Acute pain is a short-lived experience whereas chronic pain is an ongoing occurrence (Table 6.1).

Chronic non-inflammatory conditions:

- Fibromyalgia.
- Osteoarthritis.
- Whiplash.
- Chronic pain syndromes.

Table 6.1 Differences between acute and chronic pain

Acute pain	Chronic pain
Duration is transient	Duration is persistent
Location usually single site	Location is generalized
Identifiable cause	Often no identifiable cause

Reference

1. International Association for the Study of Pain (IASP) (1994). *Classification of Chronic Pain, Description of Chronic Pain Syndromes and Definitions of Pain Terms*, 2nd edn. Seattle, WA: IASP.

Further reading

Department of Health (2006). *The Musculoskeletal Services Framework. A Joint Responsibility: Doing it Differently*. London: Department of Health.

Chronic pain syndromes: understanding pain mechanisms

- In the seventeenth century, pain was seen as purely a physical phenomenon with a direct relationship between the amount of damage or 'nociception' and the pain experienced. What this theory did not explain was the variation in the pain experience for a given stimulus or injury (e.g. why some patients take longer to recover from whiplash than others) or the persistence of pain beyond the time of tissue healing.
- In 1965, Melzack and Wall revolutionized our understanding of pain mechanisms with the gate control theory of pain. This theory demonstrated that the transmission of pain messages could be modulated within the spinal cord via descending messages from the brain (our cognitions and emotions) or altered by activating another source of sensory receptor (exercise to release endorphins).[1]

Pain receptors

Pain receptors are situated in the tissues, especially the skin, synovium of joints, and arterial walls. These receptors are activated by various stimuli including:

- Mechanical changes, e.g. excess weight on a particular area.
- Temperature changes.
- Inflammatory changes—the release of prostaglandin, bradykinin, histamine, and serotonin.

The peripheral sensory nerves transmit a signal of pain from the peripheries to the CNS to enable identification of the stimulus, e.g. pain in the wrist. The alpha delta fibres (thin and myelinated) transmit the sharp pain of an acute injury and the slower C-fibres (unmyelinated) produce the dull aching pain of a more persistent problem. When these fibres are stimulated, the 'pain gate' opens and messages pass to the brain to be perceived as pain. When large fibres become activated (alpha beta) they close the 'pain gate'. Alpha beta fibres transmit the sensation of touch: consequently, electrical nerve stimulation works on the same principle and excites large fibre activity. Nerve impulses that descend from the brain can also operate 'the gate' (Fig. 6.1).

Reference

1. Doubell TP, Mannion RJ, Woolf CJ (1999). The dorsal horn: state-dependent sensory processing, plasticity and the generation of pain. In: Wall PD, Melzack R (eds) *Textbook of Pain*, 4th edn, pp. 165–81. Edinburgh: Churchill Livingstone.

Further reading

Katz J, Rosenbloom B (2015). The golden anniversary of Melzack and Wall's gate control theory of pain celebrating 50 years of pain research and management. *Pain Res Manage* 20:285–6.

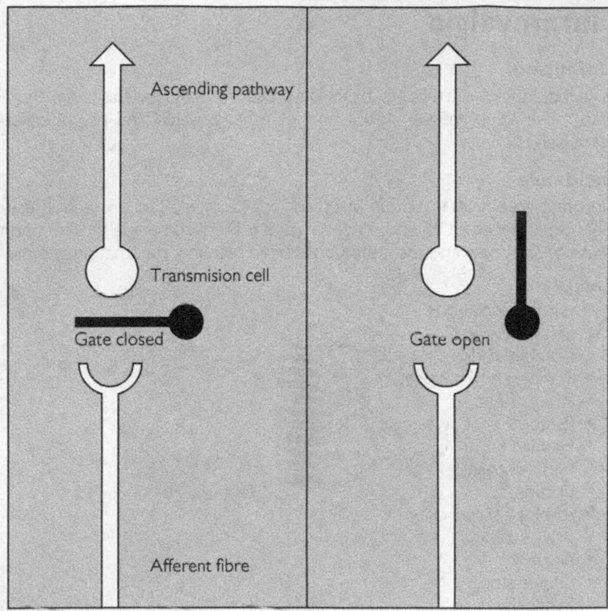

Fig. 6.1 Gate control mechanism.

Reproduced with permission from Clinical Skills Ltd.

Fibromyalgia

Definition

A condition characterized by widespread musculoskeletal pain, non-restorative sleep, fatigue, and a host of other physical and psychological associations.

Incidence

Fibromyalgia occurs in ~0.5% of ♂ and ~3.4% of ♀. The onset in ♀ usually occurs between 25 and 45 years (Box 6.1). Fibromyalgia is a common cause of joint pain and the condition is often seen in a rheumatology clinic.

Associations

- Physical associations:
  - Irritable bowel.
  - Irritable bladder.
  - Temperature changes.
  - Paraesthesia.
  - Perception of swelling.
  - Headache.
  - Muscle spasm.
  - Dizziness.
- Psychological associations:
  - Panic attacks.
  - Anxiety.
  - Depression.
  - Irritability.
  - Memory lapses.
  - Word mix-ups.
  - Reduced concentration.
  - Atypical facial pain.

Causes

Fibromyalgia can be classified as a 1° condition when it occurs on its own or as a 2° condition when it is associated with another conditions such as

Box 6.1 A typical patient

This will often be a ♀ aged 40 years who experienced neck pain 5 years ago which never resolved and who now has pain all over her body. She will experience fatigue on waking, feels 'worn out with the pain', and is tearful during the consultation. She has seen a number of other consultants in the past for various symptoms including her migraines and irritable bowel symptoms. She feels no one believes how much pain she is in and she is very anxious about her condition. She is no longer working and is finding it difficult to carry out her household chores. Physical examination reveals multiple tender hyperalgesic sites.

RA or lupus. No single pathophysiological causative mechanism has been identified and it would appear that fibromyalgia is a multifactorial syndrome.

Possible causes of fibromyalgia include:

- Abnormal central pain processing.
- Sleep disturbance.
- Genetic predisposition to pain sensitivity.
- Anxiety and depression.
- Viral infection.
- Physical trauma—road traffic accident, whiplash.
- Emotional trauma.

Diagnosis

In 2010, the ACR developed a more clinically useful and practical set of criteria for diagnostic purposes (➲ see 'Diagnosis of fibromyalgia', Chaper 6, p. 193).

Examination

The main finding is the presence of symmetrical tender/painful sites around the body (➲ see Fig. 6.2, p. 193). In patients without fibromyalgia these sites are uncomfortable to firm pressure but in patients with fibromyalgia the same pressure causes the patient to cry out and withdraw the area being examined. When patients try to stretch out a limb they find that the pain prevents them achieving full extension but when the clinician exams the same area they can achieve full extension, but the patient finds it uncomfortable.

Investigations

Limited investigations are required to exclude other causes for the symptoms, including PMR, spondyloarthropathy, and hypothyroidism—all of which can also give rise to similar symptoms.

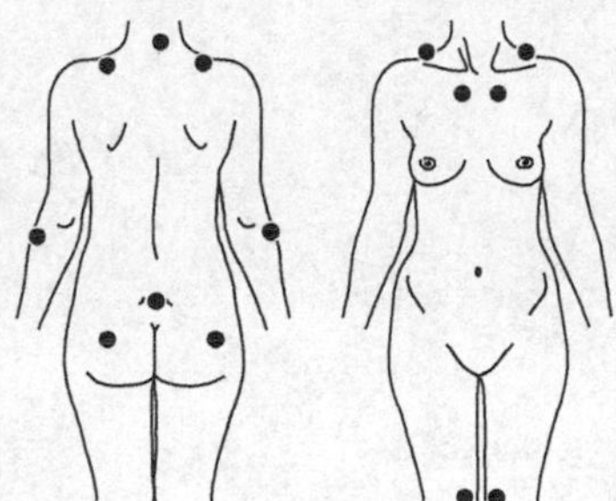

- Tenderness of skin overlaying trapezius
- Low cervical spine
- Midpoint of trapezius
- Supraspinatus
- Pectoralis, maximal lateral to the second costochondral junction
- Lateral epicondyle of the elbow
- Upper gluteal area
- Low lumbar spine
- Medial fat pad of the knee

Fig. 6.2 Some of the tender points in fibromyalgia.

Investigations include:

- FBC.
- Inflammatory markers, e.g. ESR and CRP.
- Biochemical profile—serum calcium, alkaline phosphatase, creatine kinase, and blood sugar.
- Thyroid function tests.

It is important to make a diagnosis of fibromyalgia after the clinical history and examination and explain to the patient that the blood tests are simply to ensure there is no other underlying condition. Radiological investigations are not required.

Diagnosis of fibromyalgia

See Box 6.2.[1]

Box 6.2 American College of Rheumatology diagnostic criteria for fibromyalgia

- The presence of symptoms including fatigue, waking unrefreshed, and cognitive function. The severity of these symptoms are measured on a 4-point longitudinal symptom severity scale ranging from 0 (no symptoms) to 3 (severe).
- The number of somatic symptoms (measured on a 4-point longitudinal score from 0 (no symptoms) to 3 (many symptoms) for the number of somatic symptoms in general, resulting in a symptoms severity scale ranging between 0 and 12.
- The presence of widespread pain (measured on a widespread pain index, with 1 point awarded for each anatomically painful site; 19 sites are included).
- A person will satisfy the diagnostic criteria for fibromyalgia if he or she has experienced symptoms for at least 3 months and does not have a disorder that would explain the pain and if the widespread pain index is 7 or higher, and the symptom severity score is 5 or higher, or the widespread pain index is 3–6 and the symptom severity scale score is 9 or higher.

Clinical features from the history

- Widespread musculoskeletal pain.
- Pain is a constant feature.
- Tired all the time.
- Joint stiffness.
- Non-restorative sleep.
- Difficulty carrying out normal activities.

Data sourced from Wolfe F, Clauw MA, Fitzcharles DL et al. (2010). The American College of Rheumatology preliminary diagnostic criteria for fibromyalgia and measurement of symptom severity. *Arthritis Care Research* 62: 600–610.

Reference

1. Wolfe F, Clauw MA, Fitzcharles DL, et al. (2010). The American College of Rheumatology preliminary diagnostic criteria for fibromyalgia and measurement of symptom severity. *Arthritis Care Res* 62:600–10.

Other chronic pain conditions

There are similarities between patients with fibromyalgia, chronic back pain, and chronic regional pain syndrome. The causes, symptoms, and management of complex regional pain syndrome (CRPS) are discussed in this section.

Chronic pain conditions

Back pain

Back pain is frequently seen in adults between 35 and 55 years of age. Most episodes settle within 6 weeks but 7% of people will go on to develop chronic pain.

Complex regional pain syndrome

CRPS syndrome is characterized by variable dysfunction of the musculoskeletal systems. It is a condition that is not fully understood and can be difficult to diagnose. CRPS typically affects the hand or forearm, foot, ankle, or knee.

There are two types of CRPS. In type 1, symptoms occur in the absence of injury to the nerves whereas in type 2, there is a nerve injury.

Causes

In a quarter of causes there is no identifiable cause although it sometimes occurs after the following:

- Trauma.
- Emotional stress.
- Pregnancy.
- Prolonged immobilization.
- Neurological events such as a stroke or meningitis.
- MI.

Signs and symptoms

- Pain, often 'burning' in nature, that can occur even after a light touch.
- Tenderness.
- Rash.
- Warmth over the affected area.
- Sweating.
- Soft tissue swelling.
- Sleep disturbance.
- If symptoms last for several months then the affected area can change and become cool, with altered colour and abnormal sensation.
- If symptoms continue to progress, then wasting (atrophy) of the skin and subcutaneous tissue can occur.

Investigations

The diagnosis is made from the clinical history and examination. Radiological investigation may reveal osteoporosis. The use of technetium scintigraphy can show abnormal blood flow.

Management

- Reassure the patient that they can manage their own symptoms through graded exercise, pacing, minimizing anxiety, developing a structure for the day, and adopting a sleep routine.
- Due to the importance of maintaining and improving function of the affected area as soon as possible, the PT is usually involved, and hydrotherapy is a useful option for patients struggling to exercise due to the pain.
- To improve sleep and help with the pain, low-dose (10–50 mg) tricyclics may be used.
- Regional sympathetic or ganglion blocks may also be considered in extreme cases.
- All chronic pain conditions have the same management principles which are discussed in this chapter.

The use of a biopsychosocial approach ensures that all factors contributing to the pain experience will be explored.

Factors contributing to the pain experience

- Physical factors, e.g. ↓ in physical activities results in muscle wasting, muscle fatigue, and ↑ joint stiffness.
- Psychological factors, e.g. low mood and anxiety.
- Cognitive factors, e.g. how a patient feels about their pain; if a patient is fearful that movement could cause damage, they are less likely to engage in exercise.
- Social factors, e.g. how the pain is impacting work, leisure, and relationships.

➲ Also see 'Education, social, and psychological issues', Chapter 10, pp. 336 and 339; ➲ 'Assessing pain', p. XX; ➲ Chapter 9, 'Symptom control: using pharmacological and non-pharmacological methods', pp. 307–328.

Further reading

Clunie G, Wilkinson N, Nikiphorou E, Jadon D (eds) (2018). Chronic pain syndromes. In: *Oxford Handbook of Rheumatology*, 4th edn, pp. 623–41. Oxford: Oxford University Press.

Miller C, Williams M, Heine P, et al. (2017). Current practice in the rehabilitation of complex regional pain syndrome: a survey of practitioners. *Disabil Rehabil* 11:1–7.

NICE (2016). Low back pain and sciatic in the over 16s: assessment and management (NG59). ➚ http://www.nice.org.uk/guideline/ng59

Education in chronic pain management

The patient will often need guidance, support, and motivation from a health professional before feeling able to take an active role in the management of their symptoms.

Patient-centred management goals need to be realistic, achievable, and meaningful for the patient to engage in. Patients who utilize active rather than passive coping strategies report less pain-related disability and distress, better general health, and use fewer healthcare services and medications.

Active strategies are those that involve some action by the individual to manage their pain through their own efforts, whereas passive strategies refer to an individual who is more reliant on the efforts of others or who depends on medications.

The current evidence advocates the use of behavioural strategies including:

- Graded exercise.
- Pacing.
- CBT.
- Goal setting.
- Relaxation.
- Stress management.

There is no evidence that one specific behavioural approach is more effective than another, but treatment is likely to be more effective if it:

- Includes more than education alone.
- Includes teaching patients skills based on rehearsal or practice.
- Is aimed at changing behaviour and improving function.

CBT

- This is a widely used form of psychotherapy which aims to identify and change maladaptive patterns of thought and behaviour.
- CBT can help patients adjust to their illness and acquire skills that can be used in their daily lives.
- CBT can improve a patient's sense of control regarding their symptoms.
- CBT for persistent pain should be applied early in the development of problems with daily functioning and not as a last resort.

Mindfulness

- Is based on the principle that emotions can negatively influence behaviour.
- It can be an effectiveness treatment to help cope with anxiety and pain related to the pain.
- Can improve function.
- Can be used to help the person to reengage with his or her life despite the pain.

Improving sleep

Patients often experience a disturbed sleep pattern and feel unrefreshed on waking. This ↑ the perception of pain, leading to low mood, reduced cognitive functioning, and a reduced ability to manage the symptoms. Self-help measures should be advocated, including:

- Developing a sleep routine, including going to bed at the same time each night and avoiding day-time sleeping.
- Avoiding stimulants such as caffeine.
- Carrying out relaxation techniques to clear the mind.
- Ensuring that the bedroom is quiet and well ventilated.

Tricyclics can improve sleep quality by improving non-rapid eye movement (REM), sleep which is restorative sleep. Number needed to treat = 4. The most commonly prescribed tricyclic is amitriptyline. This is prescribed in small incremental doses ranging from 10 to 50 mg and should be taken 2–3 hours before settling. The decision regarding dosage will be based on efficacy and side effects. Tricyclics should help to improve sleep within 2–3 weeks but take 3–4 months before modifying pain perception.

Exercise

Many patients become less physically active due to pain and are fearful that movement will ↑ the symptoms of pain and fatigue. Graded exercise is advocated to recondition the body and to improve muscle stamina, strength, stiffness, and generalized fitness. Graded exercise involves gradually ↑ activity over a period of time. Several sessions of supervised exercise by the PT may be required to provide motivation, education, reassurance, and feedback.

Relaxation

The patient can be taught relaxation techniques to help with:

- Muscle tension.
- Anxiety.
- Sleep.
- Fostering a sense of control over symptoms.

Pacing

Pacing involves breaking down everyday activities into achievable components. Patients tend to exert themselves on a 'good day' and under-exert on a 'poor day'. If patients can plan their activities, e.g. cleaning one room in the house a day instead of doing all the rooms in one go, they will still achieve their goal and be active every day. Patients should always be encouraged to remain in the workplace and apply the principles of pacing in the work situation.

➲ Also see Chapter 19, 'Non-pharmacological therapies', pp. 584–594 ; ➲ Chapter 10, 'Holistic and patient-centred care', pp. 329–350.

Further reading

Ryan S (2013). Care of patients with fibromyalgia: assessment and management. *Nurs Stand* 28:37–43.

Ryan S, Campbell A (2010). Fibromyalgia syndrome. In: Adebajo A (ed), *ABC of Rheumatology*, 4th edn, pp. 47–50. London: BMJ Publishing.

Managing depression in chronic pain syndromes

Symptoms of depression are common in chronic musculoskeletal pain conditions:

- For mild depression, CBT, exercise, relaxation, and pacing techniques can all be considered.
- For moderate to severe depression antidepressant drug therapy may be required including citalopram or duloxetine. Patients should be told that it will take 2 weeks before the drug becomes effective. Antidepressants also have analgesic effects which can be very useful when treating this group of patients. If a patient does not respond to antidepressant treatment then a psychiatric referral should be considered.

Other pharmacological options for the management of chronic musculoskeletal pain

- Paracetamol may be useful for joint pain in OA but for non-organic pain such as fibromyalgia there is often a poor response.
- Pregabalin and gabapentin can be used for widespread chronic musculoskeletal pain.
- Specific antidepressant drugs can work on pain pathways such as duloxetine.
- Low-dose amitriptyline can be used to improve sleep and pain.
- Tramadol may be considered but there is little evidence to support the use of strong narcotics. Tramadol should be used with caution in patients who have a history of dependence or addiction. It can also interact with the serotonin-specific reuptake inhibitor (SSRIs) and the tricyclics to cause convulsions.

Complementary/alternative medicine (CAM)

While few studies have examined the benefits of CAM, patients often use numerous types of CAM including massage therapy, chiropractic treatment, and acupuncture.

Roles of the MDT

- Nurse or OT for pacing, relaxation, goal setting, education, and self-management.
- Nurse/OT or psychologist for CBT.
- PT for graded exercise.
- Doctor/nurse or therapist prescriber for drug therapy.

➲ Also see 'Pharmacological management: pain relief', Chapter 15, pp. 430–444; ➲ Chapter 9, 'Symptom control: using pharmacological and non-pharmacological methods', pp. 307–328.

Further reading

Goldenberg DL (2016). Is there evidence for any truly effective therapy in Fibromyalgia. *Pain Manage* 6:325–9.

Versus Arthritis. Living with long term pain: a guide to self-management. https://www.versusarthritis.org/media/1248/back-pain-information-booklet.pdf

Regional musculoskeletal conditions: overview

A systematic classification of musculoskeletal disorders that comfortably includes everything is difficult to achieve. The scope of MSCs is so wide and diverse as it has to cover everything from CTDs to traumatic injuries, inflammatory to degenerative diseases, systemic conditions, and local conditions.

A chapter on regional MSCs might therefore be expected to cover a lot of the problems that don't fit into any of the other big disease categories. Don't be fooled, however, into thinking that the conditions outlined in this chapter are somehow less important. Many of the commonest musculoskeletal problems that occur in the community, and present in a 1° care setting, will be outlined in this chapter. Musculoskeletal problems are presented in ~25% of consultations with health professionals in 1° care. The average GP will see at least one case of back or neck pain every day, and will see at least one case of shoulder or knee pain every other day.

This chapter has set out to focus on the most common problems that you are likely to come across in daily practice but should complement the additional text outlining the less commonly seen conditions that are discussed in this handbook.

The neck and spine are discussed in ➔ 'Neck and spine', pp. 222 and 224; ➔ 'Examination of the spine', pp. 224 and 225.

The shoulder: common problems and adhesive capsulitis

Shoulder pain is common and can cause significant morbidity and functional impairment. The pain may be due to disease or injury of structures surrounding the shoulder joint, or referred from other sites (Box 6.3).

The most common problems are those caused by disease or injury of the tendons, muscles, ligaments, and capsule of the joint. Shoulder pain can be caused by capsulitis or rotator cuff tendon problems, or referred from the neck. These conditions can be differentiated by means of a careful history and examination. Possible diagnoses include:

- Adhesive capsulitis.
- Rotator cuff disease.
- Acromioclavicular joint (ACJ) dysfunction.
- Biceps tendonitis or rupture.
- Muscular neck pain or cervical spine OA.

Adhesive capsulitis (frozen shoulder)

Epidemiology

Capsulitis presents with pain and global restriction in shoulder movements. The cause is unknown, but the onset of symptoms is often associated with a previous minor injury or may follow a period of immobility of the limb. Presentation usually includes:

- Most commonly seen in 40–60-year-olds.
- Commoner in ♀ and diabetics.
- Bilateral in 15% of cases.
- Following a period of immobility such as:
  - Following a fracture which has led to immobilization.
  - After hemiplegic stroke.

Box 6.3 Shoulder pain: common problems and differential diagnoses

Pain arising from disease or injury of shoulder structures

- The joint capsule, e.g. capsulitis.
- Synovium, e.g. inflammatory arthritis.
- Bursitis.
- Tendon and muscle, e.g. rotator cuff tendinopathy.
- Bone, e.g. bony malignant metastases.

Shoulder pain referred from other sites

- Neck problems, e.g. cervical spondylosis.
- Cervical disc disease.
- Structures innervated by C3, C4, C6 segments, e.g. diaphragm (characteristically pain from an inflamed gallbladder may refer to the right shoulder).

The natural history of this condition is for symptoms to resolve slowly over 18 months to 2 years. However, even after this time there may be residual joint restriction.

Diagnosis

- Active *and* passive movements are restricted in all directions.
- Lateral rotation at the shoulder shows most restriction as the joint capsule has least laxity anteriorly.

► Differentiate this condition from rotator cuff injury—although the two conditions may coexist.

Management

The history and examination should be directed at excluding other causes of shoulder pain, in particular bony pain and referred pain.

► Don't forget to think about PMR in the elderly person with bilateral shoulder pain and stiffness.

The principles of management include:

- Pain relief:
  - Non-pharmacological measures, heat pads, transcutaneous electrical nerve stimulation (TENS).
  - Simple analgesia.
  - NSAIDs—short courses where no contraindications exist.
- Mobilization:
  - Avoid using a sling.
  - Gentle mobilization and activity.
  - Refer to physiotherapy if necessary.
  - Consider IA corticosteroid injection.
  - IA corticosteroid injected into the glenohumeral space may result in both pain relief and improved range of movement. The procedure may need to be repeated, but is not always successful.

► It is helpful to demonstrate the exercises to the patient and provide written information. Explain that pain relief is necessary to allow them to perform the exercises, which in turn will aid recovery.

➲ Also see 'Primary care: common musculoskeletal problems', p. 218; ➲ 'Primary care: first steps in the assessment of shoulder problems', p. 228.

Shoulder problems: rotator cuff, subacromial, clavicular, and biceps problems

Rotator cuff tendonitis and subacromial impingement

The 'rotator cuff' is the name given to the muscles and tendons that surround the shoulder joint. The shoulder is the most mobile joint in the body, and relies heavily on the surrounding muscles and tendons for stability. The tendons of the rotator cuff muscles pass through the small space below the acromion, and may cause shoulder pain if they become inflamed, damaged, or torn.

Subacromial impingement is the term used to describe the pattern of pain and symptoms produced by a number of problems affecting the structures of the rotator cuff. These include:

- Rotator cuff tendon damage or tears.
- Subacromial bursitis.
- Glenohumeral instability.
- Osteophytes affecting the inferior aspect of the ACJ.

All of these will result in pain, characteristically localized to the upper arm—so-called military badge pain which is aggravated by specific rotational or elevational movements of the arm.

Epidemiology

This is the commonest type of shoulder pain in adults. The diagnosis might be suggested by a history of trauma (e.g. a sports injury) or repetitive, forceful, overhead shoulder movements, and may therefore present in particular occupational groups such as painters and decorators and plasterers. The commonest tendon of the rotator cuff to be affected is the supraspinatus tendon, which is responsible for initiation of shoulder abduction. Occasionally calcium deposits may be found within the tendon (so-called calcific tendonitis). This often presents with a more severe acute pain with associated heat and redness.

Diagnosis

Movement will generally be most restricted and painful in one particular plane of movement. Classically pain is maximal through the mid part of shoulder abduction ('mid-arc pain') Passive movements are usually less painful.

Management

The initial management is similar to that for adhesive capsulitis and involves:

- Analgesia and rest in the acute phase (avoid overhead movements).
- Passive mobilization and physiotherapy exercises may assist recovery.
- A subacromial IA steroid injection can be useful in severe cases which fail to respond to conservative treatment.
- Consider surgical review if pain fails to settle with conservative management.
- Acute tendon rupture suggested by pain and weakness after trauma should prompt surgical review.

➲ Also see 'The shoulder: common problems and adhesive capsulitis', p. 188.

ACJ dysfunction

The ACJ is prone to trauma and subsequent osteoarthritic change, and may sometimes be the source of significant shoulder pain. The pain is often localized to the site of the ACJ, and results in pain particularly in the last 20° of shoulder abduction, and in movements which involve adduction the arm across the body, thus compressing the ACJ. This is the basis of the 'scarf test', which can be helpful in identifying ACJ dysfunction. Significant ACJ problems may also coexist with subacromial bursitis and rotator cuff problems. Symptoms are often chronic and ongoing, but some relief may be obtained by an IA corticosteroid injection into the ACJ, or, in severe cases, surgical excision of the lateral end of the clavicle.

Biceps tendonitis and rupture of long head of biceps

The tendon of the long head of biceps traverses the shoulder joint and travels through the bicipital groove between the greater and lesser tuberosity of the humerus. It is enclosed in a synovial sheath throughout its length, and may give rise to pain in the anterior shoulder and the anterior upper arm, aggravated by repetitive lifting. The pain can be reproduced by resisted elbow flexion. Treatment is with rest and analgesia, including NSAIDs if tolerated. Local corticosteroid injection into the tendon sheath can also be carried out. The tendon may rupture. This is more likely in older individuals, and is associated with a 'snapping' sensation and the appearance of a swelling in the upper arm—the 'Popeye sign'—which represents the contracted muscle belly. No specific treatment is required although residual weakness on elbow flexion is to be expected.

Elbow

The elbow joint enjoys good bony stability, and is often relatively spared in many of the commoner form of arthritis. However, elbow pain may often present from structures around the elbow. The commonest cause of pain around the elbow is medial and lateral epicondylitis, often referred to as 'tennis elbow' and 'golfer's elbow'. These two problems will be dealt with together as they represent a common pathological process.

Medial and lateral epicondylitis ('tennis elbow' and 'golfer's elbow')

The medial and lateral epicondyles are the bony extensions at the distal end of the humerus. The medial epicondyle acts as an anchor point for tendons of the flexor muscles of the forearm, which flex both the wrist and fingers. This point of attachment is often referred to as the common flexor origin. The lateral epicondyle is the anchor point for the tendons of the extensor muscles of the forearm and is referred to as the common extensor origin. The point at which tendons and ligaments attach to bone is called the 'enthesis'.

Epicondylitis is caused by inflammation within the entheses of the elbow. This can either be due to the enthesis being overloaded by persistent activity such as frequent, forceful, repetitive gripping, twisting, or wrist flexion and extension. Some occupations may be predisposed to this condition (painters and decorators, plasterers, joiners, electricians, or sports-related activities) or it may occur after particular unaccustomed activity. A history of any repetitive forceful forearm activity is therefore significant.

Epicondylitis can also be a symptom of inflammatory arthritis, particularly seronegative arthritis such as PsA.

Diagnosis

The pain may be reproduced by resisted wrist extension (lateral epicondylitis) or flexion (medial epicondylitis) with the elbow held straight. There may also be tenderness over the epicondyle.

Management

- Rest, the application of ice, and a short course of NSAIDs may help, but often the symptoms may recur with resumption of activity.
- Physiotherapy and the use of an epicondylar clasp may sometimes alleviate symptoms and promote resolution.
- Local corticosteroid injection around the enthesis should be avoided, as this has been shown to worsen long-term outcomes.[1]
- In instances where none of these measures produce benefit, surgery may be considered.

Olecranon bursitis

The olecranon bursa overlies the bony prominence at the point of the elbow. This structure is usually neither visible nor palpable, but in certain circumstances may fill with fluid and present as a large fluctuant lump on the point of the elbow. Causes to consider include:

- It may arise following trauma such as a direct blow to the point of the elbow. In these circumstances, a fracture must be excluded.

- Sepsis may also occur in the bursa giving rise to a painful, hot, and tender swelling.
- Occasionally an olecranon bursitis may occur in gout.

Management is usually conservative, with rest, ice, compression, and elevation (RICE) and an NSAID often settling the symptoms down. Aspiration may be warranted if the cause is uncertain:

- Gout—uric acid crystals may be seen on polarized light microscopy of the aspirate.
- ⚠ Although uncommon, septic arthritis needs to be considered as a diagnosis. Septic arthritis is an acute medical emergency requiring prompt referral to 2° care. If there is an index of suspicion, an urgent referral is made to 2° care for diagnosis and management. A septic bursitis is obviously not as catastrophic as a septic arthritis, but still has to be managed cautiously. Following aspiration, these bursae frequently recur, and occasionally surgical bursectomy may be considered.

Ulnar neuritis

The ulnar nerve is in a somewhat vulnerable position as it passes through a grove behind the medial epicondyle, the so-called cubital tunnel (symptoms relating to this nerve are experienced when we refer to 'hitting our funny bone'). The nerve may be vulnerable to more persistent entrapment at this site leading to paraesthesia and numbness affecting the palmar aspect of the fifth digit and the ulnar side of the fourth digit. Tapping over the ulnar nerve with a finger as it passes through the cubital tunnel (Hoffman–Tinel test) may precipitate or exacerbate the symptoms, thus assisting diagnosis.

Treatment includes:

- Rest and attention to posture or activities that may be contributing towards the development of the symptoms.
- Occasionally, corticosteroid injection or surgical decompression may be required.

Reference

1. Smidt N, van der Windt DA, Assendelft WJ, et al. (2002). Corticosteroid injections, physiotherapy, or a wait-and-see policy for lateral epicondylitis: a randomized controlled trial. *Lancet* 359:657–62.

Wrist and hand

Carpal tunnel syndrome (CTS)

CTS, similar to ulnar neuropathy, represents a nerve entrapment syndrome that occurs as the median nerve passes beneath the flexor retinaculum at the wrist. It is common, and results in an easily recognizable pattern of symptoms which include abnormal unpleasant sensations, often described as 'pins and needles', in the distribution of the sensory branch of the median nerve in the hand—the palmar aspect of the middle three fingers and the base of the thumb.

- Often worse at night and may cause wakening from sleep and described as affected hand as being 'dead' or 'asleep', and often try to gain some relief by shaking it vigorously.
- Pain may be referred proximally up the forearm, and in some cases even to the shoulder.

No cause may be found, but there is an association between the development of symptoms and any condition that may cause swelling or compression in the wrist, e.g.:

- Previous Colles' fracture, OA, or synovitis at the wrist.
- Pregnancy, hypothyroidism, acromegaly, and diabetes.

If the condition is untreated and progresses further, the symptoms may become constant and motor symptoms may develop with weakness of the adductor pollicis and flexor pollicis brevis muscles, resulting in weakness of thumb apposition.

Examination

- Tinel's test refers to the provocation of symptoms by tapping over the median nerve as it runs through the wrist.
- Phalen's test again provokes or reproduces symptoms by asking the patient to rest their arm on a table or chair, allowing their hand to hang unsupported with the wrist flexed. In more advanced cases, wasting of the thenar and hypothenar eminences may be apparent.
- Further investigation with nerve conduction studies may help to confirm the diagnosis, but this facility is not always readily available, and a reliable diagnosis can often be made on clinical grounds alone.

Management

- Exclusion of underlying conditions such as hypothyroidism or inflammatory arthritis.
- Rest and splinting may be helpful.
- Contributing conditions such as hypothyroidism or inflammatory arthritis should be treated appropriately.
- Local corticosteroid injection into the carpal tunnel may produce improvement in symptoms for ~70% of sufferers.
- Surgical decompression may be required in some cases.
- ➲ Also see 'The elbow', p. 204

De Quervain's tenosynovitis

This occurs when there is inflammation of the tendon and tendon sheath of the extensor pollicis longus tendon as it runs under the extensor retinaculum at the radial styloid. The anatomical landmarks are usually easily identified. Symptoms include:

- Pain over the radial border of the wrist. Pain may occasionally be accompanied with swelling and crepitus.
- Finklestein's test is usually positive—pain on forced flexion and adduction at the wrist with the thumb flexed into the palm.
- Treatment includes RICE and NSAIDs. Occasionally, corticosteroid injection of the tendon sheath is used in resistant cases.

Ganglia

These are fluid-filled swellings of the tendon sheaths usually seen over the dorsum of the wrist. They are often asymptomatic. Management is conservative. The swelling may be aspirated, but if ganglia have been present for a long time, the fluid is often gelatinous and difficult to aspirate through a standard 21-gauge green needle. Following aspiration, it may often recur. Surgical excision can be considered, but if asymptomatic it is often best to do nothing.

Trigger finger/thumb (flexor tendon nodule)

Flexor tendon nodules are most commonly idiopathic, though can occur in association with inflammatory arthritis and diabetes. Nodules within the tendon, often caused by trauma or overuse, can catch at the A1 pulley within the finger. This causes the affected finger to remain in the flexed position when the rest of the fingers of the hand are extended. The finger may be extended forcibly but this is often painful. *Treatment*: responds well to injection of corticosteroid into the tendon sheath.

Lower limb: hip problems

Lower limb symptoms may arise as part of a more widespread systemic rheumatic disease or may be referred from other sites such as the lumbar spine or sacroiliac joint. The commonest presenting complaint will be of pain in the limb or some part of the limb. Other common symptoms are abnormal sensation (numbness, burning etc.) often of a neurological origin, weakness, and clicking from around a joint.

Hip

Patients may complain of pain in the hip; this pain may arise from the joint itself, from structures around the joint, or be referred from other sites such as the back. Red flags should be excluded. High index of suspicion should be considered if there is:

- A previous history of malignancy.
- Systemic illness including weight loss, or persisting nocturnal bony pain. The hip joint itself enjoys good bony stability and is deeply situated. Pain arising from the joint is usually felt in the groin and deep within the buttock.

➲ Also see 'Neck and spine', pp. 212, 214 and 222; ➲ 'Red and yellow flags', pp. 313–314; ➲ 'Osteoarthritis of the hip and knee', pp. 20–21.

Bursitis

There are three bursae around the hip which may give rise to periarticular pain. These are the:

- Trochanteric bursa.
- Ischial bursa.
- Iliopsoas bursa.

Trochanteric bursitis

The commonest to be seen and causes pain over the lateral aspect of the hip. It is often painful to lie on the affected side. Pain may be exacerbated by adducting the hip and asking the patient to attempt to abduct the hip against resistance. Maximal tenderness usually over the greater trochanter.

Treatment: physiotherapy and analgesia. Occasionally corticosteroid injection is required.

Ischial bursitis

Causes pain on sitting. The ischial bursa is located deep to the gluteal muscles. Pain may also arise on hip flexion when standing, as in stooping forward.

Treatment: rest and analgesia, preferably with an NSAID if not contraindicated. Local corticosteroid injection can also be considered in resistant or prolonged cases.

Iliopsoas bursitis

Rare and causes groin pain. It is most often seen in association with sports, particularly jumping. It may be associated with groin strain.

Treatment: muscle sprains usually respond to rest and simple analgesia (if necessary consider short course of NSAIDs if not contraindicated).

Lower limb: injuries affecting the knee

Injuries that result in regional conditions affecting the knee include:

- Ligament strain and rupture: collateral and cruciate ligaments.
- Meniscal injury.

Causes of knee effusion include:

- Trauma—haemarthrosis if bleeding occurs into the joint.
- Inflammatory:
  - Inflammatory arthritis.
  - Crystal arthritis.
  - OA.
  - Sepsis.

➲ Also see 'Osteoarthritis of the hip and knee', Chapter 2, pp. 17–18.

► If there is ANY diagnostic uncertainty or there is suspicion of infection, synovial fluid should be aspirated for fluid analysis—culture and Gram stain for bacterial organisms. If gout is suspected, polarized light microscopy for crystals. If any suspicion of infection, steroid should not be injected. Septic arthritis should be urgently considered. ➲ See Chapter 17, 'Septic arthritis', Chapter 13, pp. 404–405.

Collateral ligament strain

The medial and lateral collateral ligaments are of great structural and functional importance.

- Injury usually occurs through direct trauma to the knee, particularly where the joint is subjected to excessive lateral force.
  - The joint will be unstable, and there may well be an associated effusion. If symptoms occur after trauma, an additional injury may be apparent depending on the force of the trauma.
- May be associated with OA knee, particularly where there is asymmetric arthritis affecting the medial and lateral compartments of the knee joint resulting in an angular deformity, or genu valgus deformity (leads to knock-kneed appearance) and asymmetry of biomechanical forces.
- May also be associated with an anserine bursitis (➲ see 'Anserine bursitis', Chapter 6, p. 211).

Examination

The collateral ligaments are palpable. The medial collateral ligament is a broad band-like structure, whereas the lateral collateral ligament is more cord-like. The pain may be reproduced on applying lateral force to the knee, and the ligament may be tender to palpation.

Treatment

- If ligaments rupture, they may require surgical reconstruction.
- Ligament strain will often resolve with rest, ice, and compression, followed by rehabilitation, under the supervision of a PT.
- A knee brace for use during sport may also be considered although there is limited evidence.
- Short-term NSAIDs (when not contraindicated) and simple analgesics may help initially.

Cruciate ligament injury

Cruciate ligaments are usually the result of injury and trauma on the sports field. Cruciate ligament rupture is a significant orthopaedic injury and will usually require surgical repair. A positive anterior or posterior drawer test is pathognomonic of this condition (Fig. 6.3).

Meniscal injury

The menisci are prone to injury during sports activity. The mechanism is usually a twisting injury to the knee, and contact sports such as football and rugby particularly give rise to this injury, where the foot is fixed in position in the studded boot, and the body rotates excessively over the joint. Similar injury can occur in snow sports or water skiing. Acute presentation may be associated with an effusion and haemarthrosis. Following initial injury symptoms may settle, but the hallmarks of previous meniscal injury are recurrent episodes of knee locking and the knee giving way without warning.

Examination

There may be joint line tenderness on palpation, and occasionally a loose cartilaginous body may be palpated along the joint line. The commonest site for meniscal damage is anteromedially. McMurray's test will often demonstrate a positive response (Fig. 6.4). MRI scanning is the investigation of choice.

Treatment: arthroscopic repair of the menisci is the preferred option.

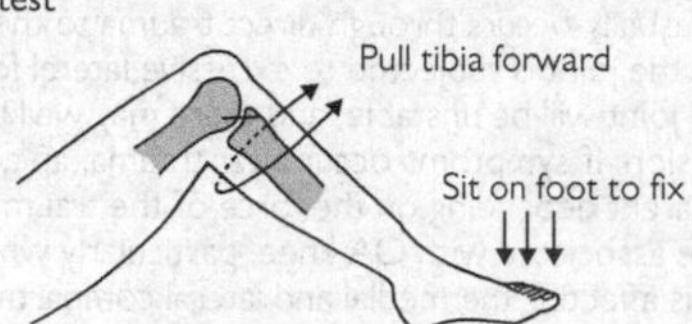
Anterior draw test
Pull tibia forward
Sit on foot to fix

Fig. 6.3 Anterior drawer test.

Reproduced with permission from Hakim A, Clunie G, Haq I (eds) (2006). *Oxford Handbook of Rheumatology*, 2nd edn. Oxford University Press, Oxford.

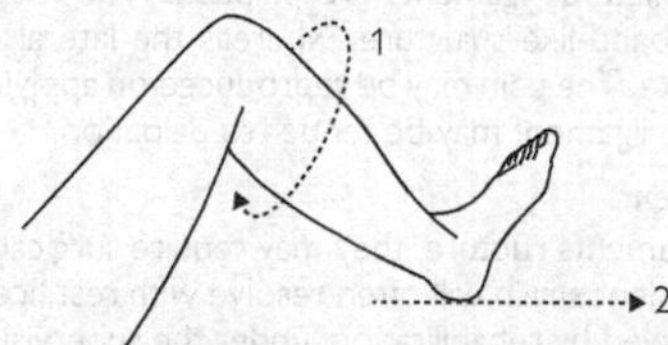
McMurray's test
1
2
Action: Hold the knee and the heel.
Internally rotate the lower leg (1) then extend it (2)
Positive test: (Palpable) clunk at joint line

Fig. 6.4 McMurray's test.

Reproduced with permission from Hakim A, Clunie G, Haq I (eds) (2006). *Oxford Handbook of Rheumatology*, 2nd edn. Oxford University Press, Oxford.

Lower limb: knee problems

► If there is a clinical suspicion of infection and a knee effusion is present, synovial fluid should be aspirated for fluid analysis—culture and Gram stain for bacterial organisms and polarized light microscopy for crystals.

➲ Also see 'Lower limb: injuries affecting the knee', pp. 209–210; ➲ 'Hip and knee', pp. 240 and 242; ➲ Chapter 17, 'Septic arthritis' pp. 404–405.

Baker's cyst

A cyst of the synovial sac in the knee which can be felt in the popliteal fossa (posterior to the knee).

- May be associated with OA in the knee.
- Occur spontaneously—rupture causes pain and swelling in the calf, mimicking DVT. If associated knee effusion, aspiration from knee joint often helps resolve the problem.

Anserine bursitis

The pes anserinus (or the 'goose's foot') is the name given to the area where the three tendons of gracilis, semitendinosus, and sartorius muscles join and insert into the medial aspect of the tibia ~3–4cm below the joint line. A bursa underlies this insertion and can be the site of pain; often associated with a genu valgus deformity and OA (➲ see 'Collateral ligament strain', pp. 209–210). It is also common to note a degree of ankle and foot pronation or 'flat footedness'. The pathology may be a bursitis or simply an enthesitis at the insertion of the pes anserinus.

Treatment

- RICE and NSAID.
- Physiotherapy if symptoms fail to settle.
- Local corticosteroid injection may help resistant symptoms.

Prepatellar/infrapatellar bursitis (housemaid's knee, parson's knee)

This is akin to the olecranon bursitis at the elbow. It presents with a large fluid-filled swelling which is palpable and lies in front of the patella. It is often associated with kneeling (hence the lay term housemaid's or clergyman's knee). Nowadays it is more often seen in trades people who kneel as part of their occupation, particularly carpet fitters.

Treatment

- RICE and NSAID.
- Avoidance of kneeling, use of knee pads.
- Bursitis may recur and can be reduced by injection of corticosteroid into the bursa.

Patellofemoral knee pain (PFKP)

Patellofemoral pain is an umbrella term to cover a wide range of disorders. Anterior knee pain is a frequently reported symptom, often insidious in onset but can occur acutely. It is common, and rarely associated with significant disease; one-third of young adults experience this type of pain at some stage. Diagnosing the underlying cause of PFKP can be challenging. PFKP is commonly seen in adolescence. In the older person, PFKP can be divided into three broad categories:

- Patellofemoral pain with instability.
- Patellofemoral pain with malalignment but no episodes of instability.
- Patellofemoral pain without malalignment or instability.

The clinical features may include tenderness in the retro- or infrapatellar area, small effusions, crepitus, and stiffness. There may be wasting of the vastus medialis obliquus. General symptoms reported may also include:

- Vague aching pain over anterior aspect of the knee.
- 'Giving way', 'clicking', or 'grating'.

Although rare, there are some key issues that may highlight important red flags that require prompt further investigations to eliminate tumours of the soft tissue and bone. These include:

- Night pain.
- Pain unrelated to activity or failing to respond to conservative treatment and with no obviously malalignment.

A detailed assessment by a physiotherapist to identify underlying mechanical issues should be undertaken before treatment can be planned.

An algorithm can be used to aid in diagnosis and subsequent approaches to management: evidence suggests that only 2–3% of those presenting with PFKP will require surgery.

Patellar tendonitis

Commonly seen in sports that involve kicking (e.g. football). The knee on the dominant side is most often affected. There is anterior knee pain localized below the patella, and the lower pole of the patella is tender. Crepitus may be palpable over the tendon.

Treatment

Rest, compression, ice, and anti-inflammatory drugs are the treatment of choice. Occasionally local corticosteroid injection may be considered.

Osgood–Schlatter disease

The pathological term given to this is a 'traction apophysitis or periostitis'. It is seen in teenage ♂ and is related to kicking sports (e.g. rugby and football). The infrapatellar tendon attaches to the tibia at the tibial tubercle. Trauma and separation may occur at this point particularly if excessive strains are applied to the area before complete fusion of the epiphysis. Attempted healing occurs through bony reaction and overgrowth at the site of injury resulting in the appearance of a tender, firm, bony mass at the tibial tubercle. The vast majority of cases settle with conservative management.

Treatment

RICE and an NSAID. Physiotherapy may help in resistant cases.

Further reading

MacAuley D (2012). *Oxford Handbook of Sport and Exercise Medicine*, 2nd edn. Oxford: Oxford University Press.

Pierce N (2016). Patellofemoral/extensor mechanisms disorders. In: Hutson M, Ward A (eds) *Oxford Textbook of Musculoskeletal Medicine*, 2nd edn, pp. 420–35. Oxford: Oxford University Press.

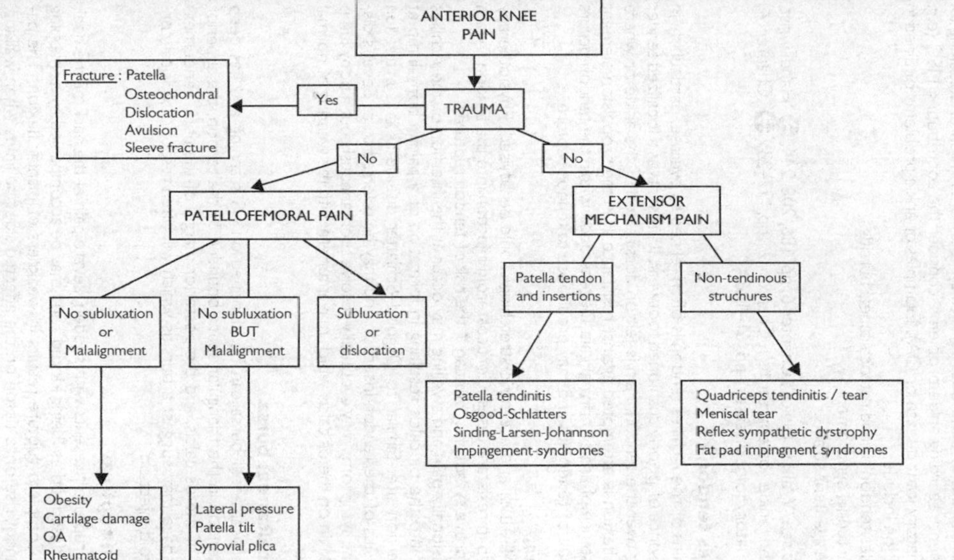

Fig. 6.5 Anterior knee pain algorithm.

Reproduced from Patellofemoral/extensor mechanisms disorders (Figure 37.1) M. Hutson and A. Ward, (2016) *Oxford Textbook of Musculoskeletal Medicine*, with permission from Oxford University Press.

Ankle problems

Ankle and foot problems often occur in conjunction with knee, hip, and back pain, and may contribute to such symptoms; ∴ when undertaking an assessment regarding ankle problems, consider the contributing MSC (e.g. inflammatory joint disease or OA). Examples of ankle problems outlined in this section include:

- Achilles tendonitis and retrocalcaneal bursitis.
- Tarsal tunnel syndrome.
- Ankle ligament strains.

➲ Also see 'Walk-in clinics', Chapter 6, pp. 186, 208, 244; ➲ 'Hand, wrist, foot, and ankle osteoarthritis', Chapter 2, pp. 22–23; ➲ Chapter 4, 'Inflammatory joint diseases', pp. 61–126.

Achilles tendonitis

Tendonitis of the Achilles tendon is often related to overuse, particularly in the presence of poorly cushioned footwear. It presents as a localized tender swelling over the tendon. Pain is felt on dorsiflexion of the ankle or where plantar flexion is attempted against resistance as in the propulsion element of the stance phase of normal gait. Degeneration within the tendon occurs as a result of tendonitis and may predispose to tendon rupture.

Treatment

RICE, NSAIDs, and eccentric stretching should be advised. Physiotherapy may help in resistant cases. Corticosteroid injection into the tendon sheath may improve symptoms, but can ↑ the risk of tendon rupture.

Occasionally pain and swelling may occur at the insertion of the Achilles tendon into the os calcis resulting in formation of a painful bony lump at the insertion site. Similar to Osgood–Schlatter disease as it is a traction apophysitis of the tendon insertion and may be referred to as Sever's disease. The symptoms may eventually resolve spontaneously but a bony lump may remain on the os calcis which may interfere with the wearing of normal footwear.

Retrocalcaneal bursa

The retrocalcaneal bursa can be identified on US scanning and lies deep to the tendon in the triangular space bounded by the tendon, the superior surface of the os calcis, and the posterior margin of the tibia. Tenderness in this space may suggest a bursitis which will often respond to local corticosteroid injection.

Tendon rupture

Tendon rupture presents with sudden, severe pain at the back of the heel, may be described as 'being kicked', and may be accompanied by a snapping sound. Complete rupture results in weakness of plantar flexion. The patient cannot rise onto tiptoe on the affected side and limps when walking. A palpable gap is often present in the tendon. With the patient lying prone on a couch, squeezing the calf muscles will cause a degree of plantar flexion at the foot if the tendon is intact, but no movement will be seen in the foot if the tendon is ruptured.

Treatment

Surgical repair or immobilizing the foot in partial plantar flexion in a cast.

Partial rupture

In some circumstances, the tendon may remain intact but may have a partial tear of the gastrocnemius muscle. This may present in a similar way to tendon rupture but the area of tenderness is more proximal, at the musculotendinous junction or in the belly of the muscle. Bruising may be apparent at the site of the rupture and may track distally under gravity to appear as bruising around the ankle joint.

Treatment

Acute treatment is with RICE. Physiotherapy should be started promptly after these measures to reduce the rare but present risk of myositis ossificans (calcification occurring within the damaged muscle).

Tarsal tunnel syndrome

This condition is similar to the more frequently diagnosed CTS in the wrist. It is an entrapment of the posterior tibial nerve as it passes deep to the flexor retinaculum on the medial aspect of the ankle, behind the medial malleolus. Symptoms are of numbness and burning pain in the sole of the foot, often made worse by standing, and eased by rest and massage. Tinel's test may be positive over the posterior tibial nerve. It may occur as a complication of ankle injury, sprain, or fracture, or in association with inflammatory arthritis or OA at the ankle.

Treatment

Orthotics and local corticosteroid injection frequently provide benefit.

Further reading

Reid H, Wood S (2015). Achilles tendinopathy: advice and management information for patients. Oxford University Hospitals NHS Foundation Trust. https://www.ouh.nhs.uk/patient-guide/leaflets/files/11924Ptendinopathy.pdf

Foot problems

Ankle and foot problems often occur in conjunction with knee, hip, and back pain, and may contribute to such symptoms. OA will often affect the first MTP joint, as will gout. Plantar fasciitis and Achilles tendonitis may occur as part of a seronegative spondyloarthritis or psoriatic arthropathy. Foot problems include:

- Plantar fasciitis.
- Pes planus (flat feet, fallen arches) pes cavus.
- Metatarsalgia.
- Morton's neuroma.
- Hallux valgus and hallux rigidus.

Plantar fasciitis

This is a common cause of heel pain. The pain is often worse first thing in the morning with the first few steps after getting out of bed.

Treatment should be conservative and involves addressing biomechanical factors such as excessive weight, and correction of ankle and midfoot pronation with arch supports. Well-cushioned footwear should be encouraged, with a low heel and broad forefoot, and secure means of fastening such as laces or hook-and-loop fastener straps (trainers are often ideal). Referral to podiatry may assist in obtaining the best footwear advice. Exercises to stretch the Achilles tendon and the plantar fascia are encouraged. Local corticosteroid injection into the heel can be considered if conservative measures fail, but it is a painful procedure, and carries a risk of atrophy of the heel fat pad.

Pes planus and pes cavus

Flat feet ('pes planus') and high-arch feet ('pes cavus') are normal variants and do not require intervention if they do not cause pain. Flat footedness is normal in children. The arch should be restored when the patient is asked to stand on tiptoe. Treatment is usually with arch supports and exercises to try to encourage strengthening of the intrinsic muscles of the foot, such as picking up a pencil off the floor with the toes.

Pes cavus (high arch) may arise as a complication of neurological conditions such as polio or spina bifida, but is often idiopathic. It is rarely of significant importance but may lead to clawing of the toes and premature OA of the metatarsal heads or the mid-tarsal joint. It can be difficult to obtain appropriate accommodating footwear—podiatry assessment may be helpful in this regard and may be able to slow progression of clawing metatarsal subluxation. Occasionally, orthopaedic intervention may be required to straighten clawing of the toes.

Metatarsalgia

The term metatarsalgia is not a diagnosis but simply descriptive of forefoot pain. It is commonly due to abnormal pressure on the metatarsal heads when weight bearing. Strain of the intrinsic muscles may contribute to pain, as may inflammation of interdigital bursae. This may be 2° to a number of other conditions including pes cavus, rheumatoid foot deformities, and

OA. Management is with the use of orthotics to offload the forefoot. Occasionally, surgical correction of established foot deformities may be useful.

Morton's neuroma

This is caused by entrapment of the interdigital nerve usually between the third and fourth metatarsal heads. This causes attacks of pain and paraesthesia while walking. On examination, the symptoms may be reproduced by 'metatarsal squeeze' and there is often an exquisitely tender area between the third and fourth metatarsals. Treatment is with insoles. Local corticosteroid injection around the neuroma is sometimes helpful. Rarely surgical excision may be considered but is not always curative.

There are other conditions related to OA such as hallux valgus and hallux rigidus.

➔ Also see 'Osteoarthritis', Chapter 2, pp. 12 and 22.

Primary care: common musculoskeletal problems

Musculoskeletal episodic history taking

Musculoskeletal problems are frequently seen in walk-in 1° healthcare settings. Those presenting with musculoskeletal problems can typically be placed into two diagnostic categories:

- Acute minor injuries.
- Acute inflammatory problems including 'overuse' conditions.

A fundamental activity for nurses assessing patients with musculoskeletal problems in 1° healthcare settings is to determine the exact nature of a patient's presenting problem(s) and to elicit a detailed history, together with identification of the areas affected. It may not be clear from a patient's opening statement if they have:

- Sustained an injury.
- Have an inflammatory overuse problem or symptoms relate to an exacerbation of a long-term MSC.

Further diagnostic musculoskeletal questions should include:

- The nature of the pain—exacerbating or relieving factors (e.g. does the pain ↑ on movement or not?).
- History of previous musculoskeletal problems of the affected area.
- The patient's use of any over-the-counter or prescription-only oral or topical analgesia and its perceived effect on their presenting problem.
- Any associated neurological symptoms, such as muscle weakness and paraesthesia in the both the affected joint and the area distal to the site of inflammation or injury.

All of the above history enquiries should be considered in conjunction with background history questions such as past medical history, drug history, allergies, social history, and, where relevant, family history.

The nurse should then identify:

Has the patient sustained an injury?

Ask the patient to specify exactly where the affected area is and if they can recall any recent history of trauma or do they have any underlying conditions?

- Patients presenting with acute musculoskeletal pain may often say that they have a history of trauma, as they attribute pain to injury even when there is no clear history of trauma. If injury is reported, ascertain the exact mechanism of injury and length of time since the reported injury.
- If a patient reports a history of trauma, the exact mechanism of injury should be ascertained together with the time that has elapsed since the reported injury.
- Determine if they have been able to carry on activities immediately post injury; e.g. was the patient able to weight bear on the injured side, and have they been able to continue to do so?

Do they have an inflammatory overuse problem?

If on direct questioning the patient reports a history of musculoskeletal-type pain with no actual history of trauma, it is important to establish the cause. It is likely that this is an acute inflammatory condition which has occurred as a result of overuse—consider whether there is evidence to suggest ↑ exercise patterns or repetitive exercise movements.

Take into account the potential impact on function, e.g. hand dominance in upper limb and hand problems may affect:

- Work or personal ADLs or
- Impair leisure and sporting pursuits.

Features attributed to a LTC?

Patients may not naturally attribute the presenting problems to their condition, e.g. a recently diagnosed patient with RA may fail to realize that a hot, swollen ankle is related to their RA if their clinical features of RA to date have only affected their hands.

- Ask about other medical conditions—they may require specialist advice on musculoskeletal-related complications.
- Explore any acquiescent problems that may relate to the current condition, e.g. a prior history of gout or pseudogout.
- Ask about associated symptoms, e.g. patients with RA pain typically also present with additional symptoms such as joint stiffness or persistent tiredness.
- Review any patient-held records or blood monitoring cards.
- If a LTC can be excluded from diagnosis, continue with diagnostic assessment for either a musculoskeletal injury or musculoskeletal acute inflammation.

Primary care: musculoskeletal physical assessment

A clear, accurate history and a thorough physical examination will determine the nature of the patient's presenting problem. The examination sequence outlined should be used particularly for those with limited experience in musculoskeletal examination.

Specific tests

These are confined to those that have practical application and can be relatively easily interpreted in a non-specialist setting.

General inspection

Begins as soon as you meet and greet the patient, before they realize that they are being clinically observed, e.g.:

- How does the patient get up from their chair? Do they need help?
- What is their gait like?
- Do they appear in any distress? Immediate distress *may* give an indication of the severity of the presenting problem.
- Can they weight bear unaided? If there is lower limb musculoskeletal pain patients may report an inability to weight bear but unobtrusive inspection may reveal reported 'unable to weight bear' as meaning 'unable to weight bear without pain'.

► A key observation: in patients with a clear history of a recent leg/ankle/foot injury, an observed inability to actually weight bear indicates a high index of suspicion for a possible bony injury.

Specific inspection

Specific inspection of the musculoskeletal dysfunction (e.g. painful joint or restricted movement) should always include comparisons with the unaffected side.

Ensure adequate exposure of the affected area and comparative sites, e.g.:

- The shoulder—the patient should remove their upper body clothing to underwear.
- The knee—the patient should remove their trousers/skirt to underwear.

Observe the affected area for:

- Skin redness/swelling/lumps/previous surgical/wound scars.
- Muscle wasting/ anatomical deformity/overlying skin lesions/rashes (e.g. a dermatome distribution of vesicles would indicate herpes zoster as the cause of pain).
- The integrity of the skin and any associated wounds post trauma.
- Compare of observations with the unaffected side.

Palpation

Palpation of the affected area include examining any areas for tenderness, overlying skin temperature—e.g. hot to touch, unusual lumps or swelling, loss of muscle bulk, and any bone or tendon crepitus (a palpable vibration).

In a person presenting with a musculoskeletal injury, a key concept to understand and detect in palpation is the difference between bony/point tenderness and diffuse tenderness (Box 6.4).

Box 6.4 Discriminating bony/point versus diffuse tenderness

- Bony tenderness refers to an exquisite, sharp pain elicited on palpating on an area of bony injury. Point tenderness refers to a similar pain, but one occurring only in a discreet part of the affected area.
- In contrast, diffuse tenderness refers to a generalized tenderness of the affected area on palpation, without the exquisite pain seen in bony/point tenderness.

After a musculoskeletal injury the presence of bony/point tenderness may indicate a possible bone fracture requiring X-ray investigation, while diffuse tenderness typically indicates soft tissue inflammation such as a ligament sprain or muscle strain.

Movement

Include range of active movement (ROAM) of the affected joint compared against the unaffected side. Examine to assess:

- Is the ROAM normal (e.g. smooth, pain-free, and equal on both sides)?
- Observe for the perceived degree of pain occurring on joint movement.
- Note anatomical location of any pain on movement, and any restriction of movement in comparison with the unaffected side.
- If discrepancies identified in active movement between the affected and unaffected sides, check passive movements of the affected side to identify any loss of function and compare with the normal ROAM.
- Resistance movements may also be checked to assess the quality and strength of muscles between the affected and unaffected sides and any signs of weakness.

Remember that:

- A definitive diagnosis does not need to be established at an initial consultation; instead aim for a more general impression of the problem.
- Focus on an assessment of the severity of the patient's problem, and consider the practical implications of what you can do with the patient in your consulting room, such as:
  - Can they be discharged from the clinic or is there is a clinical indication for onward referral, such as a possible fracture?
  - Remember, vital signs may be required in some instances to help exclude other presenting problems—e.g. temperature recording in patients with neck pain to exclude an infective illness as the cause of the neck pain.

Key features of 1° healthcare musculoskeletal physical assessment:

- Inspection of the patient and the affected area(s).
- Compare against the unaffected limb/joint.
- Absence/presence of warmth, tenderness, or swelling in the joint.
- Palpation of the affected area(s).
- Check range of movement of the affected area, including active, passive, and resistance movements as required.
- Selected special tests of affected joints to assess musculoskeletal function.

Primary care: assessment of neck problems

Introduction

Neck pain is a common non-specific symptom which can be attributed to a wide range of possible differential diagnoses, many of which are not musculoskeletal. The patient may have difficulty in specifically locating neck pain and hence may report that they have neck pain when in fact they have shoulder pain and vice versa; the exact location of the pain can be verified on examination.

Neck history

Neck pain history should include questions that exclude other conditions that require immediate assessment in the emergency department (ED), e.g.:

- Has there been any recent history of neck or head trauma?
- Do they have any symptoms suggestive of meningitis, e.g. neck stiffness and/or photophobia?
- Do they have any cardiac symptoms, e.g. chest pain?

More general questions to explore the nature of the problem include:

- How does the person feel otherwise?
- Have they had any recent viral illness-type symptoms?
- Do they have any ear, nose, and throat (ENT) symptoms?
- Have they had a recent fever?
- Do they have a headache?
- Do they have any persisting neck stiffness in association with the previously listed symptoms?

Neck injury: in patients with any history of significant neck trauma or associated cervical spine tenderness (on palpation), the neck should be immobilized with a stiff neck collar (if available) and the patient transferred by ambulance to the ED to exclude a possible cervical spine fracture.

Neck examination

- Inspection:
  - Ensure adequate exposure of the neck and upper back.
  - The head should be held erect and the neck straight.
  - Inspect the neck from all aspects—anterior, posterior, and lateral.
  - Note any obvious swellings, surgical scars, skin lesions, or rashes.
  - Ask the patient to indicate the area of pain.
- Palpation:
  - Palpate individual spinous processes of the cervical spine to the bony prominence of the C7/T1 junction.
  - Palpate paravertebral muscles on both sides, and trapezius, and sternomastoid muscles, noting any areas of tenderness, muscle spasm, asymmetry, or swelling.
- Movement:
  - Observe ROAM of cervical spine.
  - Flexion—bending forward.
  - Extension—bending backwards.

- Lateral bending/flexion—bending to each side.
- Rotation—looking over each shoulder.
- Also check resistance movement strength controlled by cranial nerve XI—spinal accessory.
- Turning face against resistance—sternomastoid.
- Shrug against resistance—trapezius.

- Neurological:
  - Check upper limb muscle strengths.
  - Test arm reflexes—triceps, biceps, and supinator.
  - Check the integrity of the distal sensations.

Presenting problems of neck pain

Torticollis

This is a common neck problem. Typically:

- The patient wakes with a stiff, painful neck, due to spasm on one side of the neck of the trapezius or sternomastoid muscles.
- May be precipitated by poor body posture or carrying heavy loads on one side of the body.
- Examination reveals the neck held in either right or left lateral flexion, diffuse tenderness and muscle spasm on the affected side, and painful restricted neck movements.
- Neurological examination is typically normal.

Treatment

Simple analgesia (paracetamol or ibuprofen if not contraindicated) and temporary rest from strenuous activities affecting the neck. There is a lack of evidence for the routine use of diazepam for torticollis. Encourage maintenance of normal everyday activities. Acute torticollis usually resolves within 24–48 hours, but symptoms may take up to a week to resolve. Persistent or recurrent episodes of torticollis may benefit from a referral to a PT assessment and treatment.

Whiplash neck injury

The common presentation typically follows a road traffic collision where:

- Sudden hyperextension of the neck muscles and ligaments has occurred.
- Within 1–2 days of an accident the patient complains of neck pain, muscle stiffness, and tenderness.
- Examination of the neck should include the neurological issues as outlined earlier for torticollis or factors that might indicate a need for radiological assessment in the ED.

Where there is no cervical spine bony tenderness or associated neurological impairment, treatment should be as for torticollis plus referral for PT assessment (dependent on local referral guidelines).

➲ Also see 'Neck and spine', pp. 222 and 224; ➲ Chapter 8, 'Assessing the patient', pp. 290–291; ➲ Chapter 9, 'Symptom control: using pharmacological and non-pharmacological methods', pp. 308–328.

Further reading

NICE Clinical Knowledge Summaries (2018). Neck pain—acute torticollis. https://cks.nice.org.uk/neck-pain-acute-torticollis

Primary care: assessment of common presenting problems—the back

Back problems

Back pain is a common presenting problem in 1° healthcare, both as an acute and a long-term problem. Acute low back pain is often due to:
- Indirect trauma, such as lifting heavy loads.
- Awkward body movements.
- Exercise activities.

In cases of potential direct trauma to the back, such as falls or blows to the body, any vertebral bony tenderness necessitates referral to the Emergency Department.

In cases of thoracic back pain, remember that this may be posterior chest pain and not back pain. Potential organ involvement presenting with posterior chest pain include cardiac, pulmonary, or respiratory conditions and must be excluded before focusing the assessment on musculoskeletal back pain. Consider contributing factors that may exacerbate or predicate/prolong back symptoms such as anxiety and depression; these psychological factors should be considered in assessment of patients with back pain.

Back history

Start the clinical questioning and history taking to exclude other causes of back pain such as:
- Genitourinary, abdominal, or chest pathology.
- In patients aged >55 years consider an abdominal aortic aneurysm as a possible cause of back pain; typically this pain is constant and unaffected by movement. A suspected aneurysm requires immediate assessment in the ED.
- Unintended weight loss in patients with back pain of a duration >4 weeks may indicate an underlying oncological cause.
- Sharp nerve-like pains radiating from the lower back down one or both legs as this may indicate nerve root pain or sciatic nerve irritation.

! Spinal cord compression: this is a red flag not to be missed in patients with back pain accompanied by one or more of the following symptoms:
- Disturbance or loss of urinary or stool continence.
- Perineal numbness (saddle anaesthesia).
- Lower limb weakness and/or numbness.

Differential diagnoses should consider those with solid cancer tumours or metastatic spread to the bones—a frequent cause of cord compression.

► Consider the high risks related to cancer history + back pain.

►► Back pain + symptoms of cord compression = immediate referral to orthopaedics/neurosurgery or oncology as indicated by their history.

Back examination

- Inspection (➔ see Fig. 6.6, p. 225):
  - Observe the patient's gait.
  - Ensure adequate exposure—view back from all aspects.
  - Look for rashes, lesions, curvature, deformity, and asymmetry.
  - Observe the spine bending forward, normal observation is a 'c'-shaped spinal curvature.

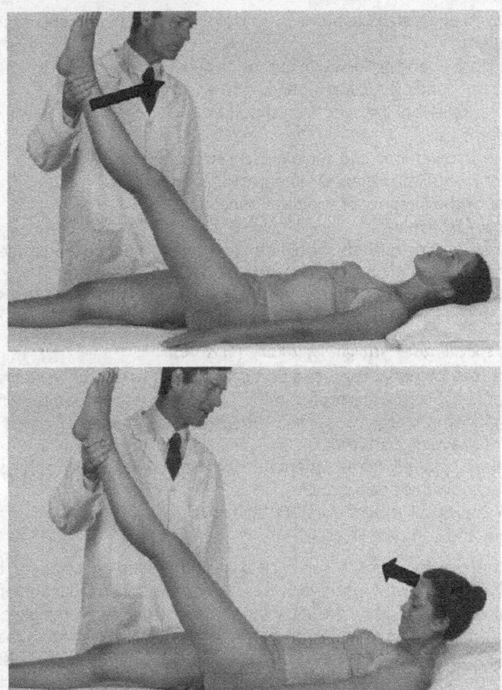

Fig. 6.6 Back examination.

- Observe iliac crest height, asymmetry may indicate pelvic tilt or unequal leg lengths.
- Note any obvious swellings, surgical scars, skin lesions, or rashes.
- Ask the patient to indicate the area of pain.

- Palpation:
  - Palpate spinous processes from T1 to S2 and paravertebral muscles on each side.
  - Note areas and levels of tenderness.
  - Check for kidney/costovertebral angle tenderness on indirect percussion to exclude renal parenchyma inflammation.
- Movement:
  - Observe ROAM of back.

- May need to stabilize pelvis by grasping the hips from behind the patient.
- Flexion—bending forward; extension—bending backwards.
- Lateral bending/flexion—bending to each side.
- Rotation—looking over each shoulder.

- Neurological:
  - Check lower limb and ankle muscle strengths.
  - Test lower limb reflexes—knee, ankle, and plantar.
  - Check the integrity of the distal sensations.
- Clinic investigations:
  - Dipstick urine analysis should be considered in order to exclude genitourinary problems as a cause of back pain.
  - Back X-rays, while often requested by patients with back pain, are unnecessary in the majority of patients.

► *Back special test—straight leg raising (SLR) test*

This is a test for nerve root irritation caused by a herniated vertebral disc. This test is especially important in low back pain with accompanying pain radiating down the leg.

- Patient in supine position.
- Examiner *passively* raises patient's straight leg up in the air to the point at which low back pain occurs.
- With the leg still raised, dorsiflex the foot.
- Repeat and compare sides.

► It is normal for slight lower back pain and stretching of hamstrings to occur during this test. A positive SLR test occurs with reproduction of sharp back pain extending down the leg. With the affected leg lowered beyond the point of pain, passive dorsiflexion of the foot normally reinforces the pain.

➔ Also see 'Neck and spine', pp. 222–224; ➔ Chapter 8, 'Assessing the patient', pp. 290–291; ➔ Chapter 9, 'Symptom control: using pharmacological and non-pharmacological methods', pp. 307–328.

Primary care: assessment of common presenting problems—treatment plans for the back

Back pain presenting problems

Low back pain (simple backache)

This the most common cause of lumbar back pain. The patient presents with a history of low back pain, sometimes associated with heavy lifting or exercise, which worsens on movement.

Examination reveals:

On palpation: localized lumbar spine tenderness with painful, restricted back movements. Neurological examination is typically normal.

Treatment plan

Low back pain can normally be adequately treated with information, reassurance, simple analgesia (NSAIDs, such as ibuprofen or naproxen first line may be considered if not contraindicated), and temporary abstinence from strenuous activities affecting the back, while attempting to maintain normal everyday activities. If the person has muscle spasm, consider offering a short course of a benzodiazepine, such as diazepam (2 mg up to three times a day for up to 5 days, if not contraindicated). If persistent or recurrent episodes of simple low back pain, consider referral for PT assessment and treatment.

Back pain with associated nerve root pain

This commonly presents as 'sciatica' where the patient complains of a sharp pain radiating from the low back or buttock and down the posterior aspect of the leg of the affected side (often sharp leg pain is perceived as more severe than the accompanying back pain).

Examination reveals: commonly the same as for low back pain + SLR test may reproduce the sharp leg pain.

Treatment plan: as for low back pain + urgent referral to PT (dependent on local referral guidelines).

► If lower limb neurological examination reveals accompanying paraesthesia, and/or muscle weakness, or altered reflexes on the affected side, further assessment in the ED should be considered.

➲ Also see 'Neck and spine', pp. 222 and 224; ➲ Chapter 8, 'Assessing the patient', pp. 290–291; ➲ Chapter 9, 'Symptom control: using pharmacological and non-pharmacological methods', pp. 307–328.

Further reading

Clunie G, Wilkinson, N, Nikiphorou, E, Jadon, D (eds) (2018). *Oxford Handbook of Rheumatology*, 4th edn. Oxford: Oxford University Press.

NICE Clinical Knowledge Summaries (2018). Back pain—low (without radiculopathy). https://cks.nice.org.uk/back-pain-low-without-radiculopathy

Primary care: first steps in the assessment of shoulder problems

Shoulder problems

Shoulder pain can provoke severe pain, in many cases with limitations in ADLs leading to heightened patient anxiety. Shoulder pain may be as a result of other non-musculoskeletal presentations (Box 6.5). The shoulder joint has a wide range of movement at the expense of relative stability, as can be seen in the shallow articulation of the humeral head in the glenoid cavity. The complex nature of the shoulder joint anatomy is dependent upon the integrity and stability of the joint including tendons and muscles of the surrounding rotator cuff (supraspinatus, infraspinatus, teres minor, and subscapularis); hence many shoulder problems seen in 1° healthcare are related to rotator cuff pathology.

Another area at the shoulder tip of frequent shoulder complaints is at the region of the subacromion. If there is inflammation, injury, or swelling rapidly at this site it rapidly presents problems due the anatomical design of the joint and limited subacromial space.

Shoulder history

A precise history should include potential causes of the pain and any limitations to the patient's current activities. They may be unable to differentiate between shoulder pain and neck pain and vice versa; the exact location of the pain can be verified on examination.

Shoulder examination

- Inspection:
  - Both shoulders and the upper chest should be exposed.
  - Inspect neck and compare both shoulders.
  - Ask patient to point to the area of pain.
  - Observe the shoulders for shape, symmetry, swelling, deformity, angulations (commonly occurs with shoulder dislocation), skin redness, muscle wasting, scars, and any skin lesions such as vesicles (occur in herpes zoster).
- Palpation: the surface anatomy of the shoulder can be used to provide a systematic approach to shoulder palpation. Carefully palpate the following bony anatomical areas:
  - Cervical spine—if indicated by the history.
  - Suprasternal notch.
  - Sternoclavicular joint/clavicle.
  - Coracoid process.
  - Acromion/ACJ.
  - Tuberosities of humerus/humerus.
  - Bicipital groove.
  - Scapula.

This bony palpation should then be followed by palpation of the following muscular areas:

- Sternomastoid (neck) and trapezius (neck).
- Pectoralis major (anterior chest).

Box 6.5 Examples of non-musculoskeletal shoulder pain

Include: ischaemia, pulmonary, and abdominal or pelvic pathologies (e.g. cardiac pain, gallbladder diseases, pulmonary embolism, and ectopic pregnancy).

Assess and exclude/refer following careful problem-focused history taking in patients presenting with non-traumatic shoulder pain.

- Biceps (anterior humerus) and deltoid (lateral humerus).
- Triceps (posterior humerus).
- Coracobrachialis (axilla/medial humerus).
- Latissimus dorsi (posterior chest).
- *Rotator cuff muscles*: supraspinatus, infraspinatus, teres minor, and subscapularis.

Examination must also include assessment of the distal neurological status of the arms and hands. This is achieved by checking the integrity of the axillary nerve at the lateral mid humerus (badge sign) and the ulnar, median, and radial nerves in their distal distribution of the hand.

- Movement: check neck movements first (if indicated from the history), followed by these active shoulder movements:
  - Flexion (forward movement) and extension (backward movement).
  - Abduction (away from midline) and lateral (external) rotation (arm tucked into chest with elbow flexed, rotating movement away from midline).
  - Medial (internal) rotation (arm tucked into chest with elbow flexed, rotating movement towards midline).
- The following compound shoulder movements can also be checked:
  - Hand touched to back of head (external rotation with abduction).
  - Hand touched to middle of back (internal rotation with adduction).

These first steps can be supported by some simple performed tests for the non-specialist (➲ see 'Primary care: specific tests for shoulder problems', pp. 230–231).

➲ Also see ➲ Chapter 6, 'Chronic non-inflammatory pain', pp. 185–187 ➲ Chapter 8, 'Assessing the patient', pp. 289–306; ➲ Chapter 9, 'Symptom control: using pharmacological and non-pharmacological methods', pp. 307–328.

Further reading

Clunie G, Wilkinson, N, Nikiphorou, E, Jadon, D (eds) (2018). *Oxford Handbook of Rheumatology*, 4th edn. Oxford: Oxford University Press.

Primary care: specific tests for shoulder problems

There are a wide range of tests for shoulder function and associated anatomical structures. In many cases these tests are for the specialist assessment of shoulder problems. The following tests are simple to perform and interpret, and are usually sufficient to assess shoulder function and the associated anatomical structures. Referral may be necessary for more complex shoulder problems.

- *Anterior and posterior drawer test.* Stabilize shoulder from behind, applying a downward pressure, and then move glenohumeral joint backwards and forwards to assess anterior or posterior instability. Compare with unaffected side looking for joint laxity in comparison with unaffected side, which would indicate anterior or posterior instability.
- *Sulcus sign.* Stabilize shoulder from the front and pull down on the patient's arm to assess inferior instability. Compare with the unaffected side, looking for a dip (sulcus) appearing below the lateral acromion, which would indicate inferior instability.
- *Active abduction test (painful arc).* Ask the patient to abduct their shoulder. Pain occurring between 70 and 140° may indicate a subacromial space problem. Pain occurring between 140 and 180° may indicate an ACJ problem (Fig. 6.7).

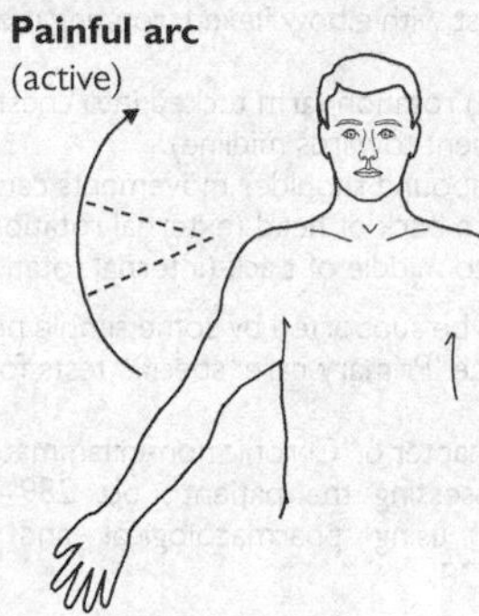
Painful arc
(active)
Action: Patient standing.
Slow arm abduction
(scapular plane).
Positive test: Pain onset (maximal)
at (variable) angular
range.

Fig. 6.7 Painful arc.

Reproduced from Hakim A, Clunie G, Haq I (eds) (2006). *Oxford Handbook of Rheumatology*, 2nd edn. Oxford University Press, Oxford with permission from Oxford University Press.

- *Passive abduction test.* Passively abduct the patient's shoulder. Pain occurring around the acromion may indicate subacromial bursitis.
- *Resisted abduction test.* Ask the patient to abduct their arm while you apply an opposing force. Compare with unaffected side. Pain occurring in the superior aspect of the shoulder may indicate supraspinatus tendinitis. Weakness on resistance may indicate a possible rotator cuff tear (supraspinatus).
- *Resisted lateral rotation test.* Ask patient to flex their elbow and press their upper arm into their lateral chest wall, and to move their forearm laterally. Apply an opposing medial force. Pain in the posterior aspect of the shoulder may indicate infraspinatus or teres minor tendinitis. Weakness on resistance may indicate a possible rotator cuff tear (infraspinatus or teres minor).
- *Resisted medial rotation test.* Ask patient to flex their elbow and press their upper arm into their lateral chest wall, and to move their forearm medially. Apply an opposing lateral force. Compare with the unaffected side. Pain in the anterior aspect of the shoulder may indicate subscapularis tendinitis. Weakness on resistance may indicate a possible rotator cuff tear (subscapularis).
- ➲ Also see 'Chronic non-inflammatory pain', pp. 185–189.

Further reading

Clunie G, Wilkinson, N, Nikiphorou, E, Jadon, D (eds) (2018). *Oxford Handbook of Rheumatology*, 4th edn. Oxford: Oxford University Press.

Primary care: shoulder pain

The most common shoulder problems presenting in 1° care are outlined in this section.

The comprehensive assessment of shoulder problems

- *Supraspinatus tendonitis*: a common problem related to overuse, particularly overarm movements (e.g. tasks undertaken by a painter/decorator). Examination reveals localized tenderness over superior aspect of shoulder, painful active abduction 70–140° and painful resisted abduction. Usually resolves after a few days; supportive measures include simple analgesia (NSAIDs if not contraindicated), and temporary rest from the strenuous activity affecting the shoulder.
- *Subacromial bursitis*: history as for supraspinatus, but no pain on resisted abduction, as no muscle or tendon involvement; instead, pain occurs on passive abduction as the subacromial space becomes compressed. Tenderness and a soft swelling may be noted at the humeral head. May be related to an inflammatory component (e.g. RA). Supportive measures include simple analgesia (NSAIDs if not contraindicated) and temporary rest from the strenuous activity affecting the shoulder. Some patients with a persisting inflammatory component may benefit from IA corticosteroid injection if not contraindicated.
- *Biceps tendonitis*: often caused by repeated lifting movements, presents with anterior humeral and shoulder pain, tenderness over biceps tendon, and resisted elbow flexion is painful. Rupture of the long head of the biceps may also occur, and presents with pain on lifting and sensation of 'something going' accompanied by palpable lump within the tendon. *Treatment*: temporary rest from lifting and simple analgesia (NSAIDs if not contraindicated).
- *Rotator cuff tear (non-traumatic)*: this may be due to fibrosis, tendonitis, or bone spurs. Often the patient is >50 years old, presenting with pain and weakness on abduction, may not be able to actively abduct or hold abduction at 90°. Orthopaedic assessment required.
- *Joint instability*: in patients <40 years of age glenohumeral instability may be seen with a history of recurrent subluxations or dislocations. Older patients (>40 years) may have feelings of shoulder joint instability, accompanied by shoulder pains and clicks; this is often related to long-term rotator cuff problems. Orthopaedic assessment required.
- *Frozen shoulder (adhesive capsulitis)*: this long-term condition is more common in ♀, diabetics, and people aged 40–60 years old. Presents with shoulder pain (occasionally debilitating) and limitation in movement, accompanied by diffuse joint tenderness. Compound external/internal rotation movements are painful and restricted which causes difficulty with everyday activities such as dressing and grooming. Initial treatment includes simple analgesia (NSAIDs if not contraindicated), physiotherapy, and sometimes local steroid injection. The natural course of the condition is usually about 18 months when it usually resolves spontaneously.

Shoulder injury presenting problems

- *ACJ injury*: fall onto shoulder, elbow, outstretched hand, or a blow to the shoulder tip may cause ACJ injury, ranging from a sprain of the ACJ ligament to disruption of the joint. The patient presents with superior shoulder pain and painful ↓ shoulder movements, particularly noted on abduction. A bulge or step may be noted in the ACJ articulation. Refer to the Emergency Department or Minor Injures Unit for X-ray and further management.
- *Rotator cuff tear*: severe blow or fall on outstretched hand, tenderness may be noted around the acromion, active and resistance abduction will be reduced or absent. A complete rotator cuff tear may not be painful, though a lack of active shoulder movement will be evident. Orthopaedic assessment needed.
- *Traumatic effusion*: typically occurs in patients >50 years old, falling onto the arm/shoulder, which leads to bleeding/effusion in the glenohumeral joint. This is often a delayed presentation with pain and restricted shoulder movement affecting everyday activities such as dressing. Proximal humeral tenderness is noted on palpation due to accompanying humeral fracture. Refer to the ED or Minor Injuries Unit for X-ray and further management.
- *Shoulder dislocation*: this is a relatively common shoulder injury, which normally occurs after falling on the arm or shoulder, or if the arm is pulled sharply. Anterior dislocation of the humeral head is more common than posterior dislocation. The patient appears in discomfort, clasping the affected arm against the body, with a flattening of the anterior outer edge of the shoulder evident. Make the patient comfortable and arrange for immediate transfer to the ED for X-ray and reduction of the dislocation.
- *Clavicular fracture*: this typically occurs after a fall on the outstretched hand. The patient complains of pain and swelling of the injured clavicle, and examination reveals a bony step in the fractured clavicle with associated tenderness and sometimes bony crepitus. X-ray in the ED or Minor Injuries Unit is required to confirm the clinical diagnosis and for fracture clinic review. Most fractures of the clavicle can be successfully managed with a broad arm sling and simple analgesia.

Note: LTCs such as IJDs may present with shoulder problems such as subacromial bursitis as a result of juvenile arthritis, gout or pseudo-gout, RA, PsA, and AS.

➲ Also see 'Chronic non-inflammatory pain', pp. 186–187.

Further reading

Clunie G, Wilkinson, N, Nikiphorou, E, Jadon, D (eds) (2018). *Oxford Handbook of Rheumatology*, 4th edn. Oxford: Oxford University Press.

NICE Clinical Knowledge Summaries (2017). Shoulder pain. https://cks.nice.org.uk/shoulder-pain

Primary care: musculoskeletal chest pain

Common causes of musculoskeletal chest wall pain are intercostal muscle sprain caused by minor chest wall trauma; intercostal muscle inflammation caused by repeated coughing; and pain at the sternal junctions caused by inflammation of the costal cartilages.

Chest history

Patients with musculoskeletal chest wall pain typically complain of an intermittent sharp pain which worsens on coughing or sneezing, inspiration, and movement. It is important to ask about the use of simple analgesia as many will have taken minimal analgesia believing such treatment will produce little benefit and are anxious that the pain is cardiac in nature even when they are young and have no risk factors for cardiac chest pain. Careful reassurance, once cardiac problems have been excluded, will help alleviate this anxiety.

Chest pain of musculoskeletal origin should only be considered as a differential diagnosis when other, more serious causes of chest pain have been excluded, such as cardiac and respiratory or pulmonary problems, with careful problem-focused history taking, including potential red flags, such as cardiac-type pain, haemoptysis, dyspnoea, and fever.

In patients presenting shortly after a potentially significant history of chest trauma, the risk of associated hepatic and splenic trauma should be considered.

Chest examination

- Inspection:
  - Ask the patient to indicate the area of their perceived pain.
  - Note shape of chest and tracheal alignment in the midline.
  - Observe for any deformities or asymmetry of the chest wall.
  - Respiratory pattern—rate, rhythm, depth, and effort.
  - Use of neck and chest accessory muscles or intercostal muscle space retraction.
  - Impaired or unequal respiratory movements.
  - Bruising or other traumatic marks on the chest wall.
  - A dermatome distribution of vesicles would indicate herpes zoster as the cause of the chest wall pain.
- Palpation:
  - Palpate ribs, sternal junctions, and intercostal spaces.
  - Palpate anterior and posterior in turn—remember lateral chest walls.
  - Identify areas of tenderness, particularly noting any areas of bony tenderness or bone crepitus, which could indicate a potential rib fracture.
  - The sternum can be compressed with one hand on the sternum and the other on the spine; in cases of musculoskeletal chest wall pain, particularly rib fractures, a sharp pain will noted at the point of inflammation or injury.

► *Respiratory and cardiac examination*

- In patients presenting with musculoskeletal chest wall pain, vital signs (blood pressure, pulse, respiratory rate, temperature, oxygen saturations) should always be recorded and interpreted.
- A chest respiratory examination should be undertaken to exclude respiratory pathology, such as a pleural rub or a respiratory tract infection.
- The precordium should be auscultated to exclude abnormal heart sounds such as a pericardial friction rub.
- *Abdominal examination* should also be considered in patients presenting with chest injuries, in order to exclude any associated liver and spleen trauma.

Treatment for musculoskeletal chest wall pain

- Chest X-rays are usually unhelpful in minor chest wall trauma and would not significantly alter treatment plans even if a rib fracture is identified on X-ray. However, the decision must be made based upon the individual assessment of need and whether clinical signs may warrant a chest X-ray
- Regular simple analgesia (NSAIDs if not contraindicated) is the mainstay of treatment; patients may be reluctant to take such analgesia, but should be gently encouraged to do so, as an effective reduction in pain symptom severity is often seen.
- The patient should be warned that the chest pain may persist, to some degree, for 4–6 weeks after its initial occurrence. Accordingly, strenuous activities affecting the chest, such as lifting, should be avoided during this time period.
- Respiratory movement may be reduced when the patient is in pain, so daily deep breathing exercises should also be recommended, in order to reduce the risk of a respiratory tract infection occurring. Do not repress coughing, as coughing can help remove phlegm, even though that may be painful to do.

➲ Also see 'Respiratory investigations', Chapter 17, pp. 525–526 and Chapter 13, p. XX; ➲ 'Respiratory complications', pp 408–412; Chapter 17, pp. 517, 525 Chapter 12, p. 390.

Primary care: elbow problems

The synovial hinge joint of the elbow is a common site of musculoskeletal inflammation. In relation to injuries, the elbow joint is prone to subluxation, dislocation, and fracture due to its relatively superficial overlying soft tissues.

Elbow history

In adults with inflammatory-type problems, any history of elbow joint overuse should be elicited. Elbow fractures/dislocations may occur after a fall on the outstretched hand or with direct injury to the elbow. In young children, traction force on the elbow can displace the radial head.[1]

Elbow examination

Inspection

- Observe the elbows for shape, symmetry, swelling, deformity, skin redness, muscle wasting, scars, skin lesions, bruising, and any wounds post trauma.
- A fractured elbow is typically held in a degree of flexion supported by the arm of the unaffected side.

Palpation

- As the overlying soft tissues of the elbow are superficial, most of the joint can be easily palpated.
- Start palpation at the lateral edge of the distal humerus, followed by the lateral epicondyle, the recess between the lateral epicondyle and radial head, the radial head, the medial epicondyle, the ulnar nerve behind the medial epicondyle, the medial edge of the distal humerus, and finally the olecranon process.

Movement

- Flexion and extension.
- Forearm rotation (elbows flexed to 90° and held against the lateral chest walls, patient then supinates and pronates their forearms).
- These movements may also be checked on resistance.

Elbow pain presenting problems

Olecranon bursitis

Inflammation of the burse overlying the olecranon may occur spontaneously or as a result of repeated pressure over the olecranon. Presents as an egg-shaped swelling over the elbow tip, which is red, hot, and tender. Pain occurs on elbow movement.

Examine the overlying skin carefully to exclude a potential entry site for bacteria such as an insect bite or a small break in the skin, and any corresponding tiredness or fever; such signs of infection would require oral antibiotics in addition to simple analgesia. Otherwise, most simple cases of bursitis can be treated with rest of the affected elbow and regular simple analgesia (ideally an NSAID if not contraindicated). Aspiration of the fluid may introduce infection, and should be reserved for either cases of traumatic bursitis, where signs of bleeding are evident, or if septic bursitis is suspected—aspirate the bursal fluid using an aseptic technique and treat with an flucloxacillin or clarithromycin (if penicillin allergic). If aspiration is not possible in 1° care, the procedure should be undertaken in the ED.

Epicondylitis

Describes inflammation of the tendons of the lateral or medial aspects of the elbow as a result of overuse or repeated movements. *Lateral epicondylitis (tennis elbow)* presents with pain and tenderness over the lateral epicondyle and pain over the lateral epicondyle on resisted wrist extension. *Medial epicondylitis (golfer's elbow)* presents with pain and tenderness over the medial epicondyle and pain over the medial epicondyle on resisted wrist flexion. Both problems respond to rest from the causative activity and simple analgesia (NSAIDs if not contraindicated). Persistent or recurrent episodes of epicondylitis benefit from PT assessment and treatment. Advice on reviewing the grip size of a racquet or golf clubs may be helpful as the condition may be exacerbated by the wrong grip size.

Elbow injury presenting problems

- *Fractured radial head*: this is caused by a fall on the outstretched hand or direct injury to the elbow. The patient presents with the affected elbow held in flexion, bony tenderness of the radial head, and painfully reduced elbow extension. Requires referral to the ED or Minor Injuries Unit for X-ray and further management.
- *Fractured olecranon process*: this is typically caused by a fall onto the elbow tip. The patient present with pain, bony tenderness, and swelling over the olecranon process and an inability to straighten the elbow. Requires referral to the ED or Minor Injuries Unit for X-ray and further management.
- *Dislocated elbow*: this painful injury normally occurs after a fall on the outstretched hand. The patient presents in discomfort with a swollen and fixed elbow, most commonly caused by dislocation of the radial head and fracture of the proximal ulna. Requires urgent assessment in the ED.
- *Pulled elbow (subluxation of radial head)*: this occurs in children <6 years old when traction is applied to the child's forearm, such as being swung by the arm. The child presents with reluctance to use the affected arm, and the carer often saying they think there is a history of direct elbow trauma, even though they have no knowledge of a history of direct trauma. Reduced movement of the elbow is the main clinical sign. In the absence of a direct history of observed or remembered trauma, X-ray is unnecessary. The subluxation can be easily reduced by applying direct pressure to the radial head while supinating and extending the forearm.
- *Supracondylar fracture*: in this type of fracture, the humerus fractures just above the elbow. These fractures usually occur in children <8 years old. This is the most common type of elbow fracture, and one of the more serious because it can result in distal neurovascular impairment. Requires immediate referral to the ED.

Reference

1. NICE Clinical Knowledge Summaries (2016). Olecranon bursitis. https://cks.nice.org.uk/olecranon-bursitis

Primary care: wrist and hand problems

The complexity of the wrist and hand joints must be carefully considered when assessing patients with wrist and hand problems. It is important to have a low threshold for onward referral for expert advice.

Wrist and hand history

The wrist and hand are prone to inflammation or trauma. Consider:

- Any history of overuse or repeated movements should be elicited.
- The patient's occupation may have an impact on the presenting problem.
- Finger, wrist, or hand fractures. Hand fractures typically occur after a punch-type injury, which the patient may initially be reluctant to reveal. Finger fractures usually occur after crush injuries or from forced flexion or extension of the interphalangeal joints. Remember that accompanying wounds in hand and finger injuries may have associated tendon and/or nerve injuries.

Wrist and hand examination

Inspection

- Observe the wrists, hands, and fingers for shape, symmetry, swelling, deformity, skin redness, scars, skin lesions, bruising, and any wounds post trauma.

Palpation

- *Wrist*: palpate the distal radius, ulna, radial and ulnar styloids, and carpal bones. Pay particular attention to tenderness in the anatomical snuffbox (scaphoid bone). Note any crepitus of the wrist extensor tendons.
- *Hand and fingers*: palpate the metacarpals, the MCP joints, the proximal phalanx, IP joint, and distal phalanx of the thumb and the proximal phalanges, PIP joints, middle phalanges, DIP joints, and distal phalanges of the fingers. Palpate the thenar and hypothenar eminence at the base of hands for swelling and tenderness.

Movement

- *Wrist*: check the active range of wrist flexion, extension, and radial and ulnar deviation.
- *Hand*: check the active range of thumb abduction, adduction, extension, flexion, and opposition. Flexion and extension of the MCP and IP joints should also be checked. Comparative resistance movements of the IP joints can be checked to assess extensor and flexor tendon function. Resistance movement testing is particularly important to assess with finger lacerations and forced extension/flexion finger injuries.
- *Neurological*: check the integrity of the ulnar, median, and radial nerves in their distal distribution of the hand.

Wrist and hand pain presenting problems

- *Tenosynovitis (tendonitis)*: is relatively common at the wrist in the extensor and flexor tendons. Patients present with wrist pain on movement and slight swelling over the affected tendon, tenderness and crepitus is noted on palpation. This responds well to rest from the causative activity and regular simple analgesia (an NSAID if not contraindicated).

Wrist and hand injury presenting problems

- *Colles' fracture*: most often occurs in older people, falling on their outstretched hand. The injury sustained is a displaced fracture of the distal radius and ulnar styloid. The patient presents with pain, swelling, and reduced movement of the wrist. Requires urgent further assessment in the ED for X-ray and reduction of the fracture.
- *Scaphoid fracture*: a fracture of this small carpal bone is normally sustained from a fall on the outstretched hand. The patient presents with a painful wrist and ↓ movement. Examination reveals slight swelling and bony tenderness in the anatomical snuffbox (located inferiorly to the distal radius). Requires referral to the ED or Minor Injuries Unit for X-ray, immobilization, and review. Fracture may not be detectable on initial X-ray—repeat X-ray or bone scan 2–3 weeks later. Clinical signs of fracture are sufficient for a diagnosis.
- *Metacarpal fractures*: are associated with a punch injury of the hand, the fifth metacarpal is particularly prone to fracture. The patient presents with swelling, pain, and bony tenderness of the affected metacarpal(s). Requires referral to the ED or Minor Injuries Unit for X-ray, immobilization, and review. If injury is a punch injury, human tooth wounds are sometimes also present; local guidelines on infection prophylaxis and immunization should be consulted.
- *Finger sprains and strains*: the collateral ligaments and muscles of the thumb and finger can be sprained or strained presenting with a swollen finger, pain on movement, and diffuse tenderness. The collateral ligaments should be stressed to identify any excess comparative laxity, which would require hand clinic assessment. Otherwise treat using the neighbouring finger as a support to strap together and use simple analgesia (an NSAID if not contraindicated).
- *Finger fractures*: avulsion fractures of the phalanges can occur with either forced hyperextension or forced flexion of an IP joint. The fracture occurs as result of a hyperextended flexor tendon avulsing a small piece of bone on the flexor surface (volar plate injury) or an hyperflexed extensor tendon avulsing a small piece of bone on the extensor surface (mallet finger injury). Fractures of the proximal and middle phalanges can also occur from direct trauma, such as a fall (presents with swelling and tenderness of the affected area). Mallet finger injury—a visible droop of the distal phalanx is evident. All injuries require referral to the ED/Minor Injuries Unit for X-ray, immobilization, and fracture or hand clinic review.

Further reading

Purcell D (2016). *Minor Injuries: A Clinical Guide*, 4th edn. London: Elsevier.

Primary care: hip problems

The ball and socket joint of the hip is stable particularly when compared against the shoulder. This is due to the deeper articulation of the head of the femur in the acetabulum, the rigid bones of the pelvic girdle, and the stabilizing strong femoral ligaments. In the 1° healthcare clinics, acute inflammation and injuries of the hip are less common presentations. In older people, fractures of the neck of the femur are common after simple falls.

Hip history

❗ Non-traumatic acute hip pain should be approached with caution in certain groups of adult patients as it may indicate:

- Hip infection (➔ Chapter 7, pp. 266, 276 and Chapter 12, p. 390).
- Metastatic spread in patients with cancer (solid tumours).
- Avascular necrosis in patients with risk factors such as SLE.
- Abdominal or pelvic pathologies.

Hip examination

Inspection

- The patient should be undressed to underwear.
- Observe the patient standing, noting any leg length discrepancy or asymmetry of the iliac crest heights.
- If possible, observe the patient's gait.
- Note any overlying bruising, wounds, scars, skin lesions, or redness.
- Observe for muscle wasting.
- If a fractured neck of femur is suspected, observe the affected leg for shortening and external rotation.

Palpation

- Palpate the bony landmarks—iliac crest, iliac tubercles, anterior iliac spines, pubic tubercles, and the greater trochanters.
- Palpate the femoral triangle and inguinal ligament—with the hip externally rotated and abducted.
- The ischial tuberosity may also be palpated with the patient lying on their side or prone.

Movement

- Flexion—bend hip and knee toward chest.
- Extension—returning leg to straight position.
- Abduction—move leg from midline.
- Adduction—move leg back to midline.
- Lateral (external) rotation—roll the extended leg outward.
- Medial (internal) rotation—roll the extended leg inward.

Hip presenting problems

- *Hip muscle strains*: can commonly occur at the adductor longus and magnus (groin tenderness and pain on resisted adduction); gluteus medius (iliac tubercle tenderness and pain on resisted abduction); iliopsoas (anterior tenderness and pain on resisted flexion); gluteal and biceps femoris (posterior tenderness and pain on resisted extension when prone). These muscle strains respond to rest and simple analgesia (ideally an NSAID if not contraindicated).

- *Hip bursitis*: can occur with overuse in greater trochanter bursa (pain on adduction in lateral hip); iliopsoas bursa (pain on flexion in anterior hip); and the ischial bursa (posterior pain, pain on sitting). Hip bursitis normally responds to rest and simple analgesia (an NSAID if not contraindicated). In patients with significant pain, soft tissue corticosteroid injection may be considered.
- *Iliotibial band syndrome*: typically seen in runners, is an overuse injury of the connective issues that are located on the lateral aspect of the femur and knee, causing pain on the outside part of the knee and sometimes the hip, especially during running when the heel strikes the ground. Responds to rest and NSAIDs.
- *Fractured neck of femur*: typically occurs in an older person after a fall. The patient complains of a painful thigh and hip and is unable to weight bear. With the patient supine, shortening and external rotation of the affected leg is evident. Requires immediate ambulance transfer to the ED.

➲ Also see 'Osteoarthritis of hip and knee', Chapter 2, pp. 20–21; ➲ 'Chronic non-inflammatory pain', p. 186; ➲ Chapter 8, 'Assessing the patient', pp. 289–306; ➲ Chapter 9, 'Symptom control: using pharmacological and non-pharmacological methods', pp. 307–328.

Further reading

Clunie G, Wilkinson, N, Nikiphorou, E, Jadon, D (eds) (2018). *Oxford Handbook of Rheumatology*, 4th edn. Oxford: Oxford University Press.

NICE Clinical Knowledge Summaries (2016). Greater trochanteric pain syndrome (trochanteric bursitis). https://cks.nice.org.uk/greater-trochanteric-pain-syndrome-trochanteric-bursitis

Primary care: knee problems

The condylar joint of the knee, despite being a significant weight-bearing joint, is dependent on its cruciate and collateral ligaments for its stability; hence problems with these ligaments give rise to many knee presenting problems.

Knee history

❗ If any of the post-knee injury problems noted here are found during the examination, refer to the ED for further assessment: dislocated patella, inability to weight bear, inability to flex/extend the knee, a grossly swollen knee (large effusion), inability to raise leg (SLR), bony tenderness of the patella or head of fibula, any distal neurovascular deficit, and any knee injuries in people >55 years old.

Knee examination

Inspection

- Exposure—knees, pelvis, lower legs.
- Inspect and compare.
- Walking, standing, sitting, supine.
- Standing—is pelvis level? Knees symmetrical, anterior/posterior, leg lengths.
- Swelling, erythema, scars/wounds.

Palpation

- Patella/patellar ligament/prepatellar bursae.
- Quadriceps.
- Check for effusion with patellar tap.
- Medial/lateral femoral epicondyles.
- Medial/lateral menisci.
- Medial and collateral ligaments.
- Gastrocnemius area (posterior).

Movement

- Active SLR.
- Flexion.
- Extension.

Knee special tests

As with the shoulder, there is a wide array of special tests for assessing knee dysfunction and instability. The following selected special tests are simple to perform and interpret, and are usually sufficient to diagnose specific knee problems.

- *Valgus stress test*: for assessing the integrity of the MCL. With the patient supine, test knee in extension and flexed to 15–20°. Push knee medially with one hand while applying an opposing lateral force at the ankle with the other hand. Laxity in extension indicates MCL disruption felt as separation of the tibia and the femur. Flexion stress—isolates MCL, looking for ↑ laxity in comparison with unaffected side.
- *Varus stress test*: this assesses integrity of LCL. Opposite manoeuvre to valgus stress test. Push knee laterally with one hand while applying an

opposing medial force at the ankle with the other hand. Again looking for ↑ laxity in comparison with unaffected side.

- *Anterior/posterior drawer test*: for ACL, anterior drawer test, where patient is supine with knee flexed to 90°.Grasp tibia just below joint line and pull forward with both hands. An intact ACL will move forward a few mm and then stop abruptly/hard end point. An injured ACL will have more forward movement and a 'soft' end point. With the knee in the same position, a reverse posterior movement can be applied to assess the PCL.
- *Apley/grinding test*: to assess the menisci. Is joint line pain meniscal or ligamentous? Patient prone, affected knee flexed 90°, apply external/ internal rotation, with downward force—pain indicates meniscal damage. Repeat external/internal rotation, with upward force—pain indicates collateral ligament injury.
- *McMurray's test*: an alternative to the Apley test. Patient supine and the knee fully flexed. Fingers placed on the medial or lateral joint line, and the knee is slowly extended with the tibia externally rotated for medial meniscus or internally rotated for lateral meniscus. Look for a painful clicking at medial or lateral joint line.

Knee presenting problems

- *MCL injury*: the MCL is the most commonly injured knee ligament. Valgus (lateral) stress, or external rotational stress with leg firmly planted. If force great, ACL also often damaged. History findings—effusion <12 hours after injury, localized swelling and tenderness over injured area, typically at the superior origin of the MCL. If there is no excessive ligament laxity: rest and simple analgesia (an NSAID if not contraindicated) is normally sufficient. Excessive laxity on stress testing ED/orthopaedic referral is required.
- *ACL injury*: second most commonly injured knee ligament. Non-contact pivoting/twisting with foot planted, non-contact hyperextension, sudden deceleration, forced internal rotation, sudden valgus (lateral) impact. There is often an accompanying meniscal injury. The patient is normally unable to continue activity, has extreme pain at time of injury, feels a 'pop' in knee or a tearing sensation, swelling 1–2 hours after injury, knee tense and painful, and has episodes of 'giving way'. Requires further assessment in the ED.
- *Meniscal injuries*: medial more common as the lateral is more fixed. Normally occurs as a result of rotational force to flexed knee. Often with ACL injury. Typically can continue activity, 'popping' sound at time of injury, effusion >12 hours after injury, painful locking or 'giving way' of knee, followed by stiffness. A clicking sensation often accompanies meniscal problems. Requires orthopaedic referral.

➲ Also see 'Anterior knee pain (patellofemoral syndrome)', pp. 211–213; ➲ 'Baker's cyst', Chapter 6, p. 211; ➲ 'Osteoarthritis', Chapter 2, p. 12; ➲ 'Septic arthritis', Chapter 13, pp. 404–405; ➲ 'Gout', Chapter 4, p. 118.

Further reading

NICE Clinical Knowledge Summaries (2017). Knee pain—assessment. https://cks.nice.org.uk/knee-pain-assessment

Primary care: lower leg and ankle problems

Ankle and foot pain/swelling are frequent presenting complaints in 1° healthcare. Pain is often due to musculoskeletal causes, whether this be injury, acute inflammation, RA, gout, or vasculitis. However, wider systemic causes of ankle and foot pain/swelling such as endocrine, cardiac, hepatic, or renal pathologies must also be considered.

Lower leg/ankle/foot history

Until definitively proven otherwise, patients presenting with non-traumatic calf pain should be presumed to have a DVT and referred either to the ED for further assessment, or managed by the local pathway for assessing patients at risk of DVT.

In patients presenting with ankle or foot injuries with accompanying malleolar pain or midfoot pain, the following clinical findings are suggestive of a possible fracture requiring referral for X-ray: bony tenderness at the posterior edge or tip of the lateral malleolus or the navicular or the base of the fifth metatarsal or alternatively an observed inability to weight bear on the injured ankle/foot.

Ankle/foot examination

Inspection

- Observe lower leg, ankle, and foot for any bruising, swelling, wounds, scars, skin lesions, redness, or anatomical deformity.
- Remember to inspect the plantar surface of the foot and the toe web spaces.
- Observe the gait; can the patient weight bear on the affected side?

Palpation

- Palpate from below the knee, including the fibular head, calf muscles, the Achilles tendon, the calcaneum, the medial and lateral malleoli, the navicular, and fifth metatarsal.
- If a foot injury is suspected, also palpate the other tarsal bones and the toe phalanges.

Movement

- Ankle dorsiflexion, plantarflexion, eversion, and inversion.
- Remember that resistance movements of the ankle will always be painful and reduced in a recently sprained ankle; so initially this may not be of clinical significance.
- Toe flexion and extension.

Lower leg, ankle, and knee presenting problems

- *Calf strain (gastrocnemius tear)*: presenting as a sudden onset of calf pain with a forceful forward leg movement such as running and stopping suddenly. Presents with tenderness and swelling over the calf muscles and pain to fully weight bear. Dorsiflexion ↑ the calf pain. Responds well to rest, ice, simple analgesia (an NSAID if not contraindicated).

Physiotherapy referral may also be useful (dependent on local guidelines).

- *Tenosynovitis (tendonitis)*: inflammation of either the Achilles tendon or extensor hallicus longus due to excessive walking or running is relatively common. Presents with pain on movement and crepitus of the affected tendon. Responds well to rest from the causative activity and regular simple analgesia (an NSAID if not contraindicated). Physiotherapy assessment may be required for persisting Achilles tendonitis.
- *Ankle sprain*: occur as a result of an inversion or eversion injury. Presents with malleolar pain, swelling, ↓ movement, and sometimes bruising. Diffuse tenderness and warmth of the affected ligaments is noted. Patients may need to be encouraged to attempt to weight bear during their examination; but this is an important observation in order to exclude a potential fracture. Treatment includes rest, elevation, and simple analgesia (an NSAID if not contraindicated).
- *Plantar fasciitis*: typically presents with unilateral calcaneum pain which worsens on standing and walking. Examination is often unrevealing; with only slight tenderness of the affected plantar surface sometimes being noted. Treatment comprises raised heel pads and simple analgesia (an NSAID if not contraindicated). May take some time to settle. Local steroid injection may be required in refractory cases.
- *Toe bruising/fracture*: a common injury, which normally occurs after 'stubbing' the end of a toe. The toes are important for foot balance when walking, so this relatively small injury can have a large impact on everyday activities. Both fractures and bruising are very painful and can be difficult to differentiate clinically. X-ray is not needed unless a dislocated toe is suspected or if there is an accompanying crush injury and subungual haematoma. Treatment includes neighbour strapping of toe and sufficient analgesia (codeine may be required in some cases). The patient should be advised that pain may continue for 2–3 weeks post injury even with regular analgesia.

Further reading

NICE Clinical Knowledge Summaries (2016). Sprains and strains. https://cks.nice.org.uk/sprains-and-strains

Primary care: skin and wound infections

Introduction

In patients presenting with musculoskeletal injuries, there can often be accompanying skin or wound infections. In patients with possible musculoskeletal acute inflammation, local infection should always be considered as an additional differential diagnosis, because the cardinal symptoms of skin redness, pain, and swelling are key features of both infection and inflammation. The commonest pathogens in skin or wound infections are *Staphylococcus aureus* and *Streptococcus pyogenes*. Fungi, yeast, and the herpes group of viruses may also cause local skin infections and should therefore be considered in clinical decision-making.

The following types of traumatic wounds carry a high risk of infection and should be considered with caution: delayed presentation (>12 hours) of wounds requiring closure; dirty wounds, e.g. those contaminated with soil, grit, or grease/oil-like substances; penetrating and/or puncture wounds; wounds with areas of non-vascularized tissue; wounds overlying potential bony injuries, which should be treated as compound fractures; and animal or human bites. These types of wounds are ideally treated in the ED or Minor Injuries Unit.

It should also be remembered that patients who are possibly immunocompromised, by virtue of their medical and/or drug history, are at a higher risk of developing skin or wound infections, and there should be a lower threshold for diagnosis and treatment of skin/wound infection in at-risk immunocompromised patients.

Cellulitis

Cellulitis typically describes an acute bacterial infection of the skin, which may present in isolation or else in conjunction with a traumatic wound. Symptoms include a defined area of redness, swelling, and pain of the affected skin area, often accompanied by general malaise and sometimes associated regional lymphadenopathy. On examination, the affected erythematous skin is hot and tender on palpation, most often with a well-defined border.

The patient should be examined for signs of spreading cellulitis, which may require hospital assessment: fever, tachycardia, red tracking marks/ascending lymphangitis, and a worsening malaise.

If signs of spreading cellulitis are not present, most patients can be successfully treated with oral flucloxacillin, or co-amoxiclav (if facial cellulitis), or clarithromycin (if penicillin allergic) as per *BNF* dosage schedules and local guidelines, in conjunction with simple analgesia, rest, and advice regarding worsening and persisting signs of infection. The area of skin redness can be marked with a pen to monitor the progression/regression of local infection.

Wound care in musculoskeletal injuries

Musculoskeletal injuries with accompanying wounds require careful inspection and thorough cleansing, so as to ↓ the chances of cellulitis occurring or developing further, if already present.

- Any visible contaminants, such as grit or soil, should be removed from a wound. This may require wound irrigation in conjunction with wiping with saline-soaked gauze, applied with a sufficient pressure to remove wound debris. If required, topical anaesthetic gel can be applied prior to wound cleansing.
- Wound debris removal is particularly important in skin abrasions, otherwise retained pieces of grit/soil ↑ the chances of infection occurring or being prolonged, and also of causing permanent skin marking.
- If an acute wound is >2–3mm deep, some form of wound closure will need to be used, whether this is adhesive skin strips, skin glue, or suturing.
- Once cleaned, the wound should be covered an appropriate non-adherent, absorbent dressing, and reviewed at regular intervals. Bacteriological wound swabs may need to be considered in discharging wounds.

Tetanus immunization status should also be determined. Adult patients who give a clear history of five or more tetanus vaccines (three preschool, one at secondary school, and one as a young adult), most probably have lifetime immunity and so do not require any further booster dosages. If there is not a clear history of five vaccines, and the last booster dose was >10 years ago, a tetanus booster dose should be given as per *BNF* recommendations and local guidance.

In patients with no clear history of any prior tetanus immunization, a full tetanus immunization course and tetanus immunoglobulin will need to be considered. This is particularly the case in tetanus-prone wounds:

- Wounds with devitalized skin.
- Puncture wounds.
- Soil/manure contaminated wounds.
- Wounds with signs of infection.

➲ Also see 'Infections in musculoskeletal conditions', Chapter 13, pp. 400–403; ➲ 'Septic arthritis', Chapter 13, pp. 404–405.

Further reading

NICE Clinical Knowledge Summaries (2019). Cellulitis—acute. https://cks.nice.org.uk/cellulitis-acute

Chapter 7

Elective orthopaedic surgery

Orthopaedic surgery: overview

Advances in orthopaedic surgery have substantially improved the overall function and quality of life for individuals with arthritic conditions. Arthroplasties (joint replacements) are now available for almost every joint, with hip and knee arthroplasty being the most commonly performed orthopaedic operation in the UK.

Individuals who fail to gain satisfactory results from conservative management of their MSC or have a progressive disease may benefit from a surgical procedure. Assessment by a surgeon for suitability for surgery is best carried out before the patient develops joint deformity or instability, muscle contractures, or advanced muscle atrophy. Delaying surgery until these problems develop can compromise the results and ↑ the risk of surgical complications occurring.

Planning surgery involves consideration of:

- The degree of pain and functional limitation perceived by the patient.
- The joints involved. No joint can be considered in isolation.
- Possible surgical and conservative treatments, including the expected short- and long-term outcomes.
- Potential risks of surgery/anaesthetic.
- The patient's individual circumstances including an understanding of their social and occupational needs.
- An understanding of the patient's goals and expectations.
- Clarification of goals and patient expectations. These goals and expectations should be confirmed as realistic and attainable by the surgical team; unrealistic expectations of surgery can ↓ patient satisfaction with surgical outcome.
- An assessment of motivation. Some surgical procedures require patients to undergo an intensive physiotherapy/rehabilitation programme to attain the best surgical outcome.

Aims of surgical intervention

The 1° aims of any surgical procedure are to:

- Relieve pain.
- Prevent and correct deformity.
- Prevent destruction of cartilage or tendons.
- Maintain or improve function of joints by ↑ or ↓ motion.
- Enable individuals to maintain their independence.

Relief of pain and loss of function are the 1° reasons for consideration of any type of surgical intervention. If the pain cannot be controlled by conservative means and the patient's life, in particular his/her sleep, is affected, surgery should be considered. Cosmesis is not a prime consideration, but for patients with RA this can bring benefits in the form of improved self-image so should not be overlooked.

Enhanced recovery programmes (ERPs)

ERPs aim to enhance the quality of care across the continuum by improving risk-adjusted patient outcomes, promoting patient safety, ↑ patient satisfaction, and optimizing the use of resources.[1,2] In the elective orthopaedic surgery setting, ERPs have been developed particularly for patients undergoing total hip replacement (THR) and total knee replacement (TKR) surgery.

ERPs are an extension of integrated care pathways (ICPs). An ICP is a multidisciplinary outline of anticipated care, placed in an appropriate time frame, to help a patient with a specific condition or set of symptoms move progressively through a clinical experience to positive outcomes. An ICP helps to determine locally agreed, multidisciplinary practice based on guidelines and evidence where available, for a specific patient or client group. It forms all or part of the clinical record, documents the care given, and facilitates the evaluation of outcomes for continuous quality improvement.

The key points of an ERP are patient preparation and identifying and minimizing risk. Patients are required to become a partner in their care and play an active role by taking responsibility for enhancing their recovery.

Patient empowerment is central to enhanced recovery and can be promoted by:

- Good communication.
- Shared decision-making.
- Education and information.
- Support for patients/family members/carers.
- Access to advice and resources.
- Clinician engagement.
- Patient engagement.

➲ See also Chapter 10, 'Holistic and patient-centred care', pp. 329–350.

References

1. Department of Health (2011). *Enhanced Recovery Partners Programme*. London: DH.
2. Driver A, Lewis W, Haward-Sampson P, Dashfield E (2012). How enhanced recovery can boost patient outcomes. *Nurs Times* 108:18 20.

Further reading

Bandolier. Integrated care pathway. http://www.bandolier.org.uk/booth/glossary/ICP.html

Orthopaedic surgery: preoperative preparation and assessment

Preoperative preparation places the patient in the best possible condition for their surgery, and helps to identify risks and instigate rehabilitation either before admission or soon after.

Early health screening should take place in the 1° care setting and is often coordinated before referral for consideration of orthopaedic surgery, except in emergency situations.

Due to the focus on reducing hospital length of stay, it is essential that all preoperative screening is complete and the patient is fit for surgery as patients are routinely admitted to hospital on the day of surgery. The aim of screening is to detect and treat any underlying health or social problems that could affect the outcome of surgery, delay discharge, or necessitate a planned operation being cancelled. It is important to begin the process of discharge planning at this point to ensure everything is in place to facilitate a smooth discharge postoperatively (➔ see 'Discharge planning', p. 268).

Hospital-based preadmission assessment

NICE has issued guidance on the use of routine preoperative tests for all grades of elective surgery.[1] These take into account the planned procedure and co-morbidities and suggest a preoperative testing regimen that determines the patient's fitness to undergo surgery.

Preadmission assessments usually take place 14–21 days preoperatively. This may be undertaken at the initial outpatient appointment where the decision for surgery is made and often involves all members of the MDT.

Aims of preadmission assessment clinics

- Identify and treat any previously unrecognized medical/social conditions which could affect the outcome of surgery. This should include:
    - Vascular assessment.
    - Screening for the presence of methicillin-resistant *Staphylococcus aureus* (MRSA) colonization. Patients known to carry MRSA should have a course of eradication therapy prior to high-risk surgery.
    - Checking for any breech of the skin which could be infected.
    - Checking for fungal infections under the patient's nails.
- Assess fitness to undergo an anaesthetic (Box 7.1).
- Establish baseline measures of health outcomes and allow the healthcare team to anticipate and prepare a care plan unique to the individual patient's problems.
- Ensure the patient understands the surgical procedure and rehabilitation to be able to give informed consent to proceed.
- Continue to the process of discharge planning.

Smoking cessation

At every occasion, but especially before surgery, advice and support for smoking cessation should be given, applying a sensitive approach to individual preferences and needs. Smoking cessation can reduce the risk of cardiac ischaemia and postoperative chest infections, but for optimal effect should be initiated at least 2 months before surgery. Heavy smoking can ↓

Box 7.1 Anaesthetic high-risk patients

- Past history of anaesthetic problems.
- Unstable diabetes/hypertension.
- Severe obesity.
- Symptomatic emphysema.
- Difficult airway.
- Abnormal U&Es.
- Unstable ischaemic heart disease.
- Previously unidentified heart murmurs/aortic stenosis.

the oxygen-carrying capacity of the blood equivalent to the loss of 2 g/dL of Hb, ∴ giving up smoking can give a benefit of a 1–2 unit blood transfusion postoperatively.

Weight reduction

Obesity is not a contraindication for surgery but can ↑ the risk of:

- Anaesthetic complications.
- Intraoperative blood loss.
- DVT.

Current evidence supports weight loss prior to surgery if morbidly obese, yet consideration should also be given to potential improvements in quality of life of some surgical procedures.

Patient education and consent

The provision of information is central to the consent process. Patients have a fundamental legal and ethical right to determine what happens to them. Treatment options will generally be discussed well in advance of the actual procedure being carried out. This may be on just one occasion, or it might be over a series of consultations with a number of different health professionals.

Before patients come to a decision about treatment, they need comprehensible information about:

- Their condition.
- Possible treatments/investigations.
- The risks and benefits (including the risks/benefits of doing nothing).
- Potential common complications.
- Any additional procedures likely to be necessary as part of the procedure, i.e. a blood transfusion, or the removal of tissue.
- Expectations for postoperative pain relief.
- The type and extent of postoperative rehabilitation.

Verbal information should be supported by additional written or visual information to refer to after the consultation to reinforce the information provided and act as a formal record. The hospital team, or in some cases patient organizations, may offer opportunities to talk to somebody who has undergone the proposed procedure. See 'Further reading', p. 254.

Consent

Valid consent to treatment is central in all forms of healthcare, from providing personal care to undertaking major surgery.

'Consent' is a patient's agreement for a HCP[2] to provide care. Patients may indicate consent non-verbally (e.g. by presenting their arm for their pulse to be taken), orally, or in writing. For the consent to be valid, the patient must:

- Have received sufficient information.
- Be competent to take the particular decision.
- Not be acting under duress.

The consent process should be carried out in two stages:

- Stage 1. The provision of information, discussion of options, and initial (oral) decision.
- Stage 2. Confirmation that the patient still wants to go ahead.

For significant procedures, it is essential for HCPs to document clearly both a patient's agreement to the intervention and the discussions which led up to that agreement. This may be done either through the use of a consent form (with further detail in the patient's notes if necessary), or through documenting in the patient's notes that oral consent has been given.

References

1. NICE (2016). *Routine Preoperative Tests for Elective Surgery* (NG45). London: NICE.
2. Department of Health (2003). *Good Practice in Consent: Implementation Guide for Health Care Professionals*. London: DOH.

Further reading

National Rheumatoid Arthritis Society (NRAS): http://www.nras.org.uk
NICE (2018). *Stop Smoking Interventions and Services* (NG92). London: NICE.
Versus Research UK: https://www.versusarthritis.org

Orthopaedic surgery: perioperative care

Safety checklist

While surgical procedures are intended to improve lives, unsafe surgical care can cause substantial harm. The WHO surgical safety checklist[1] was developed aiming to ↓ errors and ↑ teamwork and communication in surgery.

The checklist identifies three phases of an operation, each corresponding to a specific period in the normal flow of work:

- Before the induction of anaesthesia ('sign in').
- Before the incision of the skin ('time out').
- Before the patient leaves the operating room ('sign out').

In each phase, a checklist coordinator must confirm that the surgery team has completed the listed tasks before it proceeds with the operation. By consistently following these critical steps, HCPs can minimize the most common and avoidable risks endangering the lives and well-being of surgical patients.

To ensure successful implementation, it is important to make sure the checklist is suitable for an individual surgical setting. Adaptation after local consultation is encouraged. Implementation of the checklist has shown significant reduction in morbidity and mortality and is now used by a majority of surgical providers around the world.[2]

Antibiotic prophylaxis

The shortage of new antibiotics and the ↑ problem of multidrug resistance mean there is a need to restrict the use of antibiotic prophylaxis to those operations where it is most likely to be of benefit and also to limit the duration of prophylaxis. The Scottish Intercollegiate Guidelines Network (SIGN) guideline provides comprehensive evidence-based recommendations on the benefits and risks of antibiotic prophylaxis; indications for surgical antibiotic prophylaxis to prevent infection at a range of surgical sites in both adults and children; and choice, timing dosage, and route of administration of prophylactic antibiotics.

References

1. World Alliance for Patient Safety (2009). *Implementation Manual. WHO Surgical Safety Checklist: Safe Surgery Saves Lives*. Geneva: WHO.
2. Haynes AB Weiser TG, Berry WR, et al. (2009). A surgical safety checklist to reduce morbidity and mortality in a global population. *N Engl J Med* 360:491–9.
3. Scottish Intercollegiate Guidelines Network. (2014). *Antibiotic Prophylaxis in Surgery*. Edinburgh: SIGN.

Orthopaedic surgery: postoperative care

A named professional should be responsible for the coordination of care between all members of the MDT. It is important that the patient and their carers are able to identify the key persons concerned and they should be actively involved in continuously negotiating and influencing their care.

Track and trigger

The track and trigger early warning system is used to track abnormal physiology and trigger clinical action; this allows a prompt and potentially appropriate response to the occurrence of life-threatening situations.

The score is based on routinely recorded physiological observations such as blood pressure, respiration, and heart rate. Each observation is given a score of zero if it is normal, increasing to (typically) three as the observation deviates further from the normal range. The sum of all parameter scores gives a total EWS (Early Warning Score).

The recommendations from this early warning system state:

- A clear physiological monitoring plan detailing the parameters to be monitored and the frequency of observations should be made for each patient.
- There are explicit statements of parameters that should prompt a request for review by medical staff or expert MDT members.
- Respiratory rates should be monitored at any point when other observations are made.
- Staff require education and training in the interpretation and understanding of pulse oximetry readings.

Such schemes should be backed up by 'outreach' services to support ward staff in managing patients who are 'at risk'. The early involvement of senior staff when necessary is also advised.

Prevention and treatment of potential postoperative complications

All surgical procedures, particularly those that require a general anaesthetic, have the potential for complications to develop. The most common complications, nursing instructions, and patient education requirements relevant to individual surgical procedures are covered in the sections that follow.

Haemorrhage and shock

Significant blood loss can occur with major orthopaedic procedures. Consideration needs to be made to ensure a balance is made between anticoagulation to prevent DVT and PE and the risk of haemorrhage.

Signs and symptoms of haemorrhage/shock

- Patient complains of ↑ anxiety, fatigue, and ↑ pain over wound site.
- Blood loss apparent from drain or wound site.
- Tachycardia or irregular pulse, hypotension, ↑ respiration rate, and ↓ urinary output.
- FBC shows ↓ in RBC, Hb, and haematocrit values; however, if the patient is hypovolaemic, the haematocrit may not be ↓ as it is a ratio of blood cells to serum.

- If blood loss is severe—coagulation studies to detect clotting abnormalities.

Nursing management
- Stop or minimize blood loss. Apply pressure dressing to area of bleeding.
- Blood and fluid replacement—if Hb concentration is <7 g/dL, consider treatment with blood transfusion or autologous transfusion.
- Depending on the result of the coagulation screen and the amount of blood loss, fresh frozen plasma and platelets may be administered in addition to whole blood.
- Alternative strategies to reduce the numbers of transfusions required include antifibrinolytic compounds such as aminocaproic acid and tranexamic acid.

Further reading

Clarke S, Santy-Tomlinson J (eds) (2014). *Orthopaedic and Trauma Nursing: an Evidence-based Approach to Musculoskeletal Care*. London: Wiley.
NICE (2015). *Blood Transfusion* (NG24). London: NICE.
NICE (2016). *Acutely Ill Adults in Hospital: Recognising and Responding to Deterioration* (CG50). London: NICE.

Orthopaedic surgery: pain management

Acute postoperative pain has been identified as an important factor influencing the patient's perceptions of progress and recovery. Analgesia is the mainstay of postoperative pain control and should be provided according to the patient's perceived pain level and response to medication. Given that a large proportion of orthopaedic surgery is performed on the older population, care should be taken when choosing an analgesic for an individual; both co-morbidity and other medication must be considered to minimize the chance of drug–disease and drug–drug interactions. Refer to guidance documents for more information (e.g. from http://www.nice.org.uk or http://www.bnf.org.uk).

Pain relief should be sufficient to allow mobilization, rest, and pain-free sleep but avoid drug side effects.

Signs and symptoms of pain

- Patient appears pale and clammy and is restless.
- Tachycardia and hypertension.

Management of pain: regional anaesthesia

An injection of local anaesthetic agent at some point along the distribution of a nerve to block the sensation of pain. Regional anaesthesia, particularly spinal and epidural techniques, is often used for patients who have to undergo surgery, but who may not be medically fit enough to receive a general anaesthetic.

Spinal block

Local anaesthetic is injected into the subarachnoid space, where it mixes with the cerebrospinal fluid (CSF). A spinal needle is inserted below the termination of the spinal cord, usually at the level of the third or fourth lumbar space. The local anaesthetic diffuses through the CSF and blocks the cord and nerve roots. It can diffuse both up and down therefore there is a risk of respiratory muscle paralysis if the needle is inserted too high in the column.

Epidural block

Epidural block is highly effective for controlling acute pain after surgery or trauma to the chest, abdomen, pelvis, or lower limbs. Epidural block is usually prescribed as a low concentration of local anaesthetic and opiate, injected or infused into the epidural space to achieve minimum motor block and good analgesic effect.

Preprinted prescriptions are used with standard mixtures in prefilled syringes to ↓ the risk of drug calculation errors.

Monitoring and record keeping during spinal or epidural block

Epidural analgesia can cause serious, potentially life-threatening complications; throughout the procedure observations are taken and documented more frequently (usually every 30 min/determined by local policy) during the first 6–12 hours of the infusion, and for the first hour following a top-up injection or change of infusion rate.

Observations include:

- The effectiveness of pain relief achieved at rest and on movement.

- Level of sedation.
- Level of sensory and motor blockade so that potentially serious complications can be detected early.

For epidural infusions, records must also be kept of the epidural infusion rate, inspection of epidural insertion site, patency of IV access, and integrity of pressure areas. Contemporaneous records must be kept during the infusion including consent, insertion of the catheter, prescription, monitoring, additional doses, and notes about any complications or adverse events. It is advised that patients who have undergone orthopaedic surgery must be observed for possible development of compartment syndrome (➔ see 'Compartment syndrome', p. 261).

Advantages of epidural analgesia

- Patient experiences ↓ pain and sedation ∴ can participate in their nursing care and rehabilitation.

Disadvantages relating to potential complications of the epidural

- Nerve damage.
- A dural tap.
- Epidural abscess.
- Headache and/or backache.
- Urinary retention.
- Respiratory depression/nausea/vomiting/pruritus (opioid use).

Systemic side effects of local anaesthesia include:

- Cardiovascular effects such as hypotension, bradycardia, heart block, and cardiac or respiratory arrest (ventricular tachycardia or fibrillation).
- CNS effects such as agitation, euphoria, respiratory depression, twitching, convulsions, and sensory disturbances.

Infrequent but well recognized complications also include:

- Unexpected development of high block (e.g. catheter migration).
- Local anaesthetic toxicity.
- Spinal cord ischaemia; permanent harm (e.g. paraplegia, nerve injury).

Peripheral nerve block

Topical application or injection of local anaesthetic to infiltrate peripheral tissues. Used for minor procedures. Complications are rare and usually related to overdose or accidental intravascular injection.

Nursing care during regional anaesthesia

Preoperative preparation is the same as for general anaesthesia, including careful monitoring of vital signs. Additional support is required for psychological needs of the patient who remains conscious during the procedure.

Pressure areas and superficial nerves are vulnerable to pressure damage while the patient's limbs are numb.

Patient-controlled analgesia

PCA is a method of opioid administration using a computer-controlled pump that enables the patient, following adequate instruction, to self-administer a preset dose of analgesia at the push of a button, up to a preset maximum. An initial loading dose is often administered and the pump is set with a lock-out period between doses of usually 5 min.

Advantages of PCA

- Analgesia is tailored to patient's specific needs and gives control of pain relief to the patient.
- Avoids delays from waiting for oral or IM analgesia to be given.
- Can be used if oral fluids are restricted.

Monitoring

General principles of monitoring PCA analgesia are similar to those of epidural analgesia.

The administration of regular oral/IM analgesia following the discontinuation of any form of spinal, epidural, or PCA analgesia is essential to enable mobilization/rehabilitation to progress.

Further reading

Abdulla A, Adams N, Bone M, et al. (2013). Guidance on the management of pain in older people. *Age Ageing* 42: i1–i57.

Elliott J (2009). Patient controlled analgesia. In: Smith H (ed) *Current Therapy in Pain*, pp. 73–78. Philadelphia, PA: Elsevier.

Prout J, Jones T, Martin D (eds) (2014). Pain medicine. In: *Advanced Training in Anaesthesia: The Essential Curriculum*, pp. 499–524. Oxford: Oxford University Press.

Royal College of Anaesthetists (2010). *Best Practice in the Management of Epidural Analgesia in the Hospital Setting*. London: RCoA.

Royal Collage of Nursing (2015). *Pain Knowledge and Skills Framework for the Nursing Team*. London: RCN.

Acute compartment syndrome

Acute compartment syndrome (ACS) occurs when there is an ↑ in pressure and a ↓ in the size of a muscle compartment resulting in reduced capillary blood flow leading to cell death. It is essential to recognize ACS early: if the pressure is not relieved within hours, irreversible tissue and nerve damage can occur.

Signs and symptoms: the five Ps associated with ACS

Pain

- Out of proportion to the injury.
- Unrelieved by narcotics.
- Excessive use of analgesia devices (PCA).
- ↑ by movement of distal digits.
- Described as deep or throbbing.
- ↑ with elevation of the extremity.
- May not be present if central/peripheral sensory deficits are present.

Paraesthesia—subtle first symptom

- Best elicited by direct stimulation.
- Patients complain of a burning sensation.
- Can lead to hypoesthesia (numbness) pain.

Pressure

- Involved compartment or limb will feel tense and warm on palpation.
- Skin will be tight and shiny/may look cellulitic.

Pallor—late sign

- Pale/whitish tone to the skin/feels cool to touch.
- Prolonged capillary refill >3 sec.

Paralysis—late sign

- May start as weakness in active movement of involved or distal joints.
- Leads to inability to move joints or digits actively.
- No response to direct neural stimulation due to damage of myoneural junction.

Objective measurement of compartment pressures is used as an adjunct to signs and symptoms in detecting ACS.

Treatment of ACS

If pressure is not relieved by removal of dressings/casts, a fasciotomy of the affected compartments may be required. Skin grafting following fasciotomy is common.

Further reading

Via AG, Oliva F, Spoliti M, Maffulli N (2015). Acute compartment syndrome. *Muscles Ligaments Tendons J* 5:18–22.

Postoperative complications: deep vein thrombosis

The development of DVT and PE are significant complications of major orthopaedic surgery (Boxes 7.2 and 7.3). The risk of DVT is ~40%, most of these are minor, asymptomatic, and do not require treatment. The risk of fatal pulmonary embolism (PE) is <0.1%.

Signs and symptoms of DVT

- Pain and swelling in one leg, although both legs may be affected.
- Tenderness, changes to skin colour and temperature, and vein distension.

Management

- Carry out a physical examination and review the person's general medical history to exclude an alternative cause for the symptoms and signs.
- Use the two-level DVT Wells score to assess the likelihood of DVT and inform further management.

The two-level DVT Wells score to assess the probability of a DVT

Score 1 point for each of the following:

- Active cancer (treatment ongoing, within the last 6 months, or palliative).
- Paralysis, paresis, or recent plaster immobilization of the legs.
- Recently bedridden for 3 days or more, or major surgery within the last 12 weeks requiring general or local anaesthetics.
- Localized tenderness along the distribution of the deep venous system (such as the back of the calf).
- Entire leg is swollen.
- Calf swelling by >3 cm compared with the asymptomatic leg (measured 10 cm below the tibial tuberosity).
- Pitting oedema (greater than on the asymptomatic leg).
- Collateral superficial veins (non-varicose).
- Previously documented DVT.

Subtract 2 points if an alternative cause is considered more likely than DVT.

The risk of DVT is *likely* if the score is 2 points or more, and *unlikely* if the score is 1 point or less.

Management of DVT

For people who are likely to have DVT

Refer for a proximal leg vein US scan to be carried out within 4 hours. If a proximal leg vein US scan cannot be carried out within 4 hours of being requested:

- Take a blood sample for D-dimer testing.
- Give an interim 24-hour dose of a parenteral anticoagulant calculating the dose based on the patient's weight.
- Arrange for a proximal leg vein US scan (to be carried out within 24 hours of being requested).

Box 7.2 Patient-related risk factors for venous thromboembolism

- Previous venous thromboembolism.
- Cancer (known or undiagnosed).
- Age >60 years.
- Being overweight or obese.
- ♂ sex.
- Active heart disease or respiratory failure.
- Severe infection.
- Acquired or familial thrombophilia.
- Chronic low-grade injury to the vascular wall (e.g. from vasculitis, hypoxia from venous stasis, or chemotherapy).
- Varicose veins.
- Smoking.
- Obesity (BMI >30 kg/m^2).

Box 7.3 Risk factors that temporarily raise the likelihood of deep venous thrombosis

- Immobility (i.e. following a stroke, operation, plaster cast, hospitalization, or during long-distance travel).
- Significant trauma or direct trauma to a vein (e.g. intravenous catheter).
- Hormone treatment (i.e. oestrogen-containing contraception or hormone replacement therapy).
- Pregnancy and the postpartum period.
- Dehydration.

Further reading

NICE (2018). *Deep Vein Thrombosis*. London: NICE.

Postoperative complications: pulmonary embolism

Pulmonary embolism

If part of a thrombus breaks away it may lodge in the pulmonary arteries and cause a PE. PE is the commonest cause of sudden death in hospital. The following features are present in 97% of people with PE:

- Dyspnoea.
- Tachypnoea.
- Pleuritic chest pain.
- Features of DVT.
- Other features that may be present include:
  - Tachycardia (heart rate >100 beats per minute).
  - Haemoptysis.
  - Syncope.
  - Hypotension (systolic blood pressure <90 mmHg).
  - Crepitations.
  - Cough or fever.

Management of PE

Prophylaxis

To reduce venous stasis:

- Elevate limb.
- Regular dorsiflexion of the ankle when resting.
- Early ambulation.
- Antiembolism stockings or mechanical pumps.

To reduce hypercoagulability:

- Adequate hydration.
- Anticoagulant therapy. Local or national clinical guidelines should be available to determine risk of PE and major bleeding. Prophylaxis can then be prescribed as a result of the risk assessment.
- Patients can be trained to self-administer subcutaneous low-molecular-weight heparin injections at home (usually delivered for up to 10 days postoperatively).

Treatment of suspected PE

Arrange **immediate admission** if the patient has any of the following features[1]:

- Altered level of consciousness.
- Systolic blood pressure of <90 mmHg.
- Heart rate of >130 beats per minute.
- Respiratory rate of >25 breaths per minute.
- Oxygen saturation of <91%.
- Temperature of <35°C.
- If they are pregnant or have given birth within the past 6 weeks.

For all other people, assess the two-level PE Wells score to estimate the clinical probability of PE.[1]

The two-level PE Wells score to assess the probability of a PE

- Clinical features of DVT—*3 points.*
- Heart rate >100 beats per minute—*5 points.*
- Immobilization for >3 days or surgery in the previous 4 weeks—*1.5 points.*
- Previous DVT or PE—*1.5 points.*
- Haemoptysis—*1 point.*
- Cancer—*1 point.*
- An alternative diagnosis is less likely than PE—*3 points.*

For people with a Wells score of >4 points (PE likely)

- Either arrange hospital admission for an immediate computed tomography pulmonary angiogram (CTPA).
- Or, if there will be a delay in the person receiving a CTPA, give immediate interim low-molecular-weight heparin and arrange hospital admission.

For people with a Wells score of ≤4 points (PE unlikely), arrange a D-dimer test

- **If the test is positive,** either arrange admission to hospital for an immediate CTPA or, if a CTPA cannot be carried out immediately, give immediate low-molecular-weight heparin and arrange hospital admission.
- **If the test is negative,** consider an alternative diagnosis.

Reference

1. NICE (2015). *Pulmonary Embolism.* London: NICE.

Postoperative complications: infection and pressure ulcers

Infection

Infection is a potentially serious complication of surgery and is associated with a poor outcome. Infection following joint replacement surgery can lead to an infected joint and can be a major cause of joint failure. Infections potentially prolong the patient's stay in hospital and require an intensive course of antibiotic therapy.

National guidelines detail interventions and precautions practitioners should take to prevent healthcare-associated infections.[1–3] These include recommendations for:

- Hospital environmental hygiene.
- Hand hygiene.
- The use of personal protective equipment.
- The safe disposal of sharps.
- Preventing infections associated with the use of short-term indwelling catheters and central venous catheters.

Wound dressings

To provide optimum protection a dressing must be able to:

- Absorb excess exudates.
- Prevent contamination of the wound and surrounding tissues.
- Not adhere to the healing tissues.

Multiresistant infections

MRSA is carried by 30–50% of the general population, causing a high risk of transmission to patients following orthopaedic surgery as the natural barrier of the skin has been breached. Preoperative screening for the colonization of MRSA organisms is performed during the preassessment visit. High-risk factors for colonization are:

- ♂ sex.
- >70 years old.
- Previous hospital admission.
- Nursing home residents.

Drug treatment of infections

Antibiotic resistance poses a significant threat to public health, particularly as antibiotics underpin routine medical practice in both 1° and 2° care. To help prevent the development of current and future bacterial resistance, clinicians should ensure that when they prescribe antibiotics they do so in accordance with local antibiotic formularies as part of antimicrobial stewardship.

Prevention of pressure ulcers

A constant pressure of 60 mmHg can cause irreversible tissue damage within 1–2 hours. Pressures of 4–100 mmHg have been documented over the ischial, posterior trochanter, and thigh areas when clients are sitting in a wheelchair, even when using wheelchair cushions. Bony prominences such as the sacrum, heels, spine, hips, costal margins, and occiput are especially at risk when in a lying position. Shearing and friction forces contribute to the development of pressure ulcers.

All patients being admitted to 2° care should have an assessment of pressure ulcer risk using a recognized assessment tool (e.g. Waterlow score). An individualized care plan should be developed and documented for patients who have been assessed as being at high risk of developing a pressure ulcer, taking into account:

- The outcome of risk and skin assessment.
- The need for additional pressure relief at specific at-risk sites.
- Their mobility and ability to reposition themselves.
- Other co-morbidities.
- Patient preference.

Grades of pressure ulcers

- Category 1: non-blanchable erythema of intact skin. In individuals with darker skin, discoloration of the skin, warmth, oedema, or hardness may also be indicators.
- Category 2: partial-thickness skin loss involving epidermis, dermis, or both. The ulcer is superficial, and appears clinically as an abrasion, blister, or shallow crater.
- Category 3: full-thickness skin loss involving damage to, or necrosis of, subcutaneous tissue that may extend down to, but not through, underlying fascia. The ulcer appears clinically as a deep crater with or without undermining of adjacent tissues.
- Category 4: full-thickness skin loss with extensive destruction, tissue necrosis, or damage to muscle, bone, or supporting structures. Undermining and sinus tracts may also be associated with a category 4 ulcer.

Pressure ulcer prevention and care of immobilized patients

- Regular turning/repositioning schedule (at least every 2 hours).
- Toileting regimens for incontinent patients.
- Use of positioning/pressure-relieving devices including mattresses and cushions, positioning devices, etc.

References

1. NICE (2014). *Pressure Ulcers: Prevention and Management* (CG179). London: NICE.
2. NICE (2017). *Infection Prevention and Control* (QS61). London: NICE.
3. NICE (2017). *Surgical Site Infections: Prevention and Treatment* (CG74). London: NICE.

Discharge planning following orthopaedic surgery

Following surgery, some ADLs may require adjustment depending on how surgery has affected an individual. Adjustments should be anticipated pre-operatively and form part of the discharge process. Planning for discharge should begin at the point the patient is listed for surgery and the plan should be constantly updated throughout the current episode of care.

Patients and their relatives should be informed of the anticipated length of stay in hospital for the procedure they are undergoing.

Nurse-led discharge

The nurse is often the key coordinator in a patient's discharge, making decisions regarding the patient's fitness to leave hospital and coordinating the activities that facilitate this. This involves communication with other health professionals, both in 1° and 2° care settings, and the patient's family to ensure that services are in place for a safe discharge.

Discharge plans are multidisciplinary and include:

- An assessment of physical condition including general health, recovery from anaesthetic, pain control, infection screen, and wound healing.
- An occupational therapy assessment. This focuses on personal care, ADLs, and work that may have been affected by the surgery. The need for living aids or assistive devices is assessed and these should be provided prior to discharge.
- Physiotherapy includes assessing the patient's mobility, and mobility of any affected limb/joint. General advice on the need to be active and suggestions for sensible activities to ↑ post-discharge fitness is given.
- Social factors. Ensuring any care that may be required from relatives is available such as help with shopping, cleaning, and transport.
- Falls prevention. The risk of falling should be determined based on previous and current medical status, medications taken, the environment, visual acuity, and balance.
- Arrangements for transport home.

Patient education

Due to the ↑ pressure to discharge patients from hospital as early as possible following surgery, patients will be expected to continue rehabilitation at home, ∴ the patient and their significant others need to understand their ongoing treatment plan.

Prior to discharge patients should be advised of:

- Any changes to medications that have been instituted in hospital, and in particular regarding the use of analgesics and anticoagulants.
- Details of any ongoing physiotherapy/exercises they should be doing.
- Details of follow-up care required, i.e. for removal of sutures, outpatient physiotherapy, and consultant review.
- A point of contact for use if they have any questions regarding their care or in the event of any problems, particularly if these occur out of hours.
- Any surgical-specific precautions.

- The need to inform dental practitioners of prosthetic joint replacements. Antibiotic cover is required for any dental procedures lasting >30 min.
- Following patient consent, details of the implant type and size will be registered on the National Joint Register. This is important should there be any requirement for revision of the implant at any point in the future.

Hospital at home (H@H)/supported discharge schemes

The aim of such schemes is to facilitate early discharge from hospital by providing intensive levels of care and rehabilitation in the patient's home, that otherwise would be given in hospital. This support is for a defined time period.

Detailed admission and discharge criteria for the scheme have to be agreed and patients can then be referred from the scheme to community nursing services if required. All staff working in such schemes require multiple skills as it is not cost-effective to duplicate nurses and therapist visits to an individual patient.

There are two organizational models of H@H schemes:

- *Model 1*: nursing and therapists care is coordinated by a team of specialist practitioners from the 2° care sector. The medical responsibility for care remains with the orthopaedic consultant. Advantages of this model are that the practitioners are experts in the care that some patients require, which gives the consultants confidence in utilizing such services. In addition, access to reassessment or admission to hospital if necessary can be easier.
- *Model 2*: a community-based generic H@H service for a defined geographical population. This is an extension to existing community nursing services, with community nurses providing the care, and the responsibility of that care being with the GP. For this model of care to succeed, specialist training for staff involved is essential.

Postoperative follow-up

Due to changes in healthcare delivery and, in particular, a reduction of outpatient appointments, review of patients following orthopaedic surgery may be carried out by experienced practitioners, either nurses or PTs, who work as part of the surgical team. These may be undertaken in 1° or 2° care settings.

Not all surgical procedures require a follow-up visit; some follow-up consultations may be made by telephone.

Surgery to the spine

Various disorders affect the lower back. The most common causes of low back pain that may be considered for surgical intervention include the following:

Herniated vertebral disc

The nucleus pulposus extrudes through the annulus fibrosis, exerting direct contact on neural structures. The size of the spinal canal, the location of the defect, and size of herniation play a part in the decision to operate or treat conservatively. Pain is the 1° symptom. This can be intermittent in severity and frequency. Sciatica described as numbness, tingling, or burning sensation down the limb, is present if the damage is in the L4 region. Localized epidural steroid injection can offer sustained relief of pain in some patients. Spinal decompression for people with sciatica should only be considered when non-surgical treatment has not improved pain or function and radiological findings are consistent with sciatic symptoms.

Spondylolysis

Defect or break in the neural arch between the superior and inferior articulating surfaces. May progress to spondylolisthesis.

Spondylolisthesis

Forward subluxation of one vertebrae on another. Can be congenital or degenerative. Surgical treatment is considered if there is evidence of neurological deficit, persistent pain, a progressive slip, or a slip of >50%.

Spinal stenosis

Narrowing of the spinal canal. Can be congenital or degenerative and can occur at any region in the spine. Significant neurological compromise can occur if a narrowed canal is invaded by disc material. Signs and symptoms include neurogenic claudication, presenting as leg pain after walking, which is relieved by sitting or squatting.

Long-term results of spinal surgery are comparable to conservative treatment, therefore surgery is only considered in the presence of significant neurological deficit or red flags (Box 7.4).

Box 7.4 Red flags: possible indicators of serious pathology

- Thoracic pain.
- Fever and unexplained weight loss.
- Bladder and bowel dysfunction.
- History of carcinoma.
- Ill health.
- Progressive neurological deficit.
- Disturbed gait, saddle anaesthesia.
- Age of onset <20 years or >55 years.

Conservative management of back pain includes:
- Individualized exercise regimens/pain management techniques.
- NSAIDs and regular analgesia/antidepressants.
- Heat/ice/TENs machines.

Spinal decompression

The common goal of decompression surgery is to ensure careful freeing of the affected nerves by removal of bone, disc, and facet capsule. A combination of surgical techniques including discectomy, laminectomy, and foramenotomy are used to ensure a proper decompression of the nerve elements.

Spinal fusion

Spinal fusion aims to restore stability and spinal alignment. There are several approaches to spinal fusion including an anterior, posterior, or circumferential fusion, which can be performed with or without instrumentation. Spinal fusion should not be offered for people with low back pain unless as part of a randomized controlled trial.

Factors affecting outcome of surgery

Despite initial high success rates for spinal surgery, outcomes for patients can be disappointing over time (Box 7.5).

Principles of postoperative management after spinal surgery

Patients require a period of immobility postoperatively, ∴ prevention of complications such as chest infection, wound infection, ↑ risk of DVT, and pressure ulceration are key factors in postoperative management.
- *Assessment of neurological function*: sensory and motor function should be assessed every 2 hours for the first 24 hours postoperatively. Then 4–8-hourly. Cases of neurological damage have been reported up to 36 hours after surgery.
- *Pain control*: use of PCA in the immediate postoperative period (➲ see 'Patient-controlled analgesia', p. 260). Analgesia should enable early mobilization and be tailored to the individual patient's requirements.

Box 7.5 Causes for poor outcome from spinal surgery
- Recurrent disc herniation or spinal stenosis.
- Chronic nerve injury.
- Incomplete decompression.
- Infection.
- Failure of fusion to develop or poor postoperative alignment of spine.
- Loosening of instrumentation.
- Nerve irritation from instrumentation and subsequent pain.
- Incomplete diagnosis of problem preoperatively.
- Junctional failure of the spine where there is collapse/instability of a segment of the spine adjacent to a previously operated area.

General principles of body mechanics following spinal surgery

- Sleep on the side with knees bent and a supporting pillow between the legs.
- Avoid sleeping prone.
- Place a pillow under the knees for support when sleeping supine.
- After cervical surgery, use a flat pillow only.
- When getting up from the bed, the patient should roll onto their side and use their arms to push up while allowing the legs to swing slowly over the side of the bed.
- Avoid all movements that twist the neck or lower back.
- Avoid lifting any weight >~2.5–4.5 kg (~5–10 lb) in the initial 6 weeks postoperatively.

Further reading

NICE (2016). *Low Back Pain and Sciatica in Over 16s: Assessment and Management* (NG59). London: NICE.

Surgery to the hip and knee

Arthroplasty

Prosthetic arthroplasty (joint replacement) can relieve pain and improve function for patients with moderate to severe destruction of cartilage and subchondral bone. Arthroplasty of the hip is the most common operation performed in the world, closely followed by arthroplasty of the knee.

Total hip arthroplasty/THR

The surgeon may choose to use cemented or uncemented prosthesis, or a combination of the two. Selection of prosthesis is dependent on:

- Underlying pathology.
- Associated medical conditions.
- Patient's age.
- Potential postoperative activity.
- Choice of the surgeon.
- Implant availability.

THR has demonstrated excellent function for >15–20 years after which revision may be required. Revision surgery is more complex and involves removing the prosthetic bone components plus cement, followed by reconstruction of the joint using a new prosthesis and bone graft. Complications that may lead to revision surgery include prosthesis instability, dislocation, aseptic loosening, osteolysis (bone reabsorption), infection, and prosthesis failure.

Surface replacement hip arthroplasty

Surface replacement prosthesis MoM (metal on metal) were the procedure of choice for younger patients, undertaken as a first stage with a view to revision to a full THR at a later date. However, MoM implants can fail, ↑ the amount of wear and producing small amounts of debris from particles (ions) of cobalt and chromium that make up the implant. This can trigger progressive soft tissue reactions, erosion of bone, and loosening of the implants. The UK Medicines and Healthcare products Regulatory Agency (MHRA) has issued three alerts relating to MoM implants,[1] advising a schedule of review for all patients with these implants, which includes blood testing for whole-blood metal levels and MRI or US scans to determine the need for revision surgery. There is no agreed threshold value for whole-blood metal levels that either predicts outcome or mandates revision. Decisions to revise are influenced by patient factors, blood metal levels, imaging findings, and implant type and position.

Total knee arthroplasty/TKR

TKR is the current treatment choice for bi- or tri-compartmental knee arthritis. TKR prosthesis are designed to replace only the joint surface necessitating minimal bone resection, therefore bone stock is preserved which maintains treatment options in the event of joint failure. A major factor in preventing early joint failure is that all TKR prostheses allow some rotation and unlimited flexion. TKR prostheses can be cemented or uncemented.

Contraindications to TKR

- Relative contraindications: high activity expectations and long life expectancy.
- Absolute contraindications: presence of active infection, including conditions that may produce non-healing ulcers of the ipsilateral lower extremity.

Unicompartmental knee replacement (hemiarthroplasty)

If OA is limited to the medial or lateral compartment, a unicompartmental knee replacement may be considered. The success rate of this procedure is 95% after 5 years. Hemiarthroplasty does allow conversion to TKR if necessary in the future.

Minimally invasive THR/TKR

Minimally invasive THR and TKR surgical techniques have been developed using a much smaller incision and an approach that aims to reduce damage to the muscles and tendons around the joint than conventional THR/TKR surgery. The overall rate of complications is not significantly different between patients treated by minimally invasive surgery, however this approach has the potential to reduce the length of stay in hospital.

For TKR, it has been reported that achievable flexion was significantly greater in knees treated by mini-incision surgery, however the mean time to revision surgery was significantly shorter than patients treated by a standard approach.

High tibial osteotomy (HTO) of the knee

Due to the success rate of knee arthroplasty, HTO which involves resection of a wedge of bone from either the lateral or medial side of the upper tibia is rarely undertaken; however, in the future, this procedure may be combined with osteochondral allografting techniques or autologous meniscal transplantation which are currently under development.

Arthrodesis/fusion of the knee

This is the treatment choice for pain control in:

- Young active or heavy patients with end-stage unilateral disease.
- Those with relative or absolute contraindications for arthroplasty.

Surgery involves trimming of the articular surfaces of the distal femur and proximal tibia to provide flat surfaces across which fusion can occur. Postoperatively, the joint is immobilized usually in an Ilizarov external fixator frame for a period of up to 3 months. Partial weight-bearing may be necessary during this time.

Knee fusion results in an immobile joint fixed in extension, with a shortening of the limb by ~1 cm. This procedure is performed rarely and is poorly tolerated by patients.

Arthroscopy and debridement

Arthroscopy involves the visualization of the inside of the joint with the aid of an arthroscope. NICE guidelines indicate this procedure for continued locking and giving way of the knee joint.[2]

Autologous cartilage transplant

This is a two-stage procedure, involving taking cartilage cells from a non-weight-bearing aspect of the patient's joint and transplanting these cells 4–6 weeks later onto the defective area of the joint. This procedure has the potential to provide pain relief while at the same time slowing down the progression or considerably delaying partial or total joint replacement surgery. Common serious adverse events have been described in up to 5% of patients, and include symptomatic hypertrophy, disturbed fusion, delamination, and graft failure.

References

1. Medicines and Healthcare products Regulation Agency (2017). *Metal-on-Metal Hip Replacements: Updated Advice for Follow-Up of Patients* (MDA/2017/018). London: MHRA.
2. NICE (2007). *Arthroscopic Knee Washout, With or Without Debridement, for the Treatment of Osteoarthritis* (IPG230). London: NICE.

Further reading

NICE (2010). *Mini-Incision Surgery for Total Knee Replacement* (IPG345). London: NICE.
NICE (2010). *Minimally Invasive Total Hip Replacement* (IPG363). London: NICE.
NICE (2014). *Osteoarthritis: Care and Management* (CG177). London: NICE.
NICE (2014). *Total Hip Replacement and Resurfacing Arthroplasty for End-Stage Arthritis of the Hip* (TA304). London: NICE.
Niemeyer P (2008). Characteristic complications after autologous chondrocyte implantation for cartilage defects of the knee joint. *Am J Sports Med* 36:2091–9.

Principles of postoperative care for total hip/knee arthroplasty

ICPs are often used to provide a framework for planning and delivering care during a surgical episode of care.

Nursing management

- Management of pain.
- Assessment of neurovascular status in both lower limbs.
- Monitoring fluid balance and vital signs.
- Assessment of dressings/drains for excessive output.
- Chest physiotherapy.
- Encouragement of leg exercises to ↓ risk of DVT.
- Initiating mobilization and return to independence.

Common postoperative complications of THR/TKR

DVT

Follow locally accepted guidelines for the prevention of DVT/PE.

Dislocation of THR prosthesis

Occurs most commonly 2–5 days postoperatively. Signs and symptoms of dislocation include:

- Severe pain.
- Internal rotation of the limb.
- Limb shortening.

Infection

Risk ↓ in the immediate postoperative period to ~1% due to modern surgical techniques and the use of prophylactic antibiotics and antibiotic-infused bone cement.

Late complications

- Late sepsis around the prosthesis. Can occur 6–24 months postoperatively in 1–4% of THR prosthesis. Delayed infections in TKRs have been reported in 4.1% of patients, an average of 7 years postoperatively. Treatment of joint infection usually requires a two-stage operative procedure to remove the infected prosthesis and treatment with IV antibiotics for at least 6 weeks before insertion of a new joint.
- Long-term prosthetic loosening—may necessitate revision surgery. Failure rate of THR revision surgery is 10% at 5 years.
- Leg length discrepancy—may require orthotic shoe raise to correct.

Postoperative education for THR and TKR

Discuss the use of prophylactic antibiotics for future surgical dental procedures that can cause transient bacteraemia and ↑ the risk of joint infection.

Precautions following THR

Avoid extreme positions until surrounding soft tissue is healed—up to 6 weeks postoperatively (Box 7.6).

Patient education following TKR

- Optimum recovery may take up to 12 months.
- Swelling of the leg up to 1 year postoperatively is normal.
- Continued exercise is vital to achieve potential range of movement.
- Surgeons usually suggest patients do not kneel for 6 months following TKR although it is not an absolute contraindication. Numbness of the knee may result in hesitancy to kneel. Patients should be taught to kneel on a soft surface and to rise from kneeling using the unaffected leg.

Box 7.6 Precautions following total hip replacement

- Avoid bending >90°:
  - Dress operated leg first, and undress last.
  - Do not bend at the waist to tie shoes.
  - Use high chair with supportive arms/raised toilet seat.
  - Use long-handled aids to pick things up from the floor.
  - Lead with unoperated leg when ascending stairs.
  - Lead with operated leg when descending stairs.
- In the absence of pain, sexual intercourse may be resumed 6 weeks postoperatively, unless advised otherwise by the surgeon.
- Avoid crossing operative leg past the body's midline (adduction):
  - Get out of bed on the operated side.
  - Sleep on your back (6 weeks); may need to use pillow to maintain abduction.
- Avoid twisting the leg in or out (internal/external rotation):
  - Lead with your feet when changing direction, avoid twisting your body.
- Use correct walking aid.

Ankle and foot surgery

Ankle surgery

Treatment of end-stage ankle arthritis remains controversial. Treatment options include the following:

Arthrodesis (fusion) of the ankle

Normally carried out using internal fixation methods. If performed relatively early in the hindfoot for significant flat foot deformity, a simple subtalar fusion may suffice. With longer established deformities and subluxation of the talonavicular joint, a triple arthrodesis may be required. This involves fusion of the talonavicular, calcaneocuboid, and subtalar joints. The planned outcome of the surgical procedure is ensuring that the foot is plantigrade or flat to the ground. Postoperative rehabilitation requires a period of non-weight-bearing for up to 6 weeks, often in a short leg cast, followed by a further 6 weeks in an ambulatory cast.

Arthroplasty/replacement of the ankle

The advantage of arthroplasty is that when successful, it maintains motion and reduces strain on adjacent joints. Problems such as wound healing complications and implant subsidence have improved with newer designs of prosthesis in recent years; however, if the joint fails, salvage can be difficult, particularly after deep infection, which if painful and non-responsive to treatment may require a below-knee amputation.

Foot surgery

Excision arthroplasty

Surgical reconstruction of the forefoot is performed to:

Correct hammertoes

The proximal joint is fixed in flexion while the distal and MTP joints are extended. The pressure of shoes over the deformity causes painful callosities, which if the skin becomes broken, and can be a potential source in infection.

Dorsal dislocation of the lesser MTP joints

Often occurs in patients with RA. Patients complain of callosities under the metatarsal heads and pain is described as 'walking on pebbles'. Excision of the metatarsal head is performed to allow realignment of the forefoot.

Severe hallux valgus deformity (bunion)

This is a static subluxation of the first MTP joint in which there are three features:

- The first toe angulates laterally towards the second toe.
- The middle portion of the first metatarsal head enlarges.
- The bursa over the medial aspect of the MTP joint becomes inflamed and thick walled.

This may be asymptomatic or a source of chronic pain and disability. Conservative management includes advice on good footwear and padding of the deformity. Surgery involves metatarsal osteotomy, or excision of the proximal phalanx. Arthrodesis of the MTP joint is also considered an option for advanced hallux valgus deformity.

Nursing management

- Foot surgery can be extremely painful, ∴ adequate pain management is essential.
- Knowledge of the postoperative plan of care is essential to enable patients to take an active part in their recovery.
- Mobility may require the use of crutches or alternative walking aids. Practice preoperatively may help to allay anxiety.

Wrist and hand surgery

Good hand function is essential for performing most ADLs and leisure pursuits. The wrist and hand joints are prone to both OA and inflammatory arthritis; however, surgical intervention is more commonly performed for patients with inflammatory arthritis. In RA, erosive damage to hand joints can occur very early in the disease process.

Common deformities of the hand as a result of RA have ↓ in frequency over the past 10 years as a result of improved medical management, but can include:

- Ulnar drift caused by damage at the MCP joint, aggravated by normal activities.
- Swan neck deformities: hyperextension of the PIP joint with flexion of the MCP and DIP joint.
- Boutonnière deformity: flexion if the PIP joint and hyperextension of the DIP joint.
- Z deformity of the thumb: instability of the MCP or IP joint. Fusion of the thumb is usually the procedure of choice, giving the patients a stable thumb and ↑ the strength of the pinch grip.

➲ See Chapter 4, 'Rheumatoid arthritis', pp. 64–80.

Surgical interventions to the hand and wrist

Carpal tunnel decompression

Carpal tunnel decompression is the most common compression neuropathy affecting the hand. Pain is caused by compression of the median nerve as it passes with the flexor tendons, through the carpal tunnel at the wrist. Symptoms can vary from a mild tingling on the palmer aspect of the thumb and first three fingers, to loss of motor function and intense pain that disrupts sleep. There can also be a loss of grip strength and wasting of the thenar muscle.

Surgical decompression is usually carried out as a day case. Normal activities are encouraged as soon as comfortable postoperatively. Grip strength and endurance may take 3–6 months to achieve, and for some may remain incomplete.

Arthrodesis (fusion) of the wrist

Advanced degenerative disease of the IP joints, carpus, and wrist is commonly treated by arthrodesis which affords long-term pain relief and stability.

Arthroplasty of the wrist

Total wrist replacement (TWR) aims to create a stable, pain-free joint with a functional range of movement. There is evidence that TWR relieves pain, but there is insufficient evidence of its efficacy in the long term ∴TWR should be undertaken only on carefully selected patients, who understand the possible alternatives to TWR and the uncertainty about its efficacy in the long term, as further surgery may be required, including fusion of the wrist joint.

Synovectomy of the wrist

Synovial proliferation can destroy articular cartilage, causing instability and ∴ deformity. When the articular cartilage is intact, early synovectomy can be of benefit.

Tendon rupture/transfer

The loss of extension at the MCP joint, due to rupturing of the extensor tendon—particularly of the little finger—requires urgent surgical attention as direct repair of the tendon can only be undertaken in the acute phase.

Prophylactic tenosynovectomy

If it is clinically suspected that the extensor tendons are at risk, prophylactic tenosynovectomy may be performed. This is often undertaken with resection of bony prominences at the distal radioulnar joint (➔ see 'Synovectomy and excision of the radial head', p. 283).

MCP joint arthroplasty

Silicone MCP implants may be used for hands that are painful and have fixed deformities. Patients generally report a subjective functional improvement and improved appearance postoperatively; however, reported rates of fracture of implant can vary between 0% and 50%.

Nursing management and common postoperative complications

- *Pain relief*: usually managed with oral analgesia.
- *Assistance with self-care and ADLs*: the ability to wash and dress and carry out other self-care tasks may be impaired postoperatively. Referral to the OT preoperatively may result in the provision of aids to help in the performance of such activities. Help may be required on discharge and assessment of self-care should form part of the discharge planning process.
- *Splintage*: splintage to help pain control and support the operated area in an acceptable position is common following all types of hand/wrist surgery while healing is taking place.
- *Altered body image*: disfigurement of the hand and wrist can have a profound effect on an individual's body image. Surgery may be corrective; however, limiting a person's ability to self-care and the use of sometimes prolonged splintage can have a negative impact on body image. Good preoperative information and the opportunity to discuss and view the splintage may avoid unnecessary distress.

Further reading

NICE (2005). *Artificial Metacarpophalangeal and Interphalangeal Joint Replacement for End-Stage Arthritis* (IPG110). London: NICE.

NICE (2008). *Total Wrist Replacement* (IPG271). London: NICE.

Elbow surgery

OA of the elbow is usually mild as the elbow joint is a slight weight-bearing joint when compared to the lower limb joints. However, individuals who extensively overuse their upper extremities, e.g. labourers or athletes, can experience disabling pain and loss of movement as a result of OA of the elbow.

Elbow arthroplasty

Total elbow arthroplasty (TEA) is more often carried out as a result of 2° OA following an injury to the humeral, ulnar, or radioulnar joints, or for patients with RA or haemophilia. Results of TEA for 1° OA and those of a younger age group can be poor due to the heavier loading applied on the replaced joint. However, the results for surgery for individuals with RA are comparable to THR/TKR, in that 90% of patients report dramatic pain relief. Functional improvements of 90% ↑ in strength of flexion and 60–70% ↑ in pronation and supination have also been reported. These ranges include the functional arcs of movement required for ADLs.

Presenting symptoms

- Pain and stiffness at the elbow.
- Limitations in ADLs, e.g. difficulty in:
  - Lifting or receiving an item onto the hand (supination).
  - Writing (pronation).
  - Eating, dressing, or grooming which require flexion at the elbow.

The aim of surgery is to provide a stable, painless range of movement during ADLs.

Two types of prosthesis are commonly used:

- An unconstrained surface replacement—main problems postoperatively relate to joint instability in 20–50% of cases.
- A linked semi-constrained prosthesis—the ulnar and humeral components are linked to reduce the risk of dislocation, but the linkage allows a degree of laxity that permits the soft tissue to absorb some of the stresses that would normally be applied to the prosthesis–bone interface and reduces the risk of joint loosening.

Nursing management/common postoperative complications

- Pain control.
- Assessment of neurovascular status. Risk of temporary/permanent ulnar nerve injury during surgery. Evaluate motion and sensation of fourth and fifth fingers on operated side. Immediately postoperatively, oedema may minimize the patient's ability to abduct/abduct the fingers. Some numbness may continue for 6–8 weeks post surgery.
- Assessment of dressings/drains. As the skin around the elbow is thin with little subcutaneous tissue, the wound may be prone to complications including infection or wound breakdown. Infection rates have been reported to be between 2% and 5%.
- Assistance with aspects of ADLs. Post surgery, the joint is protected in 90% flexion with a back-slab or firm padding and crepe bandaging. This may be replaced with a polyurethane splint after 48 hours. This splint may be used for up 6 weeks except when exercising.

Exercise

- Gentle, active, assisted elbow flexion, passive gravity extension, and forearm rotation are commenced 1–3 days postoperatively.
- Gradual strengthening exercises for triceps and biceps are added as healing progresses.
- Avoid extension >30% to prevent subluxation or dislocation.
- Encourage extension after 6 weeks.

Patient education

- Normal activities, such as light housework, can be resumed after 4–6 weeks.
- Light gardening after 6 weeks.
- Driving after 8 weeks.
- Strenuous activities such as carrying heavy shopping and contact sports should be avoided.

Synovectomy and excision of the radial head

More commonly performed in individuals with 2° OA, as a result of RA or haemophilia. (➔ See 'Prophylactic tenosynovectomy', p. 281.)

Presenting symptoms

- Persistent synovitis around the elbow.
- ↓ ROM, particularly extension.
- Pain particularly on supination and pronation.
- On examination, clinical involvement of the radiohumeral or radioulnar joint.

Nursing management and patient education

Mild, active assisted motion of the elbow is commenced 4 days postoperatively, progressing to active motion as pain allows. Pain usually improves as strength improves.

Pain can continue to reduce over the initial 3–6 months postoperatively. ROM can continue to improve for 6 months.

Shoulder surgery

The shoulder is the most mobile joint in the body. OA of the shoulder often occurs from either significant trauma, 2° to RA, or a chronic tear in the rotator cuff. Shoulder motion is provided by the rotator cuff and deltoid muscles ∴ any tear in the rotator cuff can be associated with significant ↓ in ROMs which can compromise the results of any chosen surgical option.

Surgical repair of torn rotator cuff

The commonest cause of rotator cuff damage is from repetitive injury. Commonly presents in patients >40 years of age. Surgery may not lead to any improvement in pain, compared to exercise. Some large rotator cuff tears may not be repairable. In this instance, decompression and debridement may be the treatment of choice.

Presenting symptoms

- Pain.
- Limitation of active abduction beyond 25°. If the arm is passively abducted, the patient may then be able to hold it in that position due to the action of the deltoid muscles.
- Limitation of backwards extension and external rotation. This affects activities such as putting the arm into a sleeve.

Surgical repair can be undertaken using an open or arthroscopic approach. Long-term outcomes of arthroscopic surgery are comparable to open surgery and recovery may be quicker.

Nursing management

- Immobilization of the affected joint, to promote tissue repair.
- A poly-sling is worn when not exercising to provide support and pain relief.
- Passive elevation and external rotation exercises are commenced while in hospital and continued for 6 weeks postoperatively.
- Patients are encouraged to lift the arm with the elbow bent to create a short lever and less stress in the first 3 months post surgery. The arm must not be lifted above shoulder level.
- Active exercises are commenced after 6 weeks with the aim of mobilizing the shoulder and strengthening muscles when the tendon has healed.

Common postoperative complications

- Deltoid detachment or failure of the repair.
- Deep infection.

Patient education

- Postoperative rehabilitation including the ability to fully self-care can be prolonged. This must be fully understood preoperatively. In some instances, support with ADLs may need to be organized on discharge.
- Driving can be recommenced after 6 weeks.

Shoulder resurfacing arthroplasty (SRA)

Primary OA and RA account for ~85% of all SRAs. The main indication for surgery is relief of pain, particularly night pain. Restoration of movement and strength is dependent on the condition of the rotator cuff. Patients need to be motivated and understand that it can take up to 12 months before the full benefit of surgery is obtained.

The aim of SRA is to replace only the damaged joint surfaces, with minimal bone resection. The surface of the humeral head is exposed and reamed to restore its shape. Fixation of the articular prosthesis, which may cover the whole or part of the humeral head, is made using morcellized bone or cement. A prosthesis may be used to cover the glenoid surface of the scapula if necessary. Adverse events to SRA include loosening of the prosthesis, impingement, and overstuffing during implant if the prosthesis had been incorrectly sized. Other adverse events include infection, nerve injury, DVT, fracture, failure needing revision, and stiffness.

Nursing management and common postoperative complications

- Pain control: may necessitate the use of PCA analgesia. Step-down analgesia is essential to enable patients to take part in rehabilitation. A poly-sling is worn when not exercising for support.
- Neurovascular assessment: risk of damage to axillary nerve and brachial plexus during surgery.

Assessment of nerve function

- Motor function of the radial nerve: assess the patient's ability to abduct the thumb.
- Motor function of the ulnar nerve: assess the patient's ability to abduct or spread the fingers apart against pressure.
- Axillary nerve function: ask the patient to push the elbows out against resistance.
- Assistance with ADLs: patients require help with most care activities in the initial postoperative period.

Exercise

- 48 hours postoperatively—passive motion exercises. Aim to achieve 140° of forward elevation and 40° of external rotation.
- 10 days post surgery—assisted exercises to gain rotation and isometric exercises to strengthen the rotator cuff and deltoid muscles Followed by active abduction and flexion.
- 3 weeks post surgery—resisted exercise and passive stretching, commenced, to ↑ muscle power and improve active/passive ROM.
- Exercise to be continued for minimum of 6 months.

Patient education

- Avoid housework for 4 weeks.
- Driving and sedentary work can be recommenced after 6 weeks. Patients with more strenuous jobs may not be able to return to work for up to 12 weeks.

Further reading

NICE (2010). *Shoulder Resurfacing Arthroplasty* (IPG354). London: NICE.

Part II

Clinical issues

Assessing the patient: History taking and clinical examination

Assessing the patient

History taking and examining the patient are essential to making an accurate diagnosis. A thorough medical history is key to the first step towards a diagnosis and will inform the examination and determine appropriate investigations. A clinical history taking can guide the practitioner to a diagnosis whereas examination and investigations merely confirm or refute that considered diagnosis.

The essentials of good consultation and history taking

- Put the patient at ease.
- Establish a rapport with the patient.
- Use open questions to allow the patient to tell their story. Explore the presenting problem, using open and closed questions to clarify and elicit a full history.
- Use your listening skills to be attentive to the patient and the information they provide.
- Remember non-verbal communication is as important as verbal, e.g. eye contact, facial expression, posture, and position.
- Clarify, reflect back, and summarize to verify your understanding of what the patient is saying.
- Explore the patient's ideas and beliefs, concerns, and expectations.
- Establish a logical sequence of events.
- Show empathy and interest.

History taking consists of a series of topics, which move sequentially to explore the whole of the history (Box 8.1).

Presenting complaint

This is a short statement summarizing the patient's presenting symptoms that have brought the patient to seek advice.

History of presenting complaint

An exploration of the symptoms to elicit the cause and effect and factors that precipitated the problem or specific factors that brought on the symptoms. If the patient is able to recount any specific event consider factors such as trauma, overuse, or infections. Infections prior to onset of symptoms are important in viral or reactive forms of arthritis. When the symptoms are insidious in nature, they are less likely to be able to pinpoint any specific event.

Box 8.1 A sequence to use for history taking

- Presenting complaint.
- History of presenting complaint.
- Previous medical history.
- Drug history.
- Family history.
- Social history.
- Systems review—general examination.

Table 8.1 An example of using SOCRATES for exploring pain

S	Site	Where? Radiation? Numbness? Pattern
O	Onset	When and how it started? Changed factors?
C	Character	E.g. type of pain—shooting, burning, tingling?
R	Radiation	Does the pain go elsewhere?
A	Associated feature	Aggravating/relieving factors
T	Timing	Is it best or worse at different times of day?
E	Exacerbation	Exacerbating or relieving factors
S	Severity	Rated on a scale of 1–10, e.g. effect on sleep

Pain

As pain is the most common presenting complaint in MSCs, it is important to explore the nature of the pain.

A structured approach to the consultation and examination should be undertaken and mnemonics such as 'SOCRATES' may be helpful (Table 8.1).

Previous medical history

Related to an existing diagnosis/long-standing disease? Relevance of past medical history, e.g. associated diagnostic criteria. Previous blood tests, investigations, or presenting features, e.g. an asthmatic using long-term steroids leading to osteoporosis.

Drug history

Past and current medication.

Family history

Predisposing or genetic factors to aid diagnosis, e.g. a family history of IJD.

Social history

Explore the context of the symptoms and how they are affecting the patient.

Systems review

Examination of all health systems to identify any factors that might confirm or reveal signs aiding diagnostic decisions.

➔ Also see 'History taking and clinical examination', pp. 292–293.

History taking and examination: practical points

There are three key screening questions to ask the patient:

- Do you have any pain or stiffness in your muscles, joints, or spine?
- Are you able to dress or undress yourself without any difficulty?
- Are you able to walk up and down stairs without any difficulty?

In addition to the routine clinical history taking and full examination some specific factors should be considered:

- *Stiffness*—present in both IJD and degenerative joint disease. Ask the patient if there is any particular time of day when symptoms are present or worse:
  - The presence of EMS is a classic finding in IJD. Duration of stiffness is an indicator to the severity of the problem, e.g. in poorly controlled inflammatory arthritis (e.g. RA) stiffness can last all day.
  - In contrast, mechanical or degenerative joint disease (e.g. OA) stiffness is usually associated with inactivity or at the end of the day.
- *Swelling*—in the absence of trauma may be indicative of an inflammatory process:
  - Is the swelling localized or diffuse?
  - Site of swelling, e.g. on the joint line or in the periarticular structures such as tendons (tenosynovitis) or bursae (bursitis)?
  - Patterns of joint involvement aid diagnosis, e.g. distribution of joint involvement in seronegative spondyloarthropathies.
- *Tingling, numbness, or paraesthesia*—may indicate nerve entrapment, e.g.:
  - Tingling in the thumb, index, middle finger, and half of the ring finger seen in CTS.
  - Numbness and tingling down the leg below the knee—consider sciatica nerve entrapment.
- *Muscle weakness*—is this localized or generalized weakness?
  - Localized weakness indicates a focal problem, e.g. peripheral nerve lesion.
  - Generalized weaknesses—consider a systemic cause such as a myopathy.
- *Deformity*—may be associated with pain but can cause concern to the patient even if symptoms are absent, e.g. Heberden's nodes, on the DIP joints caused by OA, can be quite disfiguring, but are not always painful.
- *Systemic symptoms*—may indicate a more serious inflammatory process or sinister pathology:
  - Weight loss.
  - Anorexia.
  - Fatigue.
  - Malaise.
  - Night sweats.
  - Fever.
- *Sleep disturbance*—several factors may interfere with normal sleep patterns including anxiety and depression. Poor sleep pattern is also a feature of fibromyalgia.

Previous medical history

Are symptoms related to an existing diagnosis/long-standing disease? Explore past medical history for causal factors that may put patient at risk, e.g. an asthmatic using long-term steroids without bone protection leading to osteoporosis.

Drug history

Detailed drug history (past and present):

- Consider a drug side effect (e.g. statins causing myalgias) or precipitating problems (e.g. drug-induced lupus or diuretics precipitating an acute flare of gout).
- Review prescribed medications and if benefits of treatment were achieved. May also provide an indication of an existing diagnosis the patient has failed to mention.

Family history

Some rheumatic conditions have a familial predisposition (e.g. family history of psoriasis, uveitis, or inflammatory bowel disease may point to a diagnosis of a spondyloarthropathy).

Social history

Provides an insight into how the condition affects the patient's life. Considerations should include:

- Marital status and dependants.
- Home environment (bathroom facilities, stairs, etc.).
- Occupation and ability to maintain work with current symptoms.
- Infrastructures that maintain independence, e.g. car owner or ability to access public transport.
- ADL restrictions or problems as a result of the current problem, including hobbies and participation in social interaction.
- Psychological status including perceptions related to the presenting complaint, expectations, needs, and health beliefs/behaviours will have an effect on the individual's ability to cope with symptoms and possible treatment options. Managing expectations of the patient may need to be negotiated.

Review of systems

This is a methodical approach to examine all health systems to identify key indicators that may lead to or confirm a diagnosis.

➔ Also see 'History taking: assessing the patient', pp. 290–293.

For additional information on individual joint assessment, ➔ see Chapter 6, 'Chronic inflammatory pain', pp. 185–247.

History taking and clinical examination: systems review

The clinical examination is part of a comprehensive process necessary to identify clinical findings in relation to a patient's presenting complaint. Combined with history taking, the clinical examination should enable the practitioner to define abnormalities or indicators that build a diagnostic picture (➔ see 'Assessing the patient', pp. 290–291; ➔ 'Primary care walk-in clinics', Chapter 6, p. 218).

Systems review

A full clinical examination should always include a review of all body systems to ensure an accurate diagnostic picture. There are many common characteristics or links in MSCs, yet there are also areas where a differential diagnosis is sought between one MSC and another (e.g. scleroderma or SLE). Take note of:

- General: weight loss, anorexia, night sweats are all common systemic features of IJD.
- Cardiovascular or respiratory: episode of pleuritic or pericardial pain (SLE); breathlessness may be associated with anaemia of chronic disease (RA) or pulmonary fibrosis (seropositive arthritis); absence of peripheral pulses (vasculitis); haemoptysis (GPA).
- GI/abdominal GI symptoms such as diarrhoea (ReA or a seronegative arthritis associated with inflammatory bowel disease if chronic); oesophageal reflux and dysphagia (systemic sclerosis).
- Genitourinary/gynaecological symptoms: urethral discharge (ReA); genital ulceration (Behçet's disease); dyspareunia due to vaginal dryness (SS); late miscarriages (APS).
- Skin and mucous membranes: psoriasis, photosensitive rash (SLE or another CTD); oral ulceration (SLE); xerostomia, i.e. dry mouth (SS); symptoms of Raynaud's phenomenon worsening in later life or new-onset Raynaud's is associated with CTDs or exacerbated by medications, e.g. beta blockers.
- Eye symptoms, particularly episodes of acute red eyes: conjunctivitis (ReA); uveitis (spondyloarthropathies); episcleritis (painless); scleritis (painful); keratoconjunctivitis (RA) or xerophthalmia, i.e. dry eyes (SS); visual disturbance and blindness (temporal arteritis).

General examination including joint examination

Routine checks

All patients with musculoskeletal disease, whether being admitted to a ward or being seen in clinic, should have regular assessments that include:

- Urinalysis checked for blood, protein, and glucose:
  - Blood and protein are indicative of renal involvement; particularly important if the patient has a CTD.
  - Blood and protein may indicate an infection in a patient on immunosuppressive therapy, indicating a need for further investigation (e.g. midstream specimen of urine).

- Some drugs require monitoring of the urine for side effects (e.g. ciclosporin, cyclophosphamide).
- Glycosuria may be present and may indicate the development of diabetes (key in those treated with long-term corticosteroid therapy).

- Blood pressure:
  - ↑ blood pressure may again indicate renal involvement in CTD or hypertension requiring further treatment.
  - Regular monitoring is required for some medications of the blood pressure, e.g. ciclosporin and leflunomide.
- Weight and height should be recorded for baseline measurements:
  - Weight may be required to calculate drug dosages.
  - Height is also useful for assessing if there is a loss of height as a result of osteoporosis.

➲ See Chapter 17, 'Tests and investigations', pp. 505–535.

Further reading

Warrell DA, Cox TM, Firth JD (2019). *Oxford Textbook of Medicine*, 6th edn. Oxford: Oxford University Press.

General principles of joint examination

A good musculoskeletal examination relies on patient cooperation in order for them to relax their muscles so that important clinical signs are not missed:

- Always introduce yourself before undertaking any joint examination.
- Explain what you are going to do and gain the consent of the patient.
- Ask the patient to let you know if they experience any pain or discomfort at any time during the examination.
- Musculoskeletal examination should compare both sides of the body to assess for asymmetry in colour, deformity, swelling, function, and muscle wasting (Figs. 8.1 and 8.2).

Gait, arms, legs, spine (GALS)

GALS is a brief and sensitive way of assessing the whole of the musculoskeletal system for any signs of early disease and to identify areas where there is a problem that needs to be examined in more details. It looks at the first movements affected in any musculoskeletal disease or pathology.

Table 8.2 shows the recording of a normal GALS screen where gait is normal, and appearance and movement of arms, legs, and spine are all normal. The findings of the GALS screen can be tabulated in a shorthand form.

➲ Also see 'Musculoskeletal physical examination', Chapter 8, pp. 298–299; ➲ Primary care walk-in clinics', Chapter 6, pp. 218–219.

If an inflammatory arthritis is suspected

If an inflammatory arthritis is suspected based upon the clinical assessment and presenting signs and symptoms, patients should be promptly managed so that a firm diagnosis is made, and, if appropriate, treatment can be instigated based upon a treat to target approach. For RA this approach would require a 28 joint-count disease assessment tool (DAS28). Tender and swollen joints commonly affected are examined and scored, together with bloods for ESR or CRP and a patient global assessment of their general well-being using a VAS. The DAS28 has been validated for use with either ESR or CRP. However, whichever blood test is used, the subsequent

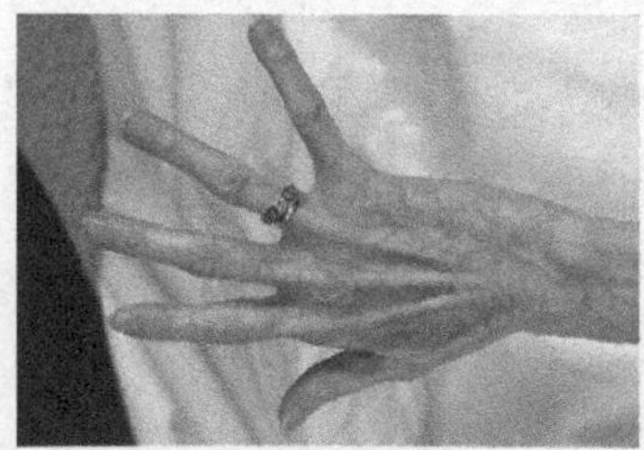

Fig. 8.1 Examination of hands.

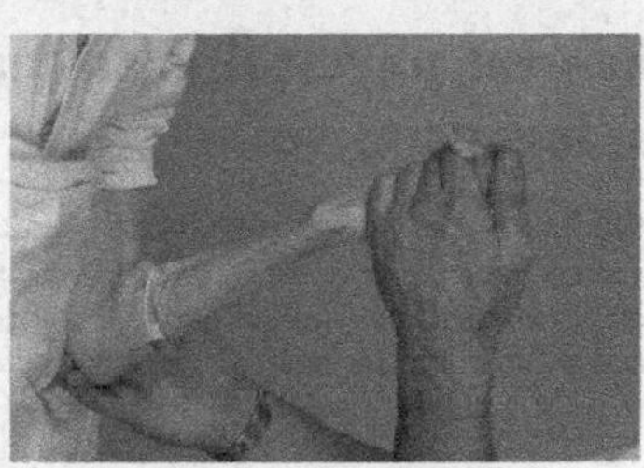

Fig. 8.2 Examination of arms.

Table 8.2 A normal GALS screen

Gait	Appearance	Movement
Arms	✓	✓
Legs	✓	✓
Spine	✓	✓

assessments should use the same blood test for calculating the DAS28 score. The calculation (using a DAS calculator) provides a composite score, e.g. 5.15, the DAS28 score. The DAS28 score for high disease activity is >5.15 with scores between 3.2 and 5.1 considered moderate disease activity. A score <3.2 is considered low disease activity and <2.6 remission.

➔ Also see 'Rheumatoid arthritis: assessing and managing the disease', Chapter 4, pp. 64–80.

Musculoskeletal physical examination: gait, arms, legs, and spine

There are three key screening questions to ask the patient

- Do you have any pain or stiffness in your muscles, joints, or spine?
- Are you able to dress or undress yourself without any difficulty?
- Are you able to walk up and downstairs without any difficulty?

Gait

Observe the patient walking, turning, and walking back:

- Look for symmetry of movement in the arms, legs, and pelvic movements; normal stride length; and the ability to turn quickly.
- Observe for an asymmetric antalgic gait where pain or deformity causes the patient to hurry from one leg onto the other.

Inspection of the patient standing in the anatomical position

- Observe from posterior, anterior, and lateral views.
- Inspect for normal muscle bulk and symmetry of shoulder girdles, spine, arms, buttocks, thighs, and calves.
- Observe for any obvious signs of swollen or deformed joints, including knees and toes or signs of flexion deformity, e.g. at the elbows.
- Inspect for normal spinal curves—cervical lordosis, thoracic kyphosis, lumbar lordosis, or signs of scoliosis in the spine.
- Look at symmetry of level iliac crests and gluteal folds.
- Signs of valgus or varus deformities in the knees or ankles, hip or knee flexion deformities, or signs of hyperextension of the knee (known as genu recurvatum).
- Signs of rheumatoid nodules of extensors surfaces of elbows and Achilles tendons.
- Signs of olecranon bursitis (at the elbow) or Achilles bursitis.
- Normal alignment and thickness of the Achilles tendon.
- Popliteal swelling, indicating a Baker's cyst.
- Loss of the medial arches of the foot.
- Ask the patient to open their jaw and move it from side to side (temporomandibular joint).
- Ask the patient to try and put their ear to their shoulder on each side (lateral flexion of cervical spine).
- Press over the midpoint of the supraspinatus muscle and roll the skin over the trapezius muscle. A wince and withdraw indicates the hyperalgesic response of fibromyalgia.
- Ask the patient to bend forward from the waist to touch the toes, place a couple of fingers over the spinous processes and see if they move together on standing upright (if they do not this may be a sign of inflammatory spine disease).
- Place the patient's hands behind their head and push their elbows back (this tests abduction and external rotation of the shoulders as well as flexion at the elbows).

- Keeping their elbows tucked in ask the patient to bring their hands up to in front:
  - Inspect the palms of the hands for swelling, wasting, or other deformity.
  - Turn the hands over, keeping the elbows tucked in to the side (this tests pronation and supination of both elbows and wrist).
  - Inspect the dorsum of the hands for muscle wasting, swelling, and deformity.
  - Inspect the nails for any signs of pitting or onycholysis (seen in PsA), nailfold infarct, or splinter haemorrhages (possible vasculitis activity).
  - Ask the patient to make a fist, test power grip.
  - Touch the pulp of each of the fingers to the thumb (opposition).
  - Squeeze across the MCP joints—pain indicates signs of inflammatory synovitis.

Examination of the patient lying on the couch

- Ask the patient to bend their knee and bring their heel as close in to their buttock as they can, one leg at a time.
- Place your hand over the knee to feel for any crepitus.
- While the knee is flexed, take the hip up to 90° and internally rotate the hip:
  - Achieved by holding the lower part of the leg and pushing the foot outwards.
  - Note how far the hip moves—in ♀ this ROM is > ♂.
  - Early disease in the hip will elicit pain radiating into the groin.
- Return the leg to the neutral straight position and test for any signs of swelling using:
  - A balloon and bulge sign.
  - A patellar tap.
- Inspect the feet for any signs of deformity.
- Inspect the toe nails (as for the finger nails).
- Inspect the soles of the feet for any signs of callus formation due to subluxation of the metatarsal heads.
- Squeeze across the metatarsals—pain on doing this is indicative of signs of synovitis in the metatarsals.

➲ See Table 8.2 for an example of a normal GALS chart, Chapter 8, p. 297.
➲ Also see 'Regional examination of the musculoskeletal system', Chapter 8, pp. 300–303; ➲ 'Primary care walk-in clinics', Chapter 6, p. 218; ➲ 'History taking and clinical examination', pp. 292–294.

Regional examination of the musculoskeletal system

Regional examination of the musculoskeletal system is a system of examination developed to ensure that examinations are conducted in a standardized way.

The key steps in any musculoskeletal examination are:

- Look.
- Feel.
- Move.
- Function.

Look

- Always start with a visual inspection of the patient at rest.
- Compare both sides for symmetry.
- Skin changes, scars, muscle bulk, and swelling in and around the joint and the periarticular structures.
- Signs of deformity in alignment and posture of the joint.

Feel

- Feel the skin for temperature using the back of the hand, in particular across the joint line and at other relevant sites.
- Any swellings should be assessed for fluctuance and mobility.
- Hard, bony swellings of OA can be distinguished from the soft, boggy swelling of synovitis in IJD.
- Tenderness is an important clinical sign to elicit both in and around the joint.
- Synovitis is detected by the triad of warmth, swelling, and tenderness around the joint line.

Move

- The full ROM of the joint should be assessed.
- Both sides need to be compared.
- As a general rule, both active and then passive movement should be assessed. (Active is where the patient moves, passive where the examiner moves the joint.)
- When examining the joint, loss of full flexion or extension should be detected, and that restriction recorded as mild, moderate, or severe restriction in ROM.
- The quality of the movement should also be noted with reference to abnormalities such as crepitus being recorded.
- In some instances the joint may move beyond the normal range—this is called hypermobility.

Function

It is important as part of a musculoskeletal examination to relate findings to function, e.g. limited elbow flexion—can the patient still feed themselves?

➲ Also see 'Musculoskeletal physical examination', pp. 298–299; ➲ 'Regional -examination of the musculoskeletal system', pp. 300–303; ➲ 'Primary care walk-in clinics', Chapter 6, p. 218; ➲ 'History taking and clinical examination', Chapter 8, pp. 294–295.

Examination of the upper limbs

Examination of the hand and wrist

Look

- With hands palm down, look for obvious swelling, deformity, posture, muscle wasting, particularly of the interosseous muscles of the back of the hand, and scarring.
- Skin for thinning and bruising (steroid use) or rashes.
- Nail changes of psoriasis (pitting and onycholysis), splinter haemorrhages, and nailfold infarct (vasculitis).
- Which joints are affected, are the changes symmetrical or asymmetrical?
- Ask the patient to turn their hands over.
- Inspect the palmar aspect of the hands, look for the same things as palms down, in particular, wasting of the thenar and hypothenar eminences, and signs of palmar erythema.

➲ Also see 'Connective tissue disease', Chapter 5, pp. 127–184.

Feel

- Assess for temperature over the joint lines of wrist and MCP, PIP, and DIP joints using the back of the hand.
- Feel for radial pulses.
- Gently squeeze across the MCP joints to assess for tenderness.
- Feel for swelling and tenderness over each of the joint lines and over the tendon sheaths.
- Test for median and ulnar nerve sensation by stroking over thenar and hypothenar eminences.
- Assess radial sensation over the web space of the thumb and index finger.
- Palpate the patient's wrists.
- Feel up the arm to the elbow to look and feel for rheumatoid nodules or psoriatic plaques over the extensor surface.

Move

- Ask the patient to straighten their fingers fully.
- Get the patient to make a fist (power grip).
- Assess wrist flexion and extension, with the patient actively doing, then passively.
- Touch finger pulp of each finger to thumb (pincer grip).
- Move each joint passively feeling for crepitus.

Function

- Ask the patient to grip two of your fingers to assess power grip.
- Ask the patient to pinch your finger to assess pincer grip.
- Ask the patient to pick up a small object such as a coin or paper clip from your hand. This is to assess pincer grip and function.

➲ Also see 'Primary care walk-in clinics', Chapter 6, p. 218; ➲ 'Regional musculoskeletal conditions', Chapter 8, pp. 300–303.

Examination of the elbow

Look

- Skin changes (scars, psoriatic plaques).
- Swelling (synovitis, bursitis over the olecranon process, rheumatoid nodules).
- Deformity or muscle wasting.

Feel

- Temperature.
- Joint line for:
  - Swelling.
  - Tenderness.
  - Crepitus on movement.
- Medial and lateral epicondyles for tenderness.
- Olecranon bursa for swelling and tenderness.

Move

- Active and passive flexion and extension, pronation, and supination.
- Compare one side to the other.

Function

- The ability to bring the hand to the mouth is an important function of the elbow.

Shoulder examination

Look

- From the front (skin changes, scars, swelling, attitude).
- From behind (wasting, deformity).
- Compare both sides, are they symmetrical?
- Is posture normal?

Feel

- Palpate in turn the sternoclavicular joint, ACJ, and glenohumeral joint for:
  - Temperature.
  - Joint line tenderness.
  - Swelling or crepitus.
- Palpate the muscle bulk of supraspinatus, infraspinatus, and deltoid.
- Identify any muscle tenderness.

Move

ROAM:

- Ask the patient to put their hands behind their head and then behind their back.
- Abduction (assessing for scapular movement and painful arc).
- Flexion and extension.

- Internal and external rotation with the elbow flexed at 90° and held by the patient's side.
- Passive range of movement, if active movement is restricted.

Function

- Includes getting the hands behind the head and behind the back as these movements are needed for washing and grooming.

➔ See 'The elbow', p. 302.

Examination of the lower limbs

Hip examination

Look

Inspection of the patient when standing:

- From the front for a pelvic tilt or rotational deformity.
- From the side for flexion deformity or scars overlying the hip.
- From behind for muscle wasting (gluteal muscle bulk in particular).
- Is there any suggestion of leg length inequality?
- Measure real leg length with a tape measure.

Feel

- Palpate over the greater trochanter.

Move

- Assess full hip flexion with the knee flexed at 90°; observe the patient's face for signs of pain.
- Assess for fixed flexion deformity of the hip by performing Thomas' test. To do this, fully flex hip while the opposite hip is observed to see if it lifts off the couch if it does this confirms a fixed flexion deformity in that hip.
- Assess internal and external rotation with the knee in 90° flexion, passively—often limited particularly in internal rotation in hip disease.
- A Trendelenburg test involves the patient standing on one leg—if there is any hip disease the pelvis dips on the non-weight-bearing side when the patient stands on the affected hip.

Function

Inspection of the walking patient:

- Do they have an antalgic gait which is a painful gait resulting in a limp?
- A Trendelenburg gait is seen when there is proximal muscle weakness and as a result the patient walks with a waddling gait.

Knee

Look

- Inspection of the patient on the couch.
- Attitude.
- Skin changes, scars, psoriasis.
- Swelling.
- Valgus or varus deformity.
- Quadriceps wasting.

Feel

- For temperature ↑ using the back of the hand.
- Palpate the borders of the patella for tenderness.
- With the knee flexed, palpate for joint line tenderness.
- Feel in the popliteal fossa for swelling (Baker's cyst).
- Insertion of the collateral ligaments.
- Effusion—include bulge sign, patellar tap, and balloon sign.

Move

- Assess full flexion and extension actively and passively.
- Assess stability of the collateral ligaments of the knee by placing the leg in 15° of flexion and alternately stressing the joint line on each side, by placing one hand on the opposite side of the joint line to that which you are testing.
- Anterior drawer test for ACLs is performed by placing both hands around the upper tibia, with thumbs over the tibial tuberosity and index fingers tucked under the hamstrings to make sure they are relaxed. Stabilize the lower tibia with the upper forearm and gently pull the upper tibia forward. If there is any laxity of the ACLs, there will be a significant degree of movement.

Function

Inspection of the patient in standing:

- From the front for genu varus and genu valgus.
- From the side for flexion deformity, posterior tibial subluxation, and genu recurvatum.
- Inspection of the walking patient.

Foot and ankle

Look

With the patient sitting on the bed:

- Observe the feet, comparing both side for symmetry.
- Inspect the dorsal surface for skin changes, nail changes, and scars.
- Observe alignment of the toes and evidence of hallux valgus of the big toe.
- Look for joint clawing of the toes, swelling, and callus formation.
- Soles of the feet for callus formation and adventitious bursae.
- Inspect the patient's footwear for any abnormal wearing or evidence of poor fit. Also look at any orthoses.

With the patient weight-bearing:

- Look at the forefoot for toe alignment and the midfoot for foot arch position.
- From behind, look at the Achilles tendon for thickening or swelling.
- Observe for normal alignment of the hindfoot; in disease of the ankle there may be varus or valgus deformity at the ankle.

Feel

- Temperature over the foot and ankle and check for peripheral pulses.
- Metatarsal squeeze for MTP joint tenderness.
- Palpate the midfoot, ankle, and sub-talar joint for tenderness.

Move

- Move actively and passively assessing for pain, crepitus, and ↓ ROM.
- True ankle joint—dorsiflexion and plantar flexion.
- Subtalar joint—abduction and adduction.
- Mid-tarsal joints—inversion and eversion.
- First MTP joint—flexion and extension.

Function

- If not already done, assess the patient's gait for the normal cycle of heel strike, stance, toe off, and swing.

Examination of the spine

Look

Look at the patient when standing:

- From the back for any signs of scoliosis, muscle spasm, pelvic tilt, and skin changes.
- From the side for normal cervical lordosis, thoracic kyphosis, and lumbar lordosis (Fig. 8.3).

Feel

Palpate the spine starting at the occiput to the sacrum and sacroiliac joints feeling for:

- Temperature.
- Swelling.
- Paraspinal muscles for spasm or tenderness.
- Spinous processes for alignment or local tenderness.

Move

With the patient standing:

- Lumbar spine flexion and extension (assess using fingers on a couple of spinous processes).
- Lateral flexion of lumbar spine, by asking the patient to run each hand in turn down the outside of the adjacent leg.

With the patient sitting:

- Thoracic spine rotation.
- Cervical spine movements of flexion, extension, lateral flexion, and rotation.
- With the patient lying as flat as possible, perform a SLR.
- Assess limb reflexes (upper and lower) and dorsiflexion of the big toe.

➔ Also see 'Neck and spine', Chapter 6, pp. 222 and 224.

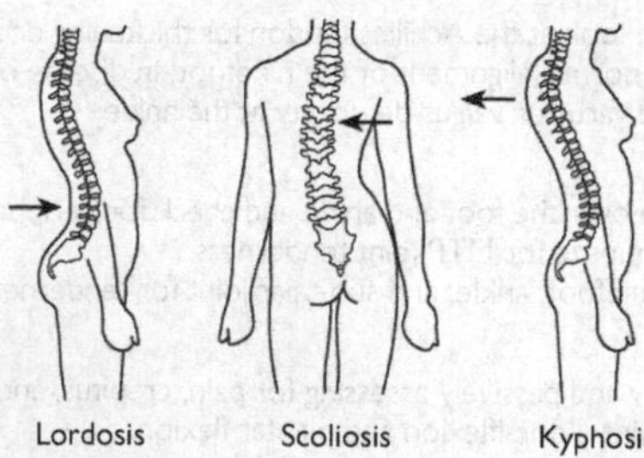

Fig. 8.3 Abnormal spine curvature.

Chapter 9

Symptom control: Using pharmacological and non-pharmacological methods

Overview

The most common presenting symptom for MSCs is that of pain. Pain is a complex phenomenon and a number of contributing factors can ease or exacerbate the perceived pain. Pain may be as a result of new trauma or a progressive deterioration of a condition. These conditions may be mild, self-limiting, or progressive. Reported symptoms other than pain may include fatigue, depression, poor sleep patterns, or deterioration in functional ability.

The essential components of achieving symptom control require a comprehensive assessment. Good clinical history taking and a thorough physical examination need to be considered in the context of symptom control and clinical assessment tools. Pain can be experienced in the joint itself, surrounding tissues, or as referred pain.

Assessment

The purpose of assessment is to identify symptoms that are impacting physical, psychological, and social function and, in partnership with the patient, to plan which symptoms to address first.

Assessment of the overall condition

- How active (acute) is the presenting condition or disease?
- Can the presenting symptoms be attributed to a chronic condition previously diagnosed?
- If presenting symptoms are related to an underlying condition, is the disease well controlled? Are medications being taken appropriately?
- Are the presenting symptoms debilitating/self-limiting or do they indicate a medical emergency such as a septic arthritis?

Factors that influence levels of perceived pain/functional changes

Following a full physical examination to elicit physical changes, other factors should be considered including key indicators that might influence the individual perceptions of pain. Consider social and psychological assessments that include:

- The level of social support and social need that may have an impact on perceptions of pain and achieving symptom control.
- Cultural and religious beliefs. In some communities, pain is to be borne and accepted as a natural phenomenon or a form of retribution.

Assessing disease activity

Some MSCs have global objective measures to assist in assessing disease activity, e.g. DAS28 is used in RA. Initially, the first approach should include:

- Examination of joint or joints affected (comparing against unaffected joint):
  - Are they tender, swollen, hot, or red?
  - Is the patient able to function normally and weight bear? With or without pain?
- Are there any indicators from blood tests such as inflammatory markers that might guide the clinical picture—e.g. CRP, ESR, uric acid, or changes in complement levels (C3 and C4)?

- How do these markers compare to recent or last investigations?
- Are there other factors that may exacerbate the condition, e.g. intercurrent infections or other poorly controlled co-morbidities (e.g. control of diabetes, chronic obstructive pulmonary disease (COPD))?

Management

On completion of the comprehensive assessment, a decision needs to be made as to whether the perceived changes in symptom control result from changes in the disease, poor understanding of the condition, or are attributed to non-disease-related factors (e.g. a lack of medication concordance, or social/psychological issues which impact the individual) which may be improved by non-pharmacological options.

Non-pharmacological options include:

- Information on the condition and understanding symptoms. Empowering the individual to self-manage is an important component of achieving symptom control.
- Non-pharmacological options include walking aids, appropriate footwear to manage load-bearing and impact, muscle-strengthening exercises, and joint protection.
- Additional non-pharmacological strategies that individuals can readily use in the home include cold and warm packs, rest and relaxation, and the use of assistive devices or splinting to protect joints.

If the assessment indicates an ↑ in the level of disease control or disease activity, consider:

- Concordance of current medication regimens—dose and frequency.
- Drug interactions that may have an effect on medication regimens—e.g. an episode of diarrhoea and vomiting will affect absorption.

If the global picture supports a change in disease control/activity with patient-reported changes, review with the prescribing clinician to review treatment options. Patients may require:

- Change in drug therapy.
- ↑ dose of current treatment or change in route of administration, e.g. subcutaneous injection for those failing to tolerate oral therapy (e.g. MTX).
- The addition of another drug therapy (combination therapy).
- Treatment to manage side effects altering bioavailability or a review of the blood picture to consider any toxicities.
- Exclusion of a new disease process or exacerbation of a co-morbidity (e.g. diabetes or GI disorders).

In some cases, the picture can be mixed with evidence of some aspects of disease exacerbation and factors that could be contributing to poor symptom control. Specialist nursing advice may be to guide management.

➲ Also see 'Assessing the patient', Chapter 8, p. 290; ➲ 'Assessment tools', Chapter 20, pp. 595–612 ➲ 'Rapid access and emergency issues', Chapter 13, pp. 399–413; ➲ 'Blood tests and investigations', Chapter 17, pp. 505–535; ➲ 'Pharmacological management', Chapter 16, pp. 445–503.

Assessing pain

MSCs cause a significant burden to the individual and society with high levels of incapacity and loss of work. The relief of pain is a basic human right yet there is still much to be done to improve symptom control for those with debilitating musculoskeletal pain. The interpretation of pain is an individual unique experience based upon perceptions of altered bodily sensations. It is a subjective, multifaceted phenomenon affecting sensory and emotional experiences that influence the perception and experience of pain. Pain can be classified in a number of ways.

- Acute or chronic.
- Chronic malignant or non-malignant pain (benign).
- Inflammatory or non-inflammatory.

Not all pain will require medications to relieve it, but a thorough assessment of the issues involved in the patient's experience of pain together with any underlying disease process that may require modification to reduce the sensation of pain is required. Factors that must be considered include physical, social, spiritual, and emotional aspects of the patient experience related to the pain.

Factors that affect pain include:

Pathophysiology

- Tissue damage, e.g. neurological damage or injury to soft tissues.
- A review of underlying disease activity, e.g. inflammatory component for IJDs such as ReA or gout.

The nature of the pain

- The patient-reported symptoms of pain including evaluation of the level of pain experienced by the individual (quality and quantity):
  - E.g. the use of a VAS to assess the level of pain.
- Relieving or exacerbating factors.
- Distribution of pain, e.g. distribution represents neurological pathways.
- Type of pain experience:
  - Intermittent or constant.
  - Trauma (sudden/acute episode) or insidious onset (relapsing and remitting).
  - Description of the pain sensation (shooting, pins and needles).
  - Effect on bodily functions/functional ability.

Pain waking the patient at night is an indicator of inflammation.

Personal interpretation of sensations

- Prior experiences of pain.
- Cultural and ethnic beliefs and interpretations of pain.
- Social and psychological factors that influence the individual's ability to interpret painful symptoms.

Consider the consultation in the context of practitioner and patient-centred models of consultation. A mnemonic to aid recall is 'PQRST':

- P = provoked by.
- Q = quality and quantity.

- R = region and where does it radiate to.
- S = severity.
- T = timing.

The nursing process

- Recognition that the pain is 'real'. Providing empathy and support.
- Listening to the patient and their experience/sensations of pain.
- Identify factors that exacerbate or relieve symptoms.
- Explore the context of the pain experience:
  - Sudden or insidious onset.
  - Interpretation of pain (attitudes, beliefs, cultural factors).
  - Exacerbating psychological factors (e.g. fear and anxiety).
- Current symptom-relieving strategies (pharmacological and non-pharmacological) and their efficacy.
- Interpreting the level of pain using tools that aid the nurse/patient therapeutic relationship—informed and shared decision-making.
- Negotiate a goal-setting approach to optimize pain control using a range of pharmacological and non-pharmacological options.
- Set an agreed review process to evaluate changes in pain sensations following planned pain-relieving strategies.

Measuring pain and its effects

The VAS is a recognized simple clinical tool consisting of a horizontal 10 cm line (Fig. 9.1). The patient is asked to mark along the 10 cm line the point which reflects their perceived pain at that time. The mark is then measured using a ruler to attribute the number along the line (e.g. 8 (8 cm) out of total score of 10 (10 cm)).

Other examples of pain assessment tools include:

- Body maps (pictorial) or verbal rating scales (the use of words to describe pain).
- Faces pain scales (pictorial—may be useful with language/communication barriers).
- Pain questionnaires such as the McGill Pain Questionnaire.
- Scales to assess for the older person with cognitive impairment/communication problems (e.g. the DOLOPLUS 2 scale).
- Other tools to assess mood, function, cognition, and health beliefs.

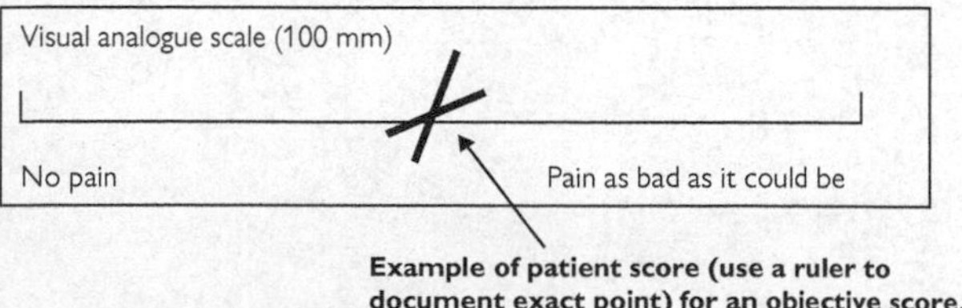

Fig. 9.1 Example of a VAS (not to scale). The cross indicates the patient's measure of their pain over the last week.

➔ See Chapter 6, 'Chronic musculoskeletal pain', pp. 186–187; ➔ Chapter 6, 'Education in chronic pain management', Chapter 6, pp. 196–197; ➔ Chapter 6, 'Management of chronic pain conditions', Chapter 6, pp. 186–199.

Assessment of pain: red and yellow flags

Introduction

The principle of using an assessment approach that refers to 'red' or 'yellow' flags has been used for some 30 years. The red and yellow flag system allows clinicians to have a rapid system of identifying high-risk indicators when undertaking a clinical examination.

Red flags—medical

A red flag approach enables treatments/assessments to be undertaken by non-medical teams provided they were able to identify those requiring rapid referral for medical examination (red flag). They are often used in a pathway approach or protocol where most of the common pathology is identified and guidance is included in the pathway—depending upon the expertise and facilities available to investigate.

The use of red flags works as a teaching aid, enhancing the need to identify key diagnostic criteria that prompt rapid screening, investigation, and treatment. There are different red flags according to the bodily system being reviewed. Red flags usually identify relatively rare but important diagnostic factors that may indicate serious disease requiring further medical examination.

Signs of symptoms that indicate serious underlying pathology might include features that indicate:

- Neurological disease.
- Malignancy.
- Infections.
- Fractures.

An example of red flags for back pain can be seen in Box 9.1.

Yellow flags—psychological

The other important indicators that need to be identified are those that indicate underlying psychological issues that may require further specialist or medical support. Yellow flags are used to identify prognostic indicators that may require further assessment and will affect outcomes or indicate an additional psychological component to the presenting condition. These factors may require further investigation/referral or require additional consideration during the consultation (Box 9.2).

Box 9.1 Examples of red flags for back pain

- Night pain.
- Pyrexia plus sweats.
- Weight loss.
- High ESR.
- History of malignancy.
- Altered sphincter disturbances plus neurological deficit/impairment.

Box 9.2 Examples of yellow flags for pain

- Family history of pain.
- Previous pain syndrome.
- Pain-related work problems.
- Poor coping skills/difficult life challenges.
- Previous history of depression/anxiety.
- Unresolved postviral symptoms.
- Poor sleep patterns.
- Significant emotional distress.

Symptom control: pain relief

Pharmacological and non-pharmacological treatments

Achieving symptom control for those presenting with a wide range of MSCs requires:

- A patient-centred consultation that includes thorough musculoskeletal examination and history taking and exploration of the patient's perspective on the condition, personal impact, expectations, anxieties, and fears.
- Information should be provided about the condition, prognosis, and treatment choices (written and verbal).
- Recognition of the value of practical aspects of symptom control that enhance self-management.
- Access or signposting to voluntary or community support that can complement healthcare support.

In some circumstances additional support may be required, such as:

- Prompt referral to specialist expertise for those with long-term systemic inflammatory conditions—such as SLE, CTDs, IJDs (e.g. RA, AS, and PsA).
- CBT.
- Referral or specific guidance on occupational health advice related to work-related functional issues.
- Advice may be required on welfare/financial issues such as those provided by the Citizens Advice network or how to claim Employment and Support Allowance.

➲ Also see 'Chronic non-inflammatory pain', Chapter 6, pp. 186–195; ➲ Chapter 10, 'Holistic and patient-centred care', Chapter 10, pp. 329–350.

Pharmacological options

Patients should be advised when effective pain relief is sought that medications should be taken at regular intervals and treatment should not be delayed until the pain becomes unbearable. Pharmacological options should be complemented by non-pharmacological options to achieve maximum treatment effect. Nurses should consider using the WHO analgesic pain ladder if it is an appropriate choice, taking into account the degree of pain experienced and previous pharmacological approach. For example, a person experiencing severe pain from septic arthritis may not achieve effective pain control using paracetamol, rest, and cold packs. Advice on dose and frequency of administration are essential for effective pain control (Box 9.3).

Non-pharmacological options

The use of non-pharmacological options should be encouraged. A wide range of options can be offered to suit to presenting problems, preferences of the patient, and ability to carry out procedures/treatment plans (Box 9.3). In some circumstances, CBT may also be helpful, particularly if higher levels of psychological support are required to aid rehabilitation.

➲ Also see 'Chronic non-inflammatory pain', Chapter 6, pp. 186–197.

Box 9.3 Pharmacological and non-pharmacological options

Examples of therapeutic options

- Simple analgesia (non-opioid): paracetamol—advise on dose and frequency.
- Compound analgesia (simple analgesia with opioid component):
  - Co-codamol—different dose regimens.
  - Co-dydramol—different dose regimens.
- Topical anti-inflammatory, rubefacients, or capsaicin:
  - Topical NSAIDs—diclofenac sodium, ibuprofen, ketoprofen.
  - Rubefacients—create a deep heat sensation.
  - Capsaicin creams—chilli pepper inhibits substance P.
- NSAIDs (including COX-2 inhibitors).
- Opioid (short or long acting):
  - Tramadol hydrochloride—short acting.
  - Transdermal fentanyl patches—long acting.

Supporting therapies

- Amitriptyline for neuropathic and chronic pain conditions—given at a lower dose than used to treat depression.
- Pregabalin, an antiepileptic therapy, may also be effective in neuropathic pain.
- Duloxetine, an antidepressant therapy for chronic pain conditions.
- Corticosteroids can aid pain relief in inflammatory condition—taken orally for systemic effect, or IA, or soft tissue injections (local benefit to swollen joint).

Non-pharmacological options

- Information, advice, and support (patient support groups) advice lines.
- Guidance on condition, prognosis, and treatment choices.
- Joint protective devices—splints, kettle tippers, walking sticks, and orthotics.
- Exercise (improves mood) and muscle strength.
- Pacing, rest, relaxation, and distraction techniques.
- Self-management programme—goal setting and problem-solving approach/stress management.
- Thermotherapy—use of hot and cold.

Further reading

NICE (2017, updated Feb 2018). Medicine optimization in long term pain (KTT21). https://www.nice.org.uk/advice/ktt21

Symptom control: depression and fatigue

Fatigue and depression are strongly associated with pain. For those with a MSC, the pivotal factor that drives them to seek medical advice is that of relieving their pain. The pain itself, the fear of pain, and what pain 'means' cause a severe burden on the individual. Unrelieved pain, changes to functional ability (such as ↓ ROMs), and disturbed sleep can build up a picture of negative attitudes and beliefs resulting in:

- Fatigue.
- A sense of vulnerability.
- Poor self-esteem and threats perceived.
- Reduced self-efficacy related to low confidence in managing symptoms.
- Depression/anger/apathy.
- Loss of motivation.

Patients require early and effective support to prevent a downward spiral of ↑ disability, fatigue, depression, and potential loss of their role in society (work, independence). Depression and fatigue are complex phenomena with a number of causes and contributing factors. Depression, fatigue, and pain are strongly linked with poor healthcare outcomes. These factors are also important to consider in the context of functional ability in MSCs.

Definition of depression

Depression is a general term to describe a negative change in mood. This change can be seen as a normal process, e.g. a short-lived low mood might be as a result of a temporary response to an event. Depression is commonly reported for those with LTCs. Social isolation and economic distress are linked to depression. Clinical depression is defined as symptoms lasting >2 weeks that are so severe they affect ADLs.

People with depression may report:

- Negative emotions—feeling of unhappiness, everything is a problem.
- Apathy—loss of interest in previous hobbies, activities, and food.
- Poor self-esteem and loss of expressions of emotions.
- Sleep disturbances—insomnia and early wakening.
- Poor concentration and irritability.
- Feelings of being 'changed'.
- May have 'real' physical symptoms, unrelieved by treatment.

Definition of fatigue

Fatigue is characterized by feelings of exhaustion or weariness which may be directly attributed to the use of excessive energy. Fatigue related to long-term MSCs can also be as a result of coping with unrelieved pain and stiffness in combination with active disease and/or an anaemia of chronic disease. Functional ability and the additional energy required to undertake normal ADLs when there is functional impairment should also be considered when assessing fatigue. The interpretation of fatigue is also a subjective state related to an awareness of ↓ capacity for physical or mental activity.

Depression and fatigue

Depression and fatigue are symptoms that can be subject to an underlying pathology but are also affected by psychosocial issues. It can sometimes be difficult to unravel the social and psychological factors when a patient with a chronic non-inflammatory condition (such as fibromyalgia) reports depression and fatigue, particularly as the diagnosis of the condition itself results chiefly upon a group of self-reported symptoms.

A nursing assessment in the context of depression and fatigue

To understand and support patients with depression and fatigue, good practice should:

- Ensure early access to a healthcare professional.
- Provide a patient-centred and holistic assessment.
- Use validated tools to measure depression (e.g. Hospital Anxiety and Depression Scale) and fatigue (SF36 vitality subscale).
- Identify contributing factors that may precipitate depression/fatigue.
- Build a framework of support that is based upon encouraging active coping styles and self-management principles.
- Avoid reliance on medication and 'quick fixes' for those conditions/patients that may have strong psychosocial issues:
  - Identify social vulnerabilities/needs.
  - Psychological factors and any prior treatments offered.
- Identify physical factors that may lead to depression or fatigue:
  - Poor disease control of inflammatory conditions—anaemia, weight loss, ↑ inflammatory markers.
  - Prior history of depression or poor mental health.
  - Functional limitations ↑ burden on ADLs.
  - Unrelieved pain which disturb sleep.
  - Adverse side effects to medications.

Useful advice

Depression and fatigue combined with poor pain control may require referral to specialist support for:

- Diagnosis and treatment of any underlying condition (e.g. RA) or management of depression.
- Prompt referral to pain management teams.
- If a long-term MSC—review of disease control.

Practical support to give the patient

- Exercise—goal-setting approach in a graded appropriate exercise programme.
- Advice on how to balance activities with rest and relaxation.
- Manage contributing factors to fatigue:
  - Review sleep patterns and encourage a healthy sleep routine.
  - Ensure good disease control.
  - Assess for anaemia, e.g. related to chronic disease.
  - Review diet.
  - Consider CBT for psychosocial factors.

Further reading

Callaghan P, Gamble C (2015). Working with specific issues and concerns. In: *Oxford Handbook of Mental Health Nursing*, 2nd edn, pp. 79–102. Oxford: Oxford University Press.

NICE (2009). Depression in adults with a chronic physical health problem: recognition and management (CG91). https://www.nice.org.uk/guidance/cg91

Supporting patients with pain

Patients who experience pain need recognition that their pain is real, and that support and guidance is available to help them achieve symptom control.

The impact of unrelieved pain

- Poor self-esteem.
- Depression.
- Fatigue.
- Disturbed sleep.
- Reduction in functional ability.
- Poor perceived self-efficacy and self-esteem.
- Negative health behaviours.
- Inability to carry out normal ADLs, e.g. changes to career progression/ redundancy.

Interpretation of pain

The unpleasant sensations associated with pain will differ from person to person based upon a range of factors including:

- Underlying disease pathology.
- Social and psychological factors related to prior experiences of pain and cultural beliefs related to pain.
- Interpretation of what the pain 'means' to the individual (fear of malignancy), level of incapacity as a result of the pain.
- Nature of the pain—relapsing, unremitting.

Patients will need information and guidance on why they are experiencing pain and what options there are to relieve the symptoms. The nursing assessment process should be used to encourage the patient to be an active participant in their management and review of how effective pain-relieving strategies have worked. Assessment tools should be used to allow a level of objective review of pain scores and treatment effect (e.g. VASs).

Common mistakes

In many cases, patients are not advised about the basic principles of how pain works. As a result, there are common mistakes that patients make in managing their symptoms. These include:

- Only taking pain relief when the pain gets really 'bad'.
- Not taking regular doses over a 24-hour period, choosing to take a large dose infrequently.
  - This may result in discarding simple analgesia given regularly (e.g. paracetamol for OA).
- Failure to advise on the non-pharmacological options, e.g.:
  - Rest and relaxation, cold packs.
  - Use of aids (walking sticks), e.g. functional problems related to knee pain.

➲ Also see 'Assessing pain', pp. 310–314; ➲ 'Chronic non-inflammatory pain', Chapter 6, pp. 186–197; ➲ Chapter 22, 'Patient's perspective', Chapter 22, p. 621.

Further reading

British Medical Association (2017). *Chronic Pain: Supporting the Safe Prescribing of Analgesia*. London: BMA.

Versus Arthritis. Living with long term pain: a guide to self-management. ✆ https://www.versusarthritis.org/media/1248/back-pain-information-booklet.pdf

Frequently asked questions

Is a goal-setting approach helpful in trying to improve symptom control?

In some cases, the patient-centred goals can be set in a structured and formal way that includes regular reviews and revision of goals but in others a more informal approach may be sufficient. (A goal may be simply by the next appointment the patient will have stepped down their paracetamol dose to 500 mg a day at lunchtime from 1 g.)

Goal setting can be effective if used as part of a patient-centred assessment. Goals should be small and achievable and may help to dispel anxieties or prior learnt health behaviours that reinforce negative thoughts about symptom control. Once positive results are achieved, it is easier to build upon these goals and increase self-efficacy (belief that they have some control over their condition and how to manage symptoms).

All treatment options can then be refined and reduced/changed according to the assessment and review following goal setting.

How do I decide which treatment options (pharmacological and non-pharmacological) are most appropriate for each patient?

Pharmacological and non-pharmacological options should be offered as an overall package. The nurse should offer the patient a range of approaches/practical tools they can use themselves to improve control and importantly enhance self-management principles. Important factors to consider include:

- The patient's health assessment and underlying risk factors (e.g. if high cardiovascular risk NSAIDs/COX-2 therapies may be contraindicated) (➔ see 'Pharmacological of management pain relief', Chapter 9, p. 316 and Chapter 15, pp. 432–443).
- Decisions should consider the patient's informed decision and preferences following education about their condition and potential risks and benefits of treatment options.
- All symptom control should consider treatments that provide the maximum benefit but most importantly with the least possible risk acceptable to the patient and the clinician. Consider advising on how to manage the side effect of medications, e.g. the use of bulking agents when patients start pain-relieving medications that may result in constipation.
- Treatment should consider the degree to which symptoms are distressing/affecting the patient and how they rate their symptoms (e.g. a high VAS score for pain).
- The healthcare professional's knowledge of the condition and guidelines/evidence related to best treatment options in the context of a disease assessment.
- Prior treatments tried and prior side effects or benefits of that treatment.
- Treatment benefits should be reviewed in the context of symptoms and benefits. Patients should be educated on how to step-up or step-down treatment wherever possible.

Practical advice for self-limiting conditions

Musculoskeletal disorders cover a wide range of conditions. It is no surprise that from time to time individuals may present with a wide range of problems related to joint or soft tissue disorders. Many of these are general short-term problems that require appropriate treatment and advice with resolution over a short time frame (treatment, surgery, or spontaneous resolution).

Conditions that require specialist support

Patients who have systemic, life-threatening, or long-term inflammatory conditions that require ongoing specialist management. These include:

- CTDs, e.g. SLE, scleroderma, and GPA.
- IJDs, e.g. RA, PsA, and AS.
- Metabolic bone diseases, e.g. osteoporosis.
- Infections, e.g. septic arthritis.
- Orthopaedic trauma.

The problems outlined in the following sections may be confined to pain or functional limitations related to a joint or the soft tissues surrounding the joint.

Examples of self-limiting conditions include:

- Back pain—early access to advice is essential for the best outcome.
- Injuries related to falls or trauma.
- Soft tissue disorders affecting tendon, ligaments, bursae, muscles, fascia, or joint capsule—occupational or sports injuries (e.g. tennis elbow).
- Musculoskeletal pain.
- Early functional limitations related to one joint such as seen in OA of the knee.

Evidence supports prompt access to:

- Symptom relief.
- Information about the problem, prognosis, and how to self-manage the condition.
- Provision of aids or devices to aid the management of functional problems.
- Regimens to return to full normal functional ability.

Practical advice on managing self-limiting conditions

- Acute soft tissue injury (Box 9.4).
- Outline the long-term prognosis of the condition.
- Identify aspects of bone healthy lifestyle—exercise, diet, and risk reduction in sports injuries by using appropriate equipment. Occupational factors such as reducing risks related to back pain.
- Encourage self-management options, including:
    - Use of walking aids, appropriate footwear or devices, e.g. insoles for plantar fasciitis.

Box 9.4 Acute phase management of soft tissue injury

- Protect.
- Rest the injured area.
- Ice (10–20 min every 2–4 hours).
- Compress.
- Elevate.
- Support.

Pain relief may also be required in the short term (e.g. oral or topical).

- Educate on appropriate use of joints and equipment, e.g. occupational issues such as equipment that exacerbates the pain and functional difficulties, such as poor posture and lack of wrist support for a typist.
- Describe pharmacological pain relief options and how pain works to ensure concordance.
- Identify non-pharmacological options that can support pain relief—thermotherapy, exercise, rehabilitation, and use of goal setting.

► Most importantly, encourage a healthy positive perspective on long-term outcome and return of normal functional ability.

Work-related issues in musculoskeletal conditions

In the UK, there are >2.2 million people receiving incapacity benefits as a result of a MSC (the highest group after mental health conditions) and the impact of work-related illness in MSC is two times higher than in those suffering from 'stress'. The introduction of biologic therapies may significantly improve these figures but rely on early proactive management if patients are to remain in employment. Some statistics from the UK include:

- >2.5 million people in the UK visit their GP with back pain every year. >80% of adults will suffer significant back pain at some time in their life.
- Almost 400,000 people have RA with 12,000 new cases each year, a quarter of who will stop work within 5 years of diagnosis. This number can significantly rise if effects of related conditions (depression, cardiac and respiratory complaints) are taken into account.
- >200,000 patients with AS visit their GP each year. Unemployment rates are three times higher in those with AS compared to the general population.

These facts are disappointing because evidence suggests significant benefits can be achieved if patients receive prompt support. Pilot studies have shown a sixfold ↑ in those actively wishing to return to work after early proactive support.

Surveys have also revealed that patients generally rate their quality of life, mood, and social factors (relationships, independences, role in society, satisfaction with care and self-esteem) more highly if they are actively employed.

The above-mentioned issues are also relevant from an international perspective. MSCs are the second most common cause of disability worldwide (measured by YLDs). Disability related to MSCs had risen by 45% in 2010. The Global Burden of Disease study estimated that in 2010, 1700 million people had problems related to MSDs. Currently, most of the evidence is collected from developed countries. Factors contributing to these figures can be seen in Fig. 9.2

➲ See Chapter 24, 'Public health awareness', pp. 639–646.

The role of the nurse

- Early intervention is essential—ensure prompt support and advice including access to multiprofessional teams (especially OTs) for advice on functional and occupational issues.
- Focus on positive issues related to capacity not incapacity of the patient. Encourage positive messages that reinforce the individual's belief that they will be able to maintain some form of employment with the right support—provide early practical guidance and information. Early referral to occupational therapy and information such as patient information leaflets on maintaining work.
- Encourage flexible working and review of work stations or other functional limitations to maintaining work.
- Flag the need to think beyond the biomedical model and highlight the psychosocial benefits of participation in society and work.

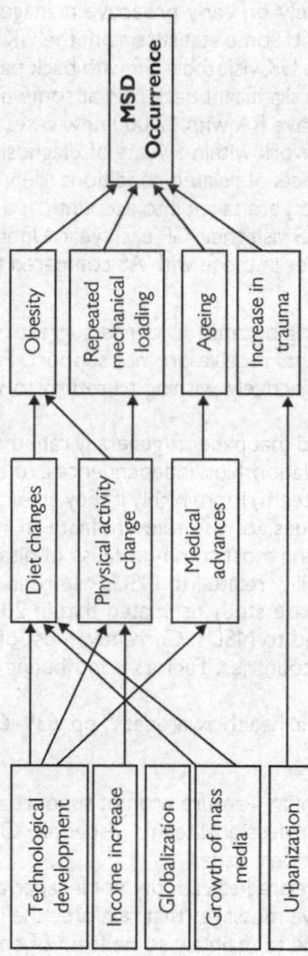

Fig. 9.2 Conceptual model relating the major determinants of musculoskeletal disorders.
Reproduced from Detels R, Gulliford M, Karim QA, and Tan CC (2015) *Oxford Textbook of Global Public Health*, Fig 8.9.2 © 2015 Oxford University Press with permission from Oxford University Press.

- Consider more than just direct costs (use of health resources) but consider indirect costs, e.g. costs to the patient, loss of social interaction, independence, financial burden, and role in society.
- Be proactive in reviewing and supporting those with MSCs.

Further reading

Barrero LH, Caban AJ (2015). Musculoskeletal disorders. In: Detels R, Gulliford M, Karim QA, Tan CC (eds) *Oxford Textbook of Global Public Health*, 6th edn, pp. 1046–60. Oxford: Oxford University Press.

National Rheumatoid Arthritis Society (2010). The economic burden of RA: survey and reports. https://www.nras.org.uk/publications/the-economic-burden-of-rheumatoid-arthritis

National Rheumatoid Arthritis Society (2017). Work matters: survey and reports. https://www.nras.org.uk/publications/work-matters

Storheim K, Zwart JA (2014). Musculoskeletal disorders and the Global Burden of Disease Study. *Ann Rheum Dis* 73:949–50.

Van Vilstern M, Boot CR, Knol DL, et al. (2015). Productivity at work and QoL in patients with RA. *BMC Musculoskelet Disord* 6:107.

Nursing care issues in the management of pain

The prevalence of pain varies considerably in published literature but ranges from 7 to 16 million people reporting musculoskeletal pain in the UK.

Patients who experience pain will require empathetic and knowledgeable support. Pain evokes fear and anxiety particularly if the cause of the pain is poorly understood. The experience of pain is debilitating, affects self-esteem, and can negatively impact the patient's ability to use positive health behaviours.

Acute or chronic pain

Although there are important factors to consider in the different management approaches for acute or chronic pain, the relief of pain for the patient is the aim of both.

Acute pain

In acute pain, the painful sensations are related to a condition that endangers other bodily functions, requiring prompt intervention of the underlying disorder causing the pain (e.g. acute prolapsed intervertebral disc).

Chronic pain

The considerable heterogeneity in definitions of chronic pain means that estimates of chronic pain range from 7% to 55% of the population in the UK. Chronic malignant pain is generally well managed with patient pathways of care and expertise readily accessible to most patients with malignancy. Chronic non-malignant pain tends to have more negative connotations with HCPs and as a result is often less well managed.

Chronic pain is a complex mix of issues that are often referred to as the biopsychosocial model of care:

- Nociception—nerve fibre impulses.
- Behavioural responses.
- Cognitive factors.

Acute on chronic pain

A classic example of acute on chronic pain is that of a patient with a LTC with an underlying pathology (e.g. IJDs such as RA). The underlying, ongoing low-grade inflammation is exacerbated by acute episodes of 'flares' of the condition, ↑ the pain sensations.

Although there are different experiences and responses to acute or chronic pain, perceived views of pain will be developed over time and prior illness experiences/health beliefs and coping styles, e.g.:

Physical

- The underlying pathology causing pain.
- Recognition of the condition.
- Ability to comprehend the diagnosis/acceptance of diagnosis.

Psychological factors
- Cognitive abilities.
- Health-seeking behaviours and beliefs.
- Coping styles whether they have a preference for:
    - Active—gentle exercise, distraction techniques.
    - Passive—bed rest, avoidance strategies.

Social factors
- Cultural or religious beliefs related to pain and treatments.
- Language barriers may add to social issues/anxieties.
- Partner/family support related to the pain/condition.
- Level of financial support and ability to manage factors associated with pain (e.g. able to purchase aids, home environment, work flexibility).
- Work-related issues.
- Additional factors that affect the emotional response to the pain at that time:
    - Death of a family member/divorce/financial worries.

Nursing issues in pain management

Prompt and empathetic approach to those experiencing pain is important:
- Undertake a holistic and patient-centred assessment:
    - Scope the patient's interpretation of pain and treatments.
    - Review medications (dosing and frequency) and efficacy of previous treatments.
- If appropriate, provide pharmacological and non-pharmacological options:
    - A review of medications may need to be discussed with prescribing/diagnosing clinician.
- Evaluate pain using a tool such as a VAS which encourages patient–practitioner communication with shared goals (reducing pain score).
- Ensure the patient understands the cause of pain (and/or diagnosis) and prognosis:
    - Try to reduce emotional distress related to pain/condition.
- Provide strategies that encourage self-management using a goal-setting approach:
    - Exercise, pacing, rest, relaxation, and distraction techniques.
- Consider CBT or pain management programme for those who require psychological treatment of pain.

Useful resources
- *The Pharmacist* is an excellent resource in medicine reviews for pain management.
- Pain management teams or psychological team (CBT).

- Specialist team dealing with underlying pathology (e.g. rheumatologist for RA).
- Consider volunteer and support groups/community health/well-being programmes.
- The British Pain Society website: ✆ www.britishpainsociety.org.

Further reading

Clunie GPR, Wilkinson N, Nikiphorou E, Jadon D (eds) (2018). *Oxford Handbook of Rheumatology*, 4th edn. Oxford: Oxford University Press.

Chapter 10

Holistic and patient-centred care

Holistic assessment

Introduction

Holistic care is that of considering the 'whole' person in the context of their physical, social, psychological, and spiritual needs. The essence of nursing is that of ensuring a holistic approach is considered for all aspects of care. Early and proactive support should focus on encouraging individuals to be informed about their condition and the treatment options. For the individual with a MSC this approach is imperative, irrespective of the condition.

A nursing consultation

If a truly holistic assessment encompassing a patient-centred approach is to be achieved, the nurse must allow adequate time in an environment conducive to exploring the factors outlined in the introduction to this topic. In a similar way to qualitative interview techniques, a framework to the consultation needs to be borne in mind. It should not be so prescriptive that it fails to enable the patient to build a therapeutic alliance with the nurse.

Holistic assessments should include:

- Social circumstances—age, sex, work-related issues, functional ability, and level of social support.
- Ethnicity or cultural needs.
- Family and clinical history.
- Health and lifestyle issues—smoking, diet.
- Psychological or educational issues/needs.
- Any impairment—visual or hearing.
- Health and illness beliefs (see Fig. 10.1 for a holistic framework to the approach to care).

Once a detailed assessment has been undertaken, the care planned and treatment required should be negotiated considering:

- The patient's condition in the context of the present symptoms and needs.
- The wider social and psychological aspects of the patient and their perceived additional needs.
- The strategy required to optimize their quality of life in the context of their perceived needs and independent state.

It is widely recognized that patient outcomes for those with LTCs can be improved if they are actively encouraged to participate in their healthcare decisions.

Further reading

Stenner K, Carey N, Courtenay M (2010). How nurse prescribing influences the role of nursing. *Nurse Prescribing* 8:29–34.

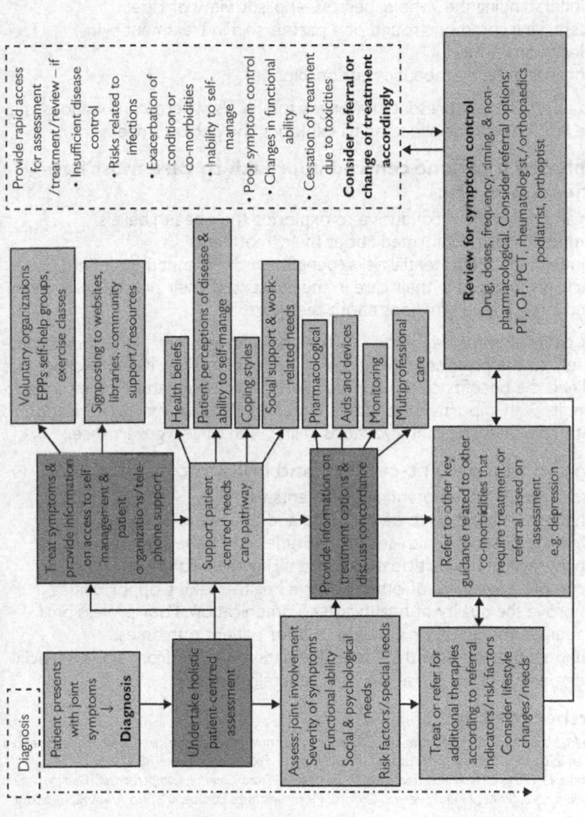

Fig. 10.1 Holistic approach to care.

Patient-centred care

Introduction

Patient-centred care theories encompass a number of domains in the consultation process. These include:

- Exploring the experience and expectations of disease and illness.
- Understanding the 'whole' person—holistic view of care.
- Identifying common ground or a partnership in treatment plans.
- Health promotion.
- Enhancing the therapeutic relationship.

This approach can present challenges for HCPs where consultations may have insufficient time allocated to exploring the patient's needs.

Achieving a patient-centred approach to care must have patients who are:

- In an environment conducive to exploring their health beliefs.
- Empowered and informed about their treatment.
- Understand the potential risks/benefits of the planned treatment.
- Actively involved in their care in the context of their holistic assessment and integral to discussions about their care.

The patient-centred approach tailors the management plan more appropriately to the priorities and needs of the patient (Fig. 10.2). Evidence has outlined the benefits of this approach and increasingly this type of consultation fits with important aspects of informed decision-making in relation to treatments or surgical interventions in line with clinical governance.

Benefits of a patient-centred and holistic consultation

This approach ↑ the potential for patients to:

- Enable health beliefs to be explored and discussed.
- Develop positive health-seeking attitudes and behaviours.
- Encourage active participation in managing their condition.
- Promote awareness of other positive health-seeking opportunities.
- Improve the quality of healthcare communication. Poor professional patient communication is linked to poor patient outcomes.
- Support the needs of the vulnerable patient (either from a psychosocial perspective or for those who are generally unwell).

Further reading

Forin M, Haggerty J, Loignon C, et al. (2012). Patient centred care in chronic disease management: a thematic analysis of the literature in family medicine. *Patient Educ Couns* 88:170–6.

Paparella G (2016). *Person-Centred Care in Europe: A Cross Country Comparison of Health System Performance, Strategies and Systems*. Oxford: Picker Institute Europe. http://www.picker.org

Patient consent and informed consent

Introduction

Before any physical investigation or any form of treatment can be given, it is the duty of HCPs to ensure that the patient consents to the treatment/investigation proposed. The duty of care is part of the statutory legal responsibilities of HCPs and as such includes the ethical principles of valid consent:

- 'The Code: Professional standards of practice and behaviour for nurses, midwives and nursing associates' by the Nursing and Midwifery Council (2018) states the essential legal responsibilities of protecting the patient.
- Employing organizations will have governance frameworks that consider ethical and professional responsibilities.

▶ Legal requirements will vary from country to country—review legal requirements before seeking patient consent to treatment.

Seeking patient consent

If in doubt about your abilities to adequately inform the patient and document decisions, guidance should be sought from the Nursing and Midwifery Council or an experienced colleague. In seeking consent, it is important to remember:

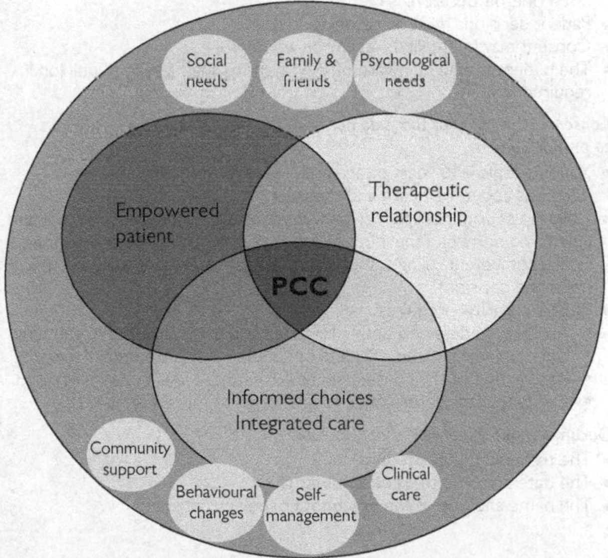

Fig. 10.2 Patient-centred care (PPC).

The responsibility of the nurse

- To act in the best interest of the patient.
- To obtain consent before treatment.
- To ensure that the process of establishing consent is rigorous, transparent, and demonstrates a clear level of professional accountability.
- To accurately record the process of consent and decisions made.

Consent must be valid

- Consent must be given voluntarily.
- The patient must be an adult.
- The patient must be presumed to be mentally competent to provide consent (or have a legally nominated guardian).
- The decision to provide consent is based upon accurate and valid information to enable a decision that reflects the risks/benefits of the treatment.
- The patient should be informed if the treatment is unlicensed or part of a research trial.

Consent-specific patient issues

- The HCP providing the treatment or undertaking the investigation should seek consent from the patient.
- It is an ongoing and continuing prerequisite of all treatment/ investigations provided throughout the patient's healthcare journey. It is not a one-off decision.
- Patient decisions must be respected.
- Consent may be implied, verbal, or written.
- The patient should be aware of their right to seek a second opinion if required.

Consent—the young or those do not have the mental capacity to provide consent

- Young people >16 years of age are presumed competent to make decisions about their care and treatments.
- Children of younger age may provide consent if seen as competent and able to comprehend the information in relation to the decision—the Gillick competent ruling (otherwise the legal parent or guardian can make the decision).
- Mental capacity—requires:
  - Ability to understand simple language and the purpose of treatment.
  - Understanding of the risks and benefits or other treatment options.
  - Recognition of the consequences if treatment was not administered.
  - Ability to retain information long enough to make a decision.

Documentation of consent should include:

- The treatment or procedure.
- The date and time that consent was given.
- The name and title of the practitioner seeking consent.

- An outline of key factors related to risks related to the treatment and the information provided.
- Any specific instructions that the patient outlines in giving consent.

Informed decision-making

The validity of consent rests with the patient's ability to make a truly informed decision based upon the information provided. There is an ↑ interest in tools that aid patients' treatment decisions. These aids vary. Some provide the detailed facts and then interpret the risk based upon visual images of risks and benefits (Fig. 10.3). Such tools may have value for those who are illiterate or have language barriers.

Further reading

Barry M, Edgman-Levitan S (2012). Shared decision making—the pinnacle of patient centred care. *N Engl J Med* 366:780–1.

British Medical Association (2013). An introduction to patient decision aids. *BMJ* 347:f4147.

Nursing and Midwifery Council (2018). The Code: Professional standards of practice and behaviour for nurses, midwives and nursing associates. ℛ https://www.nmc.org.uk/standards/code/

The Health Foundation. 'Magic' shared decision making: a UK implementation study. ℛ https://www.health.org.uk/sites/health/files/MagicImplementationofSharedDecisionMakinginPractice_presentation.pdf

Education

Education is a core component of the support nurses provide to patients. The format of delivering education may vary from a one-off information-sharing approach to a clearly defined treatment to an ongoing planned educational component for a patient-centred consultation for someone with a LTC.

In the past, delivering education was considered part of a structured training package frequently delivered in a group setting over a clearly defined time frame (e.g. a 2-hourly weekly programme delivered by a multiprofessional team delivered over 6 weeks). Increasingly, there is recognition that this approach may not be effective as tailoring education/information giving with an emphasis on tailoring information to the patient's specific needs and expectations with the aim of achieving behavioural changes.

Group education programmes delivered using cognitive behavioural approaches (i.e. ↑ motivation, self-efficacy (SE), and promoting health behaviour change) are significantly more effective than providing a series of short weekly informative lectures from members of the multiprofessional team.

However, current models of one-to-one educational approaches have had surprisingly little evaluation. Education should be tailored to meet people's information needs and enable them to make treatment decisions. To help patients make health behaviour changes, education should be structured, use goal-setting, and be supported with printed materials. Behavioural changes require practice so that the patient can recognize the benefits of change and can become confident and skilled in their new behaviours.

Patient education is strongly associated with other aspects of healthcare and should aim to:

- Endorse and empower patient self-management principles.
- Enhance patient satisfaction and perceived SE.
- Strengthen governance and reduction of risks.
- Reduce litigation.
- Support the patient to adopt new health behaviours and beliefs conducive to optimal patient outcomes.
- Improve concordance to treatment and monitoring.

The scope and depth of information/education provided may vary according to the nature of the condition and treatment offered, e.g.:

- The personal preferences of the individual in relation to informational/educational needs, e.g.:
  - Active or passive coping style.
  - Health beliefs and behaviours.
  - Cognitive abilities.
- Acute or chronic condition (one-stop rather than ongoing).
- Medical intervention (high- or low-risk treatment).
- Complexities related to treatments (e.g. risks and benefits of drug therapies).
- The mediating factors that improve outcomes (e.g. prompt treatment of infections).

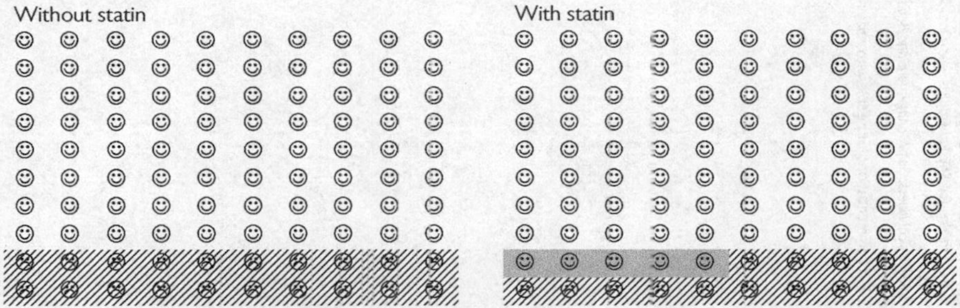

Without statin

With statin

If 100 people each take a statin (such as simvastatin) for 10 years:

- About five people will be 'saved' from having a cardiovascular event by taking the statin (solid grey face above)
- About 80 people will not have a cardiovascular event, but would not have done so even if they had not taken a statin (unshaded faces above)
- About 15 people will still have a cardiovascular event (hatched faces), even though they take a statin

Fig. 10.3 Decision aids. An example of a visual aid to improve decision making.

Adapted from Ahmed, Naik, Willoughby et al. (2012) Communicating risk. *BMJ* 2012;344:e3996 with permission from the BMJ Publishing Group.

- The level of distress or anxiety experienced by the patient (and their family).
- The rehabilitation or recovery phase.

Further reading

Hammond A, Niedermann K (2010). Patient education and self-management. In: Dziedzic K, Hammond A (eds) *Rheumatology: Evidence Based Practice for Physiotherapists and Occupational Therapists*, pp. 78–93. Edinburgh: Churchill Livingstone.

Newman S, Steed L, Mulligan K (eds) (2009). *Chronic Physical Illness: Self-Management and Behavioural Interventions*. Oxford: Oxford University Press.

Zangi HA, Nodosi M, Adams J, et al. (2014). EULAR recommendations for people with inflammatory arthritis. *Ann Rheum Dis* 75:954–62.

Social and psychological aspects of a new diagnosis

When a person receives a diagnosis, it may be perceived as a threat to health and well-being. The ability to adapt to a diagnosis and the consequences varies significantly. This ability to adjust to a diagnosis is often independent of disease severity and correlates more closely to levels of perceived confidence (SE) and active coping styles.

For some the diagnosis can result in a perceived change from (healthy) person to (sick) patient. The level of threat may rest upon:

- The perceived (or actual) threat of the diagnosis and treatment.
- Prior experiences of ill health or knowledge of the condition, e.g. family history.
- The adaptation to health and lifestyle as a result of a new diagnosis.
- The stigma attached to the continued illness, e.g. OA is a considered a disease of the elderly.
- The effect the diagnosis has upon their perceived role in society, and within the family infrastructure/community.
- The patient's psychological status and coping styles.
- Acute or chronic status of condition.
- Predictable nature of symptoms/disease changes.

Adjustment phase

The practitioner–patient relationship is frequently cited in research as an important factor in aiding the patient's ability to adjust to their diagnosis.

However, individuals differ in many ways to their diagnosis and in the length of time taken to 'come to terms' or 'adjust' to their condition.

Patients may be aware of changes in their mobility or limitation in ADLs. These losses can impact independence, self-esteem, and relationships. In acute conditions, these losses may be short lived. In LTCs, the loss can be compounded by the unpredictable yet deteriorating nature of the disease. The effects can be profound in psychological and social terms (e.g. poor self-esteem, denial, and financial losses due to work-related issues). Self-reported pain and depression in MSCs is high. Deterioration in physical ability is a contributing factor to poor outcomes in MSCs.

During the adjustment phase, patients may be in 'denial' and fail to actively participate in healthcare decisions or recall important information. This phase may also result in numerous stressors that may be socially or psychologically driven. These factors may mean that the patient's ability to retain or recall information may be suboptimal.

Key message

Educational opportunities must be taken whenever the patient appears responsive to receiving information. Education should be an ongoing aspect of nursing care and should not be considered a 'one-stop shop'.

Educating the patient and the family

Educating the patient about their condition and treatment options is a perquisite of all nursing support. Education should be delivered using a patient-centred and holistic approach, enabling a strong therapeutic relationship to develop. Patient education is the precursor to self-management.

Some MSCs are poorly understood and there are many lay perceptions about the conditions, treatment efficacy, and long-term outcomes—the commonly quoted phrase (even by some HCPs) is that 'nothing can be done to treat arthritis', for instance.

Dispelling lay perceptions and building a positive and informed approach to practical aspects of managing conditions such as 'arthritis' will start the patient on the right pathway through their healthcare journey and will enhance the patient's perceived control over their disease.

Key points and tips to educating the patient and their family

- Encourage the patient to bring a partner or family member along to the consultation.
- If the partner attends the clinic (and the patient consents to their participation), recognize the partner's role in supporting the patient and include them in the consultation where appropriate.
- Always ensure that information provided at the consultation is supported by written information for the patient to take home with them.
- For those who do not have English as their first language, a partner or family member can be very helpful in interpreting but also advising on lifestyle issues (e.g. fasting times, pain beliefs).
- A partner may provide additional importance advice about family responsibilities or functional difficulties that the patient is reticent about reporting.
- Patient support groups or volunteer activities can be mentioned which include the patient and the partner.
- Partners may aid recall and questioning of issues.
- The HCP is seen by the partner to give full recognition to the patient's condition and symptoms.
- Partners may become integral to patients' care over time and active involvement helps to build a relationship with the multiprofessional team, e.g. poor hand function may mean a partner will offer to administer subcutaneous injections.

Challenges in educating the patient and family

- The patient may decline to have the partner involved in care or there may be tensions between the patient and their partner during the consultation.
- Anxieties of a partner can be higher than those of the patient.
- Managing the consultation may be more complex.

Self-efficacy and concordance

Self-efficacy

SE is the perception or belief that a person has the confidence in their ability to undertake important activities that benefit their lives. SE focuses on the person's perception of their ability rather than the actual ability of undertaking the task. Believing someone has control over their life and the ability to undertake certain tasks in their life can improve health outcomes. SE was originally defined by Bandura in 1977.[1]

SE related to health behaviour is predictive of future health status and is amenable to change through education (unlike other psychological traits that are resistant or prove difficult to change). SE is an important outcome to focus on because:

- Beliefs can powerfully determine the level of commitment a person applies to achieve defined outcomes.
- Timely, targeted patient education interventions improve SE.
- SE can be used as a patient-centred outcome measure.
- Assessment tools can provide evidence on baseline SE for pain and other symptoms.

There are specific SE tools for arthritis:

- The Arthritis SE Scale (ASES).
- The Rheumatoid Arthritis SE scale (RASE).
- Self-Efficacy Scale (SES).

➲ Also see 'Assessment tools', Chapter 20, pp. 595–612.

Concordance

Concordance is a term used to describe an interactional decision process that creates a therapeutic partnership. Developing concordance with a patient is an effective approach to treating a patient with therapies they wish to be prescribed and feel able to take. Healthcare resources can be used more effectively, and patient satisfaction and outcomes are likely to benefit from this approach.

Concordance is an important component of:

- A holistic patient-centred consultation.
- Patient empowerment and self-management.
- Clinical governance and risk management.
- Responsible prescribing.

➲ Also see 'Holistic assessment', pp. 330–331; ➲ 'Patient-centred care', pp. 332–335.

Reference

Bandura A (1977). Self-efficacy: toward a unifying theory of behavioral change. *Psychol Rev* 84:191–215.

Further reading

Nodosi M, Johnson D, Young T, et al. (2016). Effects of needs-based patient education on self-efficacy and health outcomes in people with rheumatoid arthritis: a multi-center, single blind, randomised controlled trial. *Ann Rheum Dis* 75:1126–32.

Ryan S, Carr A (2010). Applying the biopsychosocial model to the management of rheumatic disease. In: Dziedzic K, Hammond A (eds) *Rheumatology: Evidence Based Practice for Physiotherapists and Occupational Therapists*, pp. 63–75. Edinburgh: Churchill Livingstone.

Vanden Bernt BJ, Zwikker HE, vanden Ende CH (2012). Medication adherence in patients with RA: a critical appraisal if the existing literature. *Expert Rev Clin Immunol* 8:337–51.

Self-management: what is it?

Introduction

The term self-management describes the ability of an individual to effectively manage their condition on a day-to-day basis. This ability to self-manage is the aim of all patient education and as such, these two concepts go hand in hand. These are different models for delivering education. Educational aspects also need to be considered in the context of the biopsychosocial model of health and illness (➔ see 'Patient education', pp. 336–337).

Following on from patient education, the patient should recognize the scope and potential benefit of undertaking some level of self-management of their condition. This usually comes once the patient has made an initial adjustment to their diagnosis and received sufficient education to enable them to feel confident in their ability to self-manage and to effectively cope with some aspects of their condition.

Self-management principles include:

- Taking responsibility for their lives, health, and disease states
- Recognizing the value of making informed decisions about their treatment.
- Understanding how to manage exacerbations of their condition using pharmacological and non-pharmacological treatments.
- Monitoring aspects of their treatment and potential side effects/toxicity.
- Knowing when to seek medical advice and who to go to.
- Recognizing health behaviours beneficial to general well-being.

It is important to remember that long-term MSCs are:

- Chronic—treatable but rarely curable.
- Have a very variable course—characterized by episodic exacerbations of symptoms.
- Have a variable outcome—symptoms may deteriorate slowly, a few people have infrequent, mild exacerbations, and a minority experience constant, severe symptoms.
- Access to help is not available 24 hours a day, 7 days a week, so people must learn to self-manage non-life-threatening fluctuating symptoms and problems.

The biopsychosocial model of health and illness

The biopsychosocial model of health and illness recognizes the influence of people's perspective on their physical, psychological, emotional, and social well-being. These perspectives include the individual's:

- Attitudes.
- Health beliefs.
- Understandings.
- Experiences.
- Emotions.
- Personal relationships.
- Social environment.
- Social networks.

The biopsychosocial model advocates a holistic approach to management of chronic conditions. The individual's experiences of living with the consequences of ill health (physical, social, and psychological) must be recognized to ensure appropriate strategies are provided to aid the individual adjust and learn to self-manage and enhance SE. The biopsychosocial model identifies the importance of the following:

- Positive experiences enhance appropriate health beliefs and behaviours and negative experiences are detrimental to SE.
- Psychosocial traits are key determinants of poor health behaviours ('catastrophizing' or 'fear-avoidance').
- Health behaviours (or traits) may not be easy to change. Factors that will affect the individual's ability to modify or change health behaviours include:
  - Prior health behaviours and beliefs.
  - Perceived threat to the individual's health and health beliefs.
  - Anxieties and needs of the individual.
  - Prior experiences in achieving SE.
  - The predictable or unpredictable aspects of their condition.
  - Beliefs in the ability to access support and advice when self-management principles have been exhausted.

Self-management strategies

- Challenge erroneous ill-health beliefs.
- Teaches coping skills.
- Enhances SE.
- Reduces helplessness.
- Reduces social isolation.

Achieved by:

- Information and knowledge about the condition.
- Endorsing and empowering self-management principles.
- Practising new skills.
- Encouraging alternative supportive 'non-medicalized' infrastructures (voluntary or support groups).
- Demonstrating SE principles.

Further reading

Newman S, Steed L, Mulligan K (eds) (2009). *Chronic Physical Illness: Self-Management and Behavioural Interventions*. Oxford: Oxford University Press.

Motivational interviewing and goal setting

Motivational interviewing

Motivational interviewing (MI) is an evidenced-based approach used to talk to patients about making changes in their behaviour. Living with the symptoms of a chronic MSC, including pain and fatigue, often means that changes in behaviour are required to manage these symptoms effectively, thus improving everyday life. For example, pacing out activities can help with both pain and fatigue but the patient concerned may find it difficult to adjust their behaviour to accommodate this. This is where MI can be useful.

The following questions are part of a MI approach which can be used to help the patient consider changing their behaviour and the example of managing fatigue through the use of pacing demonstrates how these questions can be used in practice:

- What do you not like about where you are now? ('I am always feeling tired.')
- What would be the consequences if you continue? ('I will keep feeling tired.')
- What might be the consequences of change? ('I might feel less tired.')
- What would you have to do in order to change? ('Try something to reduce the tiredness.')

The main emphasis of MI is that the clinician asks the questions rather than informing the patient what to do. People learn their own views and attitudes by hearing themselves talk and learn best by providing solutions as to how they might change their behaviour. The reasons for change need to be stronger than maintaining the status quo and using MI can prompt the patient to consider the advantages and disadvantages of behaviour change. During the consultation, the clinician can offer views and expertise but any decision to change needs to come from the patient.

MI promotes patient decision-making and is a key element of collaborative care and self-management. Using MI questions can improve the communication between the clinician and the patient but will often require practice as it can be a very different way of conducting a consultation.

Evidence where MI has been used effectively in MSCs includes:

- Improved function and a trend towards improved pain control in knee OA.
- ↑ engagement with exercise in fibromyalgia syndrome.
- Enhanced medication adherence, physical activity, and coping strategies for pain and fatigue in RA.

Goal setting

Goal setting is one of the most effective motivational strategies used in self-help and personal development. It is often a component of self-management programmes for people with RA, OA, and fibromyalgia syndrome to enable patients to develop the skills to manage their own symptoms. It can also be used on an individual basis.

Goal setting enables the patient to decide on an outcome that they identify as important to them, e.g. being able to walk the dog, and to plan how they will achieve the desired outcome.

The SMART model can be used with a patient to provide a structure to the goal setting. The model consists of the following aspects:

S = Specific: walking the dog.
M = Measurable: twice a week.
A = Appropriate: how important is this goal to you (1–10)?
R = Realistic: how confident are you that you can carry out this goal (1–10)?
T = Time-bound: on a Monday, Wednesday, and Friday.

It is necessary to ask the patient how important the goal is and how confident they are so that they can achieve the goal by rating both aspects from 1 to 10. If a patient cites <7, they are unlikely to achieve the goal. If this occurs, the nurse needs to revisit this goal and establish whether this is the right goal to be undertaken and what would need to occur to ↑ the patient's confidence in undertaking the goal.

There is evidence that goal setting can:

- ↑ physical activity and manage pain and fatigue in RA, OA, and fibromyalgia syndrome.
- Help patients with RA to set personal, social, and treatment goals.

Further reading

Georgopoulous S, Prothero L, Lempp H, et al. (2016). Motivational interviewing: relevance in the treatment of RA. *Rheumatology* 55:1348–56.

Strand V, Wright GC, Bergman MJ, et al. (2015). Patient expectations and perceptions of goal setting strategies for disease management in RA. *J Rheumatol* 42:2046–54.

Simple self-management strategies for symptom control

Non-pharmacological self-management strategies include a range of options. The strategies work on reducing the heightened awareness to pain sensations by distraction or changing mood. Perceived SE enhances the reduction of anxieties. A number of tools can be considered.

Heat and cold (thermotherapy)

- Some people find warming a joint relieves pain, others find cooling more effective.
- Commercial heat/cold packs are available but can be made by wrapping a hot water bottle, ice cubes, or frozen peas in a towel; a warm bath or thermal clothing coolant sprays are also effective. Advise to:
  - Position yourself comfortably so the joint is supported.
  - Place the hot/cold pack over the joint for 10–15 min.
  - Remove the pack and gently move the joint.
  - Replace the hot/cold pack on the joint for another 5–10 min.
- Gently warming or cooling a joint is very safe. The sensation of heat/ cold should not become uncomfortable. People with circulatory problems or ↓ thermal sensation (diabetes) should use it cautiously.

Transcutaneous electrical neuromuscular stimulation

TENS produces pulsed electrical stimulation using electrodes placed on the skin. The current then activates specific nerve fibres which may inhibit pain sensations to the brain. TENS may deliver:

- High frequency.
- Low frequency.
- A pulsed form of TENS that can switch between high and low frequency.

The use of TENS carries very little risk, is non-invasive, and can be self-applied using relatively cheap, readily available machines.

Massage

- Rubbing a pain is an innate reaction to pain.
- Direct human physical contact has a profoundly comforting effect, inducing relaxation and calm.
- The pain relief produced by moisturizers, oils, gels, and creams is partially due to the massaging action in applying them.
- Gently massaging painful joints or muscles for 5–10 min is a simple, effective, safe, and pleasurable (!) way to relieve pain.

Joint protection

The use of aids and devices to support, protect, or rest the affected or painful joint. Forms of joint protection include:

- Splints particularly used in inflammatory forms of arthritis or where instability or pain is present (➔ see 'Joint protection', Chapter 19, pp. 584–585; ➔ 'Why split joints?', Chapter 19, pp. 586–587).

- Aids and devices include equipment used to relieve the stressors to the joint, e.g.:
  - Tap turners, chair raisers, vegetable peelers, and kettle tippers.
  - Dressing aids and hook-and-loop fastener straps.
  - Walking aids and specific footwear.

➲ Also see 'Equipment aids and devices', Chapter 11, pp. 361–363.

Pacing, rest, and relaxation

Rest–activity cycling

'Rest–activity cycling', or pacing, encourages people to intersperse activity with periods of rest. Muscle fatigue causes abnormal movement which can lead to pain and damage. People often carry out activities (especially chores such as gardening, housework, and shopping) in spite of discomfort and pain. Adopting good habits and behaviours can avoid fatigue and pain (Box 10.1). Initially this may seem be seen an inconvenience, but gradually individuals should find that as the time of activity between rests ↑, the activity becomes easier with much less pain.

Physical activity

- Physiologically, physical activity improves joint mobility, strength, endurance, 'normalizes' motor neuron transmission, and biomechanics.
- Psychologically, appreciating what they can do makes people feel good, ↓ depression, and ↑ self-confidence, self-esteem, and independence.
- For simple ways of ↑ physical activity, see ➲ 'Exercises', Chapter 11, pp. 367–380.

Box 10.1 Advice to patients on a rest–activity cycle

- Identify activities that cause pain, e.g. gardening, hoovering, and shopping.
- Think about the way you are doing them—most people begin to experience pain after a relatively short time but continue the task until it is completed or pain forces them to stop.
- Recognize how long it takes you to begin to feel tired and some mild discomfort (e.g. after 20 min); take a break at this point (5–10 min), before returning to the task.
- Take another break if pain starts to ↑ again, or finish the task later.

Pacing, rest, and relaxation as an additional option for symptom control

For those with severe or inflammatory pain, they may need to build in a period of relaxation to enable them to cope with an otherwise full day of activity—particularly during exacerbations of their condition.

- To achieve effective relaxation, a timed period of total muscle relaxation resting on the bed listening to restful music or reading may reduce levels of fatigue and ultimately reduce pain levels.
- The time spent relaxing can be gradually reduced as the flare settles.

Self-management principles: relaxation and breathing techniques

Perception of pain is heightened by stress, anxiety, worry, and depression, ↑ muscle tension, poor shallow breathing patterns, and feelings of being helplessly controlled by pain. Left unchecked, individuals can start to 'catastrophize' based upon the learnt behaviours and beliefs.

These feelings can be modified and ultimately changed by allowing individuals to recognize the effects of their feelings on signs of stress, tension, and anxiety that result in:

- Shallow breathing, feeling uptight, and shoulders, neck, back, and leg muscle tension.
- Certain recognized situations that make the individual tense or anxious.
- Learnt beliefs or behaviours that link association to pain.

Self-management strategies encourage the individual to recognize their ability to relieve anxieties related to perceived threats to health status.

Simple relaxation and breathing strategies that can be used any time, any place, anywhere include deep breathing (Box 10.2).

Managing exacerbations of pain and inflammation for patients

- Rest, do not go to bed, but avoid or reduce activities that aggravate your pain (i.e. prolonged standing or walking) for a couple of days until the pain subsides.
- Use heat or cold therapy several times each day.
- Practise deep breathing and relaxation techniques if you feel anxious and tense.
- Resume exercising gently once the pain starts to settle; if you do not move, your joints will stiffen up very quickly and your muscles will weaken and tire quickly.
- Gradually ↑ your activity levels.

Box 10.2 Deep-breathing advice for patients

- Sit or stand up straight.
- Relax your shoulders.
- Place a hand on your tummy just below your ribs.
- Take a slow, gentle deep breath in through your nose, feel your hand and tummy rising and your chest to expand fully.
- Slowly breathe out through your mouth, feel your tummy and hand gently sink.
- Repeat this for four or five deep breaths, then rest and breathe in a normal relaxed way for a couple of minutes.
- If necessary, repeat the exercise for 5–10 min.

Expert patient and voluntary sector education and support

There are many sources of education and support in the community for people with MSCs, particularly to provide information based on a general support for problems related to LTCs or aspects of 'arthritis' (the lay term to describe all forms of joint pain). They can be helpful in providing generic information about managing the symptoms and how to cope on a day-to-day basis. The community and voluntary sector now play an increasingly important role in providing information or support for patients.

Voluntary organizations

There are numerous opportunities for a number of community-based services or voluntary organizations to complement the healthcare services. Examples include:

- The National Rheumatoid Arthritis Society (NRAS) volunteer network. Developing volunteers from the patient group who may be able to provide a 'buddy system' or be trained to provide telephone support (e.g. the NRAS Telephone Volunteer Network).
- Classes to improve their health and well-being (e.g. swimming or exercise classes provided by the local leisure centre, funded by a charity but delivered in the community).
- Dietary advice and cookery classes on healthy eating options.
- Local pharmacy programmes to encourage simple screening (e.g. of blood pressure) or information access points on medication queries.
- Facilitating meetings or events that enable people to meet with others who have the same condition or similar problems.
- Community-based education programmes providing general advice for all people with a LTC.
- Enabling patients who have become 'experts in their condition' to work as lay teachers in a structured educational programme.
- Patient educators—where patients are trained to educate HCPs on joint examination techniques.
- Regional networks where patients can become an important member of an expert panel on the needs of the local community (e.g. the national network of Arthritis and Musculoskeletal Alliance (ARMA) groups).

Support groups

- NRAS: campaigning support group with many resources, telephone support, local networks of support, and regional volunteer/coordinators (http://www.nras.org.uk/).
- Healthtalkonline (http://www.healthtalkonline.org): video and audio clips of people discussing their health experiences.
- ARMA: an alliance of patient and health professional organizations (http:arma.uk.net). The website provides many useful resources and links to patient organizations for a wide range of conditions.

Care in the community

General practice: practical tips

Painful joints

Patients will often present in 1° care with problems related to joint or muscle pain and this can be daunting for the new practice nurse with little or no experience of MSCs. Patients may also present for other investigations or treatment and may refer to their joint problems at the same time. Individuals with symptomatic conditions affecting the joints may be reticent about seeking advice as they believe 'nothing that can be done to help their joint pains'. Support and advice offered by the 1° care team will be invaluable to those who are symptomatic.

This chapter will focus on how the patient can be assessed and referred appropriately to the right HCP and help that can be offered during the consultation (Box 11.1).

The ranges of MSCs can span mild, self-limiting, acute, chronic, and re-occurring chronic conditions. In older patients, the commonest problems are symptomatic of OA or gout; the prevalence of inflammatory conditions ↑ in middle age; and in the young, systemic conditions are more likely.

➲ Also see 'Introduction', Chapter 1, pp. 4–5; ➲ 'Assessing the patient', Chapter 8, pp. 290–291.

Observe ROMs and examine the affected joint for:

- Position at rest.
- Gait.
- ROM.
- Deformity.
- Signs of active inflammation (synovitis).

➲ Also see 'Assessing the patient', Chapter 8, pp. 290–291.

Nursing/team aspects to consider

- Listen to their story and show empathy.
- Document the patient-reported experiences and problems.
- Assess the impact the pain has on their day-to-day life:
  - Consider referral to their GP; confirm diagnosis if indicated.
  - Explore current pain-relieving strategies and efficacy (pharmacological and non-pharmacological), e.g. rest position and heat/ice (➲ see 'Symptom control', Chapter 9, pp. 315–319).

Box 11.1 Questions to ask all patients with joint pain

- Which joints are affected?
- Is this a new problem?
- How long have you had the pain?
- How does it affect you day to day?
- Does the pain wake you at night?
- What have you tried to relieve it, including medications?
- What exacerbates the pain?
- Have you consulted with anyone about this before and are there any plans to deal with this?
- What is/was your occupation?

- If appropriate, consider investigations, e.g. CRP, ESR, RF, Hb, and urate.
- Offer written information or recognized website access.[1,2]

➔ Also see 'Care in the community', Chapter 11, pp. 351–383.

The team approach in primary care

In many countries, a range of new roles have been developed to support the management of patients, such as physician's assistant/associate and clinical/community pharmacists. A collaborative team approach is encouraged, and, in some practices, there are meetings at the end of morning sessions to discuss cases that require more complex review and management.[3]

Red flags in history taking and assessment

- Fever.
- Pain that wakes them at night.
- If one joint is red, very hot, intensely painful, with limited ROM, septic arthritis must be excluded—GP intervention. ❗ Septic arthritis is easy to miss with a patient with coexisting RA and may be mistaken for a flare-up of their RA.
- Patients with arm pain—might be due to other causes other than arthritis, such as angina or cervical nerve root compression. It is important to ensure that these concerns are appropriately explored.
- Patients on MTX and other specific DMARDs must have regular blood tests including LFTs, FBC, and ESR.
- Patients newly prescribed MTX may fail to understand that MTX is to be taken once a week. If possible, an early telephone check on compliance is useful.
- Ensure patient has a completed Electronic Shared Care Agreement for their management.
- Rarely can develop blood dyscrasias (➔ see 'Monitoring and treatment of side effects', Chapter 16, pp. 446–451 and Chapter 17, pp. 508–509).
- Mouth ulcers may be a sign that folic acid is not being taken.
- Patients should be aware that while they are having a flare, exercise should be continued but the time spent and intensity should be reduced.

References

1. Versus Arthritis (formed in 2018 from a merger of Arthritis Research UK and Arthritis Care): https://www.versusarthritis.org/
2. National Rheumatoid Arthritis Society: http://www.rheumatoid.org.uk
3. Denovan J, Dawe J, Loganath K. Huddles in primary care: promoting healthy team dynamics. RCGP. http://www.rcgp.org.uk/clinical-and-research/resources/bright-ideas/huddles-in-primary-care-promoting-healthy-team-dynamics.aspx

Managing patients with co-morbidities

The general health of individuals in wealthy economies has greatly improved in the last century and as a result life expectancy has ↑ significantly. However, ↑ longevity can come at a cost for the individual and society as life is extended but with a growing number of incurable conditions and additional health problems. Many of these incurable conditions are categorized as a LTC. These LTCs can affect many body systems. Examples include:

- Cardiovascular disease, e.g. peripheral vascular disease, congestive cardiac failure, and hypertension.
- Diabetes.
- Neurological conditions, e.g. dementia, Parkinson's disease, and multiple sclerosis.
- Respiratory conditions, e.g. asthma and COPD.
- Musculoskeletal, e.g. OA, RA, JIA, and scleroderma.
- Mental health, e.g. depression.

The 1° diagnosis of a LTC can be compounded by additional co-morbidities. Individuals with one or more co-morbidities face numerous challenges over the course of their disease, impacting on the individual's physical, social, and psychological well-being (Box 11.2).

➲ Also see 'Education, social, and psychological issues', Chapter 10, pp. 329–340; ➲ 'Assessing the patient', Chapter 8, pp. 290–291.

For the nurse providing care for those with LTCs, planned reviews and management are essential to ensure appropriate care is provided and treatment adheres to recognized standards and guidelines in care. These management decisions experience additional complexities particularly for:

- The frail and elderly who require additional health needs assessments.
- Those with one or more co-morbidities will present:
  - Challenges in prescribing appropriate pain relief.
  - Concordance with exercise regimens.
  - Treatment monitoring and side effects related to different drugs.
  - The additional factors related to the social and psychological impact of more than one co-morbidity.

Assessments must adequately account for patient needs, particularly as:

- Pain is the predominant reason for those with joint problems to seek advice from their doctor or nurse. Simple practical information, appropriate pain relief, and signposting to information or referral are essential aspects of nursing care.
- Functional limitations (e.g. OA of knee or hip) may be the key limiting factor in achieving exercise tolerance, weight reduction, or positive health behaviours.
- Self-efficacy can be enhanced by addressing patient-identified needs in relation to changes in functional ability, social activities, independence, and quality of life.
- Health awareness and a positive approach to achieving a bone healthy lifestyle can be enhanced by demonstrating a positive 'can do' attitude in all care settings reducing the risk of learned 'helplessness'.

➲ Also see 'Symptom control', Chapter 9, pp. 315–319; ➲ 'When to refer to the multidisciplinary team', Chapter 12, pp. 392–393.

Box 11.2 Co-morbidities and pain: management approach

- Full holistic nursing assessment and screening questions for MSCs.
- If unsure about diagnosis, seek medical opinion to confirm underlying pathology (e.g. OA not PsA or mild, self-limiting conditions). Referral, if required, to specialist teams.
- Identify aggravating or relieving factors for pain (and functional problems in relation to pain).
- Assess pain using VAS for pain—review after a 2-week treatment plan.
- Provide written and verbal information on how pain works and why regular, simple analgesia is more effective in managing pain than sporadic dosing.
- Provide information (written and verbal) on non-pharmacological self-management approaches to support pain relief (e.g. rest, pacing, joint protection, and cold packs or hot baths). Use as an adjunct to pharmacological measures (➔ see 'Symptom control', Chapter 9, pp. 315–319).
- In prescribing consider:
  - Contraindications and drug interactions/cautions in relation to current medications and proposed pharmacological options.
  - Frail/elderly/renal or liver impairments/cautions and contraindications in prescribing and reduce dosages or select most appropriate drug.
  - Analgesia (simple and compound) regular dosing and optimal doses to achieve pain relief.
  - If first step approach to achieving pain relief fails to adequately control pain, review other prescribing options (➔ see 'Symptom control', Chapter 9, pp. 315–319).
- Consider psychological and educational needs in relation to pain and underlying pathology.
- Encourage access to voluntary organizations/additional resources.
- Review pain assessments and prescribing plan/referral where necessary.
- Identify changes/benefits to LTC/co-morbidities.

Functional limitations

- Identify functional limitations in relation to lifestyle, social support, and level of need/distress/pain.
- Provide practical advice on simple aids and devices if appropriate.
- Consider referral for functional assessment with PT and/or OT (for joint protection and assessment on functional ability in the context of ADLs).
- Discuss risk factors in relation to changes in functional ability—risk of falls, loss of independence.
- Management plan and review of function/pain/goal setting.

Skin integrity, continence, and caring for carers

Some MSCs can impact normal ROMs, functional ability, and distribution of weight. Other factors include changes to tissues as a result of the disease process (e.g. scleroderma) or drug therapies (e.g. corticosteroids). These changes may affect skin integrity, continence, and function by:

- Causing friction or rubbing from abnormal movement or weight distribution (e.g. Trendelenburg gait and use of crutches).
- Inhibition (in ability or pace) to access toilet facilities or manage clothing (functional limitation to gait or manual dexterity—e.g. scleroderma changes that cause tight and contracted skin tissues).
- Poor disease control resulting in an inability to mobilize at particular times of the day (gelling after inactivity in OA or EMS in RA). Flares of the disease can result in a systemic illness with fever, pain, and systemic effects such as fatigue.
- Disease-specific changes that result in ulcerations due to autoimmune responses, e.g. vasculitis.
- Medications that affect skin integrity, e.g. corticosteroids.

Consider a formal assessment for those at risk.

Caring for the carers

The practice nurse will often have contact with carers of those diagnosed with arthritis and may find themselves in a position to counsel, advise, or perhaps just listen to the carer. Providing good support is important. Although the patient may receive enough support the carer may not and they may feel inadequate, isolated, and frustrated at not knowing how they can help.

The practice nurse may recognize psychological and emotional reactions especially at initial diagnosis of a partner or close relative.

Nursing interventions

- Encourage the carer to talk about their feelings and anxieties.
- Offer information.
- Encourage the carer to give emotional support.
- Include the carer in decision-making.
- Highlight the areas the patient might be experiencing concerns with in relation to loss of independence, altered body image, reduced self-esteem and low mood, and medication side effects.
- Encourage the carer to act as a link and information provider to others involved in the patient's care.
- Encourage the patient to acknowledge their own needs and seek appropriate guidance and support.
- Ensure patients and carers are aware of care benefits that may be available to them through the health or social care system (e.g. Carer's Allowance).

Musculoskeletal conditions in the frail and elderly

Care for the frail and elderly

The frail or elderly patient may be receiving support in a care home or sheltered housing or may be living independently. Pain and functional limitations are likely to alert the nurses to a potential musculoskeletal problem (MSC) (Box 11.3). The level of trained nursing support may also vary and patients may have inter-related health and social care needs. Pain is a common feature and is frequently under-treated in the frail and elderly.

Nurses play an important role in enabling the individual to maximize their general health status and quality of life. People who have complex needs, long-term conditions, multiple co-morbidities, or polypharmacy require a thorough assessment and review to optimize management.[1]

The assessment

Apart from the key aspects required to assess all patients (clinical history and physical assessment), there may be specific issues to consider when assessing individuals who are frail or elderly who will require a more in-depth exploration to identify those vulnerable or frail individuals who have additional complex needs. This may include:

- Functional ability in the context of:
  - Achieving optimum in quality of life and activities.
  - Risk of falls.
  - Maintaining independence.
- Cognitive ability and/or any sensory impairments:
  - Visual or hearing deficits may ↑ risks and ↓ quality of life.
- Social and psychological needs:
  - Social isolation.
  - Economic issues.
  - General physical and mental factors that affect psychological functioning, e.g. bereavement, isolation, and depression.
- Symptom control:
  - Some individuals may be more accepting of their condition (an inevitable consequence of ageing) or may not wish to be seen as a nuisance.
- Personal care needs.
  - Physical ability and cognitive aspects may reduce independence and the ability to carry out some aspects of personal care.

Box 11.3 The most common MSCs affecting the elderly

- Symptomatic and asymptomatic OA—commonly affecting hands, base of thumb, cervical spine, hip, and knees.
- PMR.
- Gout or pseudogout.
- Osteoporosis and related low-impact fractures.
- Inflammatory arthritides, e.g. RA.

- Tissue viability:
  - The ageing process and skin damage may result in fragile or friable tissues vulnerable to damage.
- Dignity and choice:
  - Individuals may require support and guidance on maintaining treatment options and their independent roles.
  - Impairment (physical or mental) should not be a barrier to maintaining choice and dignity.
- Pharmacological aspects:
  - Ageing kidneys do not excrete drugs so effectively and prescribing decisions need to take into account the patient's age and ability to absorb, metabolize, and excrete drug therapies.

Assessing pain

The assessment of pain is discussed in ➔ 'Assessing pain', Chapter 8, pp. 290–291 and pp. 310–313. Individuals with pain (particularly if cognitively or sensorial impaired) may present with agitation, disorientation, poor sleep patterns, depression, anxiety, or anorexia. Pain will frequently affect mobility and ability to self-manage, e.g. ↑ pain may present challenges for the individual in maintaining continence. In those with dementia, assessing pain presents additional challenges. Ideally, patient self-reported pain tools should be used. Evidence suggests that even those with a Mini Mental State Examination score as low as 6 are able to verbally report pain using self-report tools.

Management

➔ Refer to Chapter 6, 'Chronic non-inflammatory pain', pp. 185–197; ➔ Chapter 9, 'Symptom control: using pharmacological and non-pharmacological methods', pp. 315–318; ➔ Chapter 15, 'Pharmacological management: pain relief', pp. 436–444; ➔ Chapter 16, Pharmacological management: disease-modifying drugs, p. 445.

Key pharmacological issues in prescribing for the elderly

Generally, the majority of drug therapies result in greater and prolonged effects in those of ↑ age due to physiological changes in the older person. These changes can be seen in:

- Changes in the fat-to-muscle ratio.
- Muscle volume and power are ↓.
- Ageing heart, kidney, or liver leads to less efficient/poor function.
- ↓ in collagen, e.g. in the elasticity of the skin.
- Less acidity in the gut—acidity falls with ↑ age and motility ↓.
- Chronic kidney disease can be identified by measuring the glomerular filtration rate. Some drugs may be contraindicated with chronic kidney disease and others may require a reduction in dosing regimen to avoid the risk of drug toxicity.

Reference

1. NICE (2016). Multimorbidity: clinical assessment and management (NG56). http://www.nice.org.uk/guidance/ng56

Further reading

National Osteoporosis Society: http://www.nos.org.uk

NHS England (2014). Safe, compassionate care for frail older people using an integrated care pathway: practical guidance for commissioners, providers and nursing, medical and allied health professional leaders. http://www.england.nhs.uk/wp-content/uploads/2014/02/safe-comp-care.pdf

Royal College of General Practitioners and British Geriatrics Society (2016). *Integrated Care for Older People with Frailty: Innovative Approaches in Practice*. London: RCGP, BGS.

Scofield P (2018) The assessment of pain in older people: UK national guidelines. *Age Ageing* 47:il–22.

Versus Arthritis: https://www.versusarthritis.org/

Telephone advice line support

Telephone advice lines (sometimes referred to as helplines) provide prompt and effective support to individuals who require healthcare advice. Helplines are valued by patients, form a significant proportion of the workload for many nurse specialists, and frequently prevent hospital admissions or requests for specialist consultations.

Helpline services vary depending upon whether it is a generic rapid access service with the aim of prompt triage for those who require urgent care or is provided by a specialist team managing specific disease areas or conditions. Some examples include:

- *NHS 111.* A decision support system manned by nurses who provide generic support for a wide spectrum of individual calls in relation to all health problems.
- *Voluntary or charitable organizations.* Provide non-medical guidance and support. This is often within a specific disease area or set of conditions (e.g. continence services or RA).
- *A rheumatology or musculoskeletal advice line service.* Provided for those with a musculoskeletal diagnosis who require LTC guidance in relation to exacerbations or side effects.
- 1° *care services.* Some provide telephone triage prior to referral to a GP or rapid access support that allows a targeted triage system that enables the individual to see the most appropriate clinicians, effectively manage resources, and provide patient choice.

Individuals with a LTC value support provided by telephone advice line services because:

- Advice and support can be accessed from their own home in the context of their specific needs. This approach has the potential to enhance self-management principles if used effectively as a training tool.
- Specialist support in specific disease areas is valued by individuals who develop a therapeutic relationship with a team or service who understand the complexity of their condition.
- Continuity of care—a thorough audit trail and access to patient records allows specific advice for some patients.
- They can report side effects and problems with monitoring promptly.
- The consequences of the telephone advice line decisions are part of the overall specialist team's management plans for the specific condition.

Core principles of advice line support must include:

- Knowledge and competencies of those providing telephone advice.
- Clarity for all about the aims and objective of the service and times when available. This should include how long to wait for a return call if using an answerphone service.
- Documentation and effective communication about decisions/advice provided.
- Risk management and recognition of dangers of non-verbal prompts. This should include risks related to potential flaws in patient self-reported information and patient recall on advice given.

Further reading

RCN (2012). *Using Telephone Advice for Patients with Long-Term Conditions.* London: RCN.

Equipment aids and devices

Assistive technology: what is available to help?

There is a huge range of assistive technology including equipment, aids, devices, and support designed to help the elderly and people with disabilities maintain independence and function. Patients can have practical difficulties with a number of daily activities, e.g. personal care; household activities such as cooking, housework, and shopping; work (paid or voluntary); study; social and leisure activities (e.g. hobbies, gardening); and mobility (e.g. driving, walking, stairs, and public transport). Presume there is something that could help. Staying independent and actively engaged in work and leisure makes for a healthier person physically and psychologically.

Where can I get help with daily activities and work?

OTs have particular training in helping people remain independent through using rehabilitation and assistive technology (Table 11.1). They work in the NHS, local authority social services (LASS), housing associations, independent living equipment companies, and voluntary sector. Examples of support available in England and Wales include:

- OT assessments for functional needs and practical advice enabling aids to be reviewed before purchase: 'try before they buy'. OTs may be able to arrange free provision if the person is eligible.
- Housing adaptations and large personal care equipment, e.g. for bath, toilet, stair lift, or rails, can be provided for free by the local authority social services. Some may be means tested.
- The Disabled Living Foundation (DLF) has regional centres with extensive equipment displays from small kitchen gadgets, to bath and toilet aids, chairs, mobility aids, and stair lifts. Ring for an OT appointment in advance for independent advice.
- Environmental control systems (e.g. operating lights, curtains, doors, and electrical equipment) exist for people with more severe disabilities.
- Many small aids and devices can be purchased:
  - Increasingly, small gadgets are available in high street stores.
  - The DLF has helpful online advice and fact sheets on selecting equipment to suit all needs.

Work related issues: what help is available?

If your patient has problems coping with work because of arthritis you must act quickly.[1] OTs can provide lots of practical help—see Table 11.1.

- If the person has disclosed their condition to their employer, the OT can carry out a work visit and on-site ergonomic assessment.
- If they go on long-term sick leave or become unemployed it is much harder to get people back into work.[2] This can result in additional financial and psychological problems if not addressed as a priority.[2,3]

Table 11.1 Sources of help for aids and devices

Small gadgets for meal preparation	High street kitchen shops—look for light products, larger non-slip handles, lever action. 'Good Grips' range
Finding out about gadgets and equipment available	Any NHS OT or local authority social services OT for detailed assessment and help
	DLF centres (free professional independent advice from OTs). To locate centres and 'try before you buy' go to: 🔗 http://www.dlf.org.uk/public/findaproduct.html and also click on 'Ask SARA' for online advice and to download factsheets
	🔗 https://www.arthritisresearchuk.org/shop/products/publications/patient-information/living-with-arthritis/everyday-living-and-arthritis.aspx
	🔗 https://www.gov.uk/financial-help-disabled/home-and-housing —advice on where to get information; benefits; practical help with housing adaptations etc.
Free provision of aids and equipment	🔗 https://www.nhs.uk/conditions/social-care-and-support/equipment-aids-adaptations/—eligibility criteria may apply
Specialist shops and equipment providers	🔗 http://www.ableworld.co.uk—shops and online
	🔗 http://www.independentliving.co.uk—provides links to various suppliers
Driving and mobility (cars, scooters, and powered chairs)	🔗 http://www.drivingmobility.org.uk—independent OT advice on car adaptations/driving with a disability
	🔗 http://www.motability.co.uk—for financial assistance if eligible for mobility benefits
Work	Coping at work: refer to OT for work advice, ergonomic assessment, and getting help with changes
	🔗 http://www.gov.uk/browse/working
	🔗 http://www.gov.uk/access-to-work
	'Access To Work' scheme provides financial help with work adaptations
	Employer's occupational health department

References

1. Hammond A, O'Brien R, Woodbridge S, et al. (2017). Job retention vocational rehabilitation for employed people with inflammatory arthritis (WORK-IA): a feasibility randomized controlled trial. *BMC Musculoskelet Disord* 18:315.
2. Prior Y, Amanna A, Bodell S, Hammond A (2017). A qualitative evaluation of occupational therapy-led work rehabilitation for people with inflammatory arthritis: patients' views. *Br J Occup Ther* 80:39–48.
3. Department for Work and Pensions (2016). Improving Lives: The Work, Health and Disability Green Paper. 🔗 https://assets.publishing.service.gov.uk/government/uploads/system/uploads/attachment_data/file/564038/work-and-health-green-paper-improving-lives.pdf

Further reading

NRAS (2018). I want to work—a guide for people with rheumatoid arthritis on rights and responsibilities in the work place. ➶ https://www.nras.org.uk/publications/i-want-to-work

NRAS. Information leaflets on aids and devices: ➶ https://www.nras.org.uk/publications

Versus Arthritis. How can I get the right support? ➶ https://www.versusarthritis.org/about-arthritis/living-with-arthritis/work/

Case scenarios for the practice nurse

Case scenario 1

Mrs C comes to see you for her blood pressure check. While she is removing her coat she seems to be in significant pain from her upper arms and finds it difficult to raise her arms. She confides to you that she has had pain in her shoulders for a few months and it is getting worse—she puts it down to old age.

Questions to ask

- How does it affect you day to day?
- What have you tried to relieve it?
- How does it affect your ADL?
- What is/was your occupation?
- Any hobbies?
- Does it keep you awake at night?
- Any pins and needles?

Note the type of pain

- Location.
- Intensity.
- Frequency.
- Precipitating factors.
- Exclude referred pain or other underlying pathology, e.g. referred pain from the neck.
- Document the subjective information from the patient, in their own words.
- Note the patient's posture while talking to you.

Nursing intervention

- Temperature.
- Blood pressure.
- ESR/CRP and FBC.
- Appointment with GP after blood results are received.
- Encourage patient to take simple analgesia until their GP appointment.
- Provide information on non-pharmacological pain-relieving strategies, e.g. use of cold or heat packs.

Differential diagnosis

- PMR.
- OA in the shoulder.
- Simple muscular strain.

Case scenario 2

Ms B has recently been diagnosed with RA and started on MTX. She is 18 years old. She is being monitored at the local hospital rheumatology department. She comes to see you for her contraceptive check. She bursts into tears and after listening to her it becomes apparent she is worried about the consequences to her life; for instance, will she ever be able to have her own children or is she is going to end up in a wheelchair like her grandmother?

How can you help?

Nursing interventions

- Listen and empathize.
- Tease out all her concerns—remember she has probably been told to limit her alcohol intake which can be tricky if she is young and possibly wants to be out with her peers in clubs (➲ see Chapter 16, 'Pharmacological management', p. 445).
- Explain that the principle of intensive treatment at the start of the diagnosis is to prevent damage and complications in later life (➲ see Chapter 16, 'Pharmacological management', p. 445).
- Reassure her that RA is better understood today and treatments have changed significantly and are much more effectively targeted to achieve remission. Treatment has dramatically improved since the days when her grandmother was treated.
- Advise her that with a bit of careful planning of her treatment with her specialist team she will be able to consider having a family at some point (➲ see 'Pregnancy and fertility', chapter 14, pp. 415–418).
- Encourage exercise governed by how she feels day to day.
- Explain pacing to ensure she can manage her job.
- Encourage her to explain her problems to her friends. Reassure her that she will have good and bad days to start with when she may feel more tired, and that the medication will take a few months to reach its full potential.
- Encourage concordance related to medication and blood monitoring.
- If available, advise her of the specialist telephone advice line service.
- Suggest she contacts the specialist nurse for additional advice on her RA if indicated.

For practical advice on osteoporosis and osteoarthritis see ➲ Chapter 2, p. 12; ➲ Chapter 3, 'Osteoporosis', p. 40.

Case scenario 3

Mrs H comes to see you for a blood test as she has been prescribed MTX to help modify her recently diagnosed RA.

She is in a 'bit of a state' as she couldn't hear very well when the doctor at the hospital told her about the medication. She is very worried she is not talking her medication correctly and thought the doctor said something about cancer drugs—but she can't remember what was said.

How can you help?

- Reassure her that you will be able to help and you will be able to write down the instructions for her.
- Explain that in much larger doses MTX is used in cancer care as well as for RA.
- Explain that the MTX must only be taken once a week as a single dose on the same day each week.
- Ensure that she has also been prescribed folic acid 5 mg—also to take once a week on a different day to the MTX.
- Reinforce the message about blood tests and reasons for regular tests which are set out in national guidelines.[1]

- Advise that infections should not be left unchecked and should be treated promptly. Contact the healthcare team if in doubt.
- Check immunity status and advise about travel immunizations as responses to vaccinations may be suboptimal while on treatment. Also encourage annual influenza vaccinations. Pneumovax is recommended for patients on DMARDs.
- Ask if she has been referred to the OT for joint protection advice. If not, refer to the OT to undertake an assessment for aids and/or adaptations to the home to help maintain independence.
- Assess and ask the patient about any mobility problems they may have.
- Check that analgesia has been prescribed and that she understands how to take these to their full potential.
- Explain that the medication can take some time to modify the RA and that it is sometimes possible to have a steroid injection to settle things down while the medication is taking effect.
- Ensure Mrs H has a contact number to phone for advice—either at the surgery or the specialist nurses at the hospital.

➲ See Chapter 16, 'Pharmacological management: disease-modifying drugs', p. 445.

Reference

1. Ledingham J, Gullick N, Irving K, et al. (2017). BSR and BHPR guideline for the prescription and monitoring of non-biologic disease-modifying anti-rheumatic drugs. *Rheumatology (Oxford)* 56:865–8.

Principles of exercise for musculoskeletal conditions

The importance of muscle and physical activity

Physical activity is essential for muscle, joint, general physical, psychological, and social health, function, and well-being. Muscles play a vital role in the health and function; they:

- *Contract* to move joints.
- *Allow functional stability* so that they maintain mobility.
- *Protect* from injury by preventing excessive harmful movement.
- Act as *shock absorbers* attenuating harmful forces during gait.
- Aerobic exercises (those that cause your heart and lungs to breathe faster) help to maintain *body weight*, preserve balance, *control blood sugar*, and *improve mood*.

Prolonged inactivity is bad for joints; if a joint is not moved through its full ROM regularly:

- Movement becomes restricted.
- Muscles become weaker, tire quicker, and fail to prevent harmful movement.

For muscles to work efficiently, a combination of factors must be applied including maintaining a joint through an adequate but full ROM. When assessing patients consider:

- If adequate use of the joint is being maintained, including full ROMs.
- Can they demonstrate strength, endurance, and finely controlled movements?
- Are these abilities maintained by regular exercise or physical activity?

Table 11.2 outlines functional issues to consider.

Safety issues and how to prevent injury

For the vast majority of people sensibly planned physical activity/exercise has many health benefits and few dangers. People with serious, unstable medical conditions, or very deformed and unstable joints may need to seek guidance from a health professional before undertaking strenuous strengthening exercises, and despite advice should still be counselled to be physically active little and often, using a walking stick, etc. (Box 11.4).

Sports-related issues

Most sports injuries can be avoided:

- Through careful preparation and ensuring safe techniques.
- Warm up exercises may be helpful.
- The right equipment (including protective equipment) and appropriate shoes are imperative to safe exercising.

Sports injuries are beyond the scope of this book but consider if it is an acute or chronic problem. Prompt treatment to acute injuries includes rest, topical applications of ice packs, compression, and elevation (RICE).

Table 11.2 Functional issues to consider

Joint range of movement	Move joint frequently through its full ROM (3–4 sets of 5–10 stretches, 2–3 times a day), holding a sustained stretch (10–30 sec) at the end of ROM
Strength	Perform a few contractions (5) against a high resistance (e.g. pushing against a fixed object or lifting a heavy weight), 2–3 times a day
Endurance	Perform many contractions (10 sets of 10–20 contractions), against a low resistance (light weight) 5–10 times a day
Controlled movement	Frequent practice of specific activities so that muscle activity patterns that make up a movement become automatic

Box 11.4 To exercise safely, effectively, and regularly people should:

- Always ensure they are stable and safe when exercising.
- Start a new exercise/activity cautiously.
- Set simple, challenging, but realistic, achievable goals—pursue them in a very focused way.
- Write an 'action plan' of *exactly* what, when, where, and how they will exercise.
- Progress slowly the time, frequency, and intensity of exercise.
- Work within their capabilities but 'nudge the boundaries 'of their capabilities.
- Exercise moderately—they should feel slightly warm and their heart should beat a little faster but they should be able to hold a conversation while doing an activity. Blood, sweat, and tears are not essential—or desirable.
- If an activity causes prolonged pain, discomfort, or swelling lasting more than a couple of days or wakes them at night, rest for a couple of days. As the pain settles, resume exercising gently, gradually building up the exercises as before but leave out activities that previously caused pain or add them cautiously.
- Monitor progress. If they can't achieve a goal, make it easier.
- When their goal is achieved—recognize and encourage—appreciate their achievements and benefits. Encourage them to reward themselves. Revise goals and action plans, setting more challenging goals to improve further or maintain the improvement.
- Plan for relapse—think about what might stop them exercising and how to overcome these barriers.
- Get support from their family and friends.

Exercise: health benefits

As health benefits are 'dose related', the more people do, the better. In fact, our usual daily physical activities—manual work, walking, gardening, shopping, housework, a day out—are 'informal' exercises that have health benefits. Almost anything that ↑ activity is good. Patients may wish to attend organized classes, such as yoga and tai-chi. Equally, they can choose individual activities, such as walking or cycling.

However, attaining health benefits:

- *Does not require* long bouts of exhausting, strenuous exercise.
- *Does not require* joining a gym, supervision, or expensive equipment.
- Occurs by accumulating 30 min of physical activity most days of the week.

So, health improvements =
1 × 30 min activity = 2 × 15 min activity = 3 × 10 min activity

It is essential to incorporate normal health benefits of exercise using a practical approach to improve functional ability. This can be achieved by:

- Undertaking a patient-centred assessment:
    - Consider current health status and functional ability.
    - Cognitive abilities.
    - Health beliefs and behaviours.

Identify a goal-setting approach with an aim of progressively improving functional ability in the context of the patient's abilities and aims.

Walking is a safe, simple physical activity that can be integrated into normal routine. Provide simple practical advice for those with mild self-limiting conditions or conditions where evidence demonstrates benefits of walking. Encourage simple options such as:

- Walking rather than driving.
- Getting off a bus/train earlier and walk the last bit.
- The use of stairs rather than the lift.

Exercise is effective whether it is performed at home alone, at a leisure centre, or in an exercise class. The important thing is to find something that the patient finds comfortable, enjoyable, achievable, affordable, and available, and that they can integrate into their lifestyle.

Exercise: nursing issues

Encouraging exercise in joint disease

An often-neglected area in management of arthritis and especially in OA and RA is exercise and the practice nurse is well placed to encourage and motivate patients. Cardiovascular risk prevention is an important factor especially for patients with RA who are four times more likely to suffer from cardiovascular events compared with the general population.

A gradual ↓ in functional mobility and ↑ in pain and stiffness can have a negative impact on physiological, psychological, and social aspects of an individual's life. As with many MSCs the condition itself can confer risks that will result in a functional decline, e.g.:

Rheumatoid disease confers a heightened risk of:

- Cardiovascular disease.
- Depression.
- Mood disturbance.
- Osteoporosis.
- Muscle wasting.
- 2° degenerative arthritis.
- Fatigue.
- Anaemia of chronic disease.

These are all good indications for an exercise regimen. Patients will often ask the practice nurse 'Is it ok for me to exercise?' Most forms of exercise are safe and effective in improving function, especially if appropriately advised and gradually developed.

Exercise can be self-supervised but follow-up will encourage adherence

- Aerobic—walking.
- Strengthening—upper and lower limb exercise, swimming, and cycling.
- Gentle stretching and education about use of ice after exercise to reduce any post-exercise inflammation is important.

Patients will need:

- Reassurance.
- Encouragement and support.
- May require involvement of therapist to support concordance for those failing to achieve goals.
- Optimization of regular analgesia especially for those who are having trouble mobilizing.
- Encouragement to keep an exercise diary.

Exercise examples for patients

The following exercises should be started gently and ↑ gradually.

Knees

See Fig. 11.1.

Hip

See Fig. 11.2.

Back

See Fig. 11.3.

Neck

See Fig. 11.4.

Shoulders

See Fig. 11.5.

Further reading

Versus Arthritis. Exercise leaflets. https://www.versusarthritis.org/about-arthritis/managing-symptoms/exercise/

Simple exercises

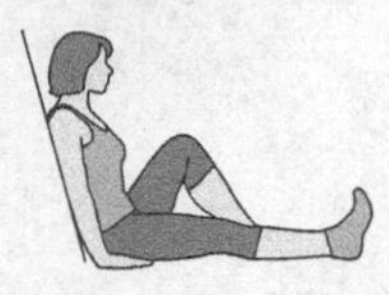

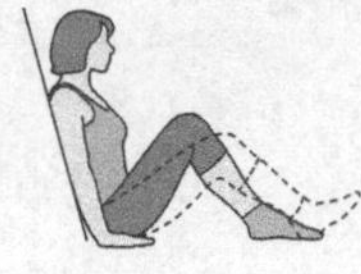

Leg stretch

Sit on the floor with your legs stretched out in front. Keeping your foot to the floor, slowly bend one knee until you feel it being comfortably stretched. Hold for 5 seconds. Straighten your leg as far as you can and hold for 5 seconds. Repeat 10 times with each leg.

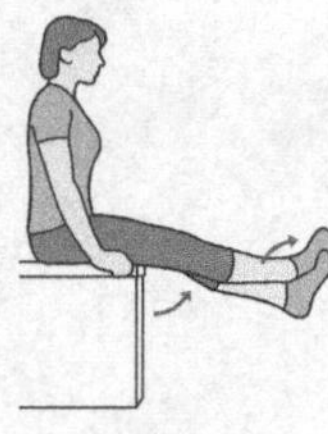

Leg cross

Sit on the edge of a table or bed. Cross your ankle sover. Push your front leg backwards and back leg forwards against each other until the thigh muscles become tense. Hold for 10 seconds, then relax. Switch legs and repeat. Do 4 sets with each leg.

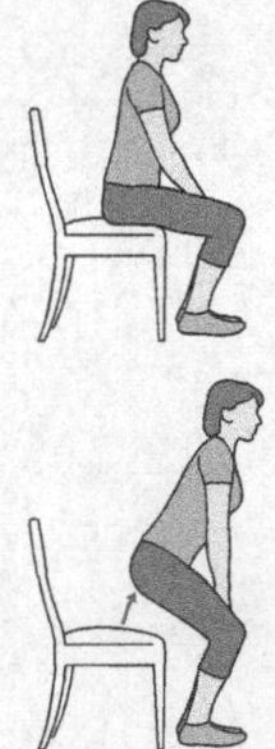

Sit/stands

Sit on a chair. Without using your hands for support, stand up and then sit back down. Make sure each movement is slow and controlled. Repeat for 1 minute. As you improve, try to increase the number of sit/stands you can do in 1 minute and try the exercise from lower chairs or the bottom two steps of a staircase.

Thigh muscle (quadriceps) exercises

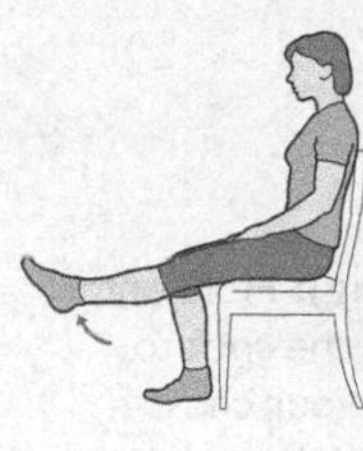

Straight-leg raise (sitting)

Sit well back in the chair with good posture. Straighten and raise one leg. Hold for a slow count to 10, then slowly lower your leg. Repeat this at least 10 times with each leg. If you can do this easily, try it with light weights on your ankles and with your toes pointing towards you. Try doing this every time you sit down.

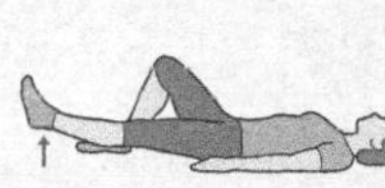

Straight-leg raise (lying)

Bend one leg at the knee. Hold the other leg straight and lift the foot just off the bed. Hold for a slow count of 5, then lower. Repeat 5 times with each leg. Try doing it in the morning and at night while lying in bed.

Fig 11.1 Simple exercises for the knees and upper thighs.

Reproduced from Knee Pain 2304/P-KNEE/12-9: Arthritis Research UK with kind permission from Versus Arthritis.

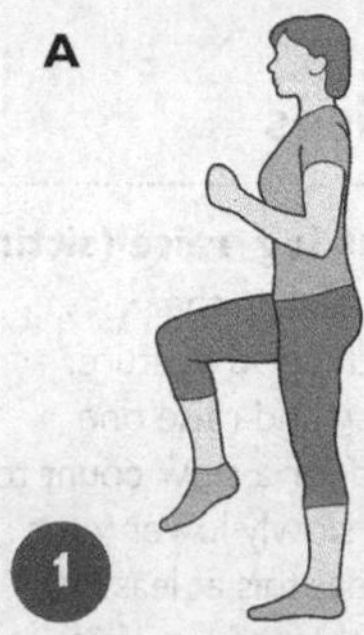

Hip flexion (strengthening): Hold onto a work surface and march on the spot to bring your knees up towards your chest alternately. Don't go above 90 degrees.

B

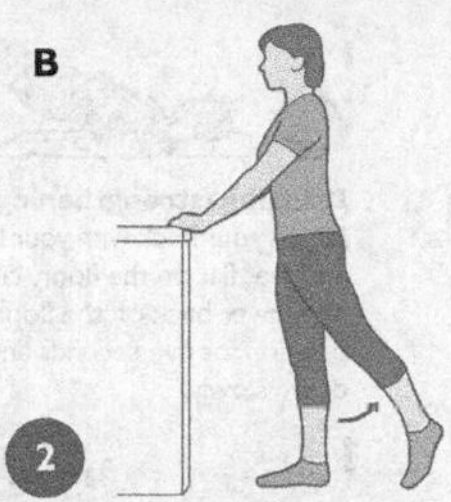

Hip extension (strengthening): Move your leg backwards, keeping your knee straight. Clench your buttock tightly and hold for five seconds. Don't lean forwards. Hold onto a chair or work surface for support.

C

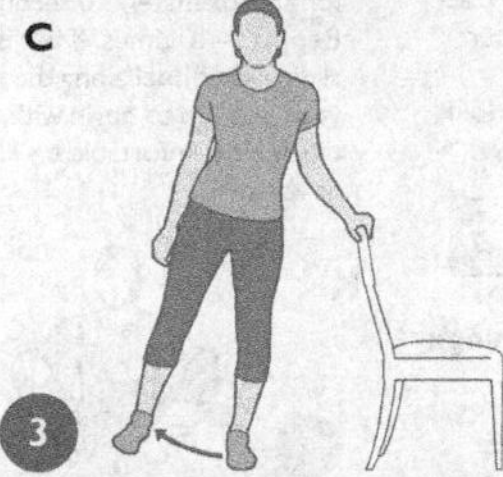

Hip abduction (strengthening): Lift your leg sideways, being careful not to rotate the leg outwards. hold for five seconds and bring it back slowly, keeping your body straight throughout. Hold onto a chair or work surface for support.

D

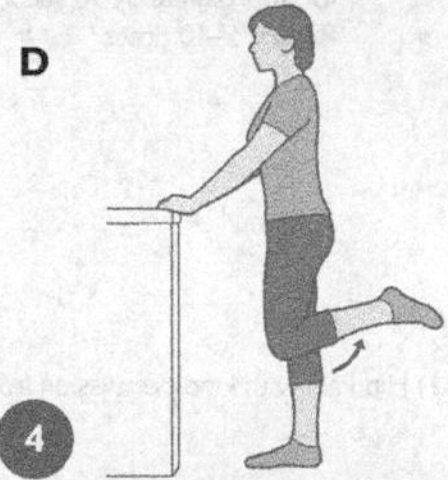

Heel to buttock exercise (strengthening): Bend your knee to pull your heel up towards your bottom. Keep your knees in line and your kneecap pointing towards the floor.

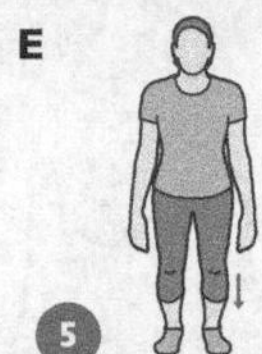

Mini squat (strengthening): Squat down until your knees are above your toes. Hold for a count of five if possible. Hold on to a work surface for support if you need to.

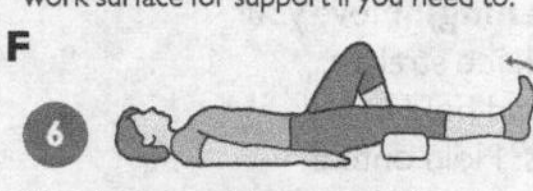

Short arc quadriceps exercise (strengthening): Roll up a towel and place it under your knee. Keep the back of your thigh on the towel and straighten your knee to raise your foot off the floor. Hold for five seconds and then lower slowly.

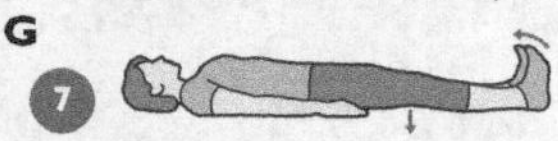

Quadriceps exercise (strengthening): Pull your toes and ankles towards you, while keeping your leg straight and pushing ypur knee fiemly against the floor. Ypu should feel the tightness in the front of your leg. Hold for five seconds and relax. This excercise can be done from a sitting position as well if this is more comfortable.

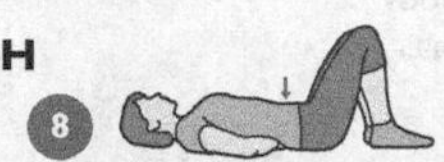

Stomach exercise (strengthening/ stabilising): Lie on your back with your knees bent. Put your hands under the small of your back and pull your belly button down towards the floor. Hold for 20 seconds.

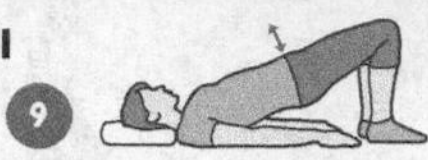

Bridging (strengthening/stabilising): Lie on your back with your knees bent and feet flat on the floor. Lift your pelvis and lower back off the floor. Hold the position for five seconds and then lower down slowly.

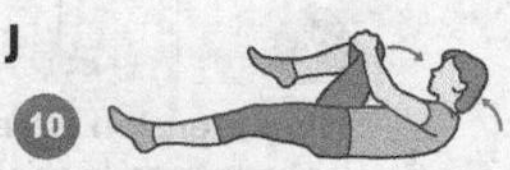

Knee lift (stretch): Lie on your back. Pull each knee to your chest in turn, keeping the other leg straight. Take the movement up to the point you feel a stretch, hold for approximately 10 seconds and relax. Repeat 5–10 times. If this is difficult, try sliding your heel along the floor towards your bottom to begin with, and when this feels comfortable try lifting your knee as above.

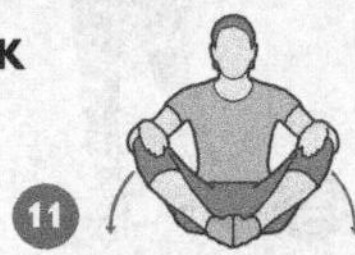

External hip rotation (stretch): Sit with your knees bent and feet together. Press your knees down towards the floor using your hands as needed. Alternatively, lie on your back and part your knees, keeping your feet together. Take the movement up to the point you feel a stretch, hold for approximately 10 seconds and relax. Repeat 5–10 times.

Fig 11.2 Exercises for hip pain.

Simple exercises

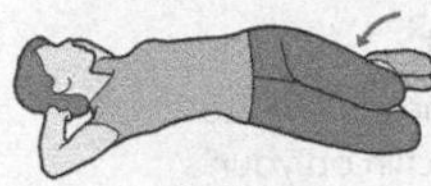

NB. Upper knee should be directly above lower knee.

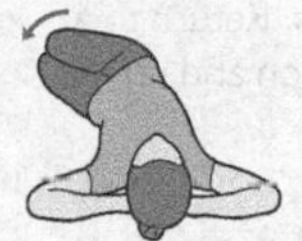

Back stretch

Lie on your back, hands above your head. Bend your knees and roll them slowly to one side, keeping your feet on the floor. Hold for 10 seconds. Repeat 3 times on each side.

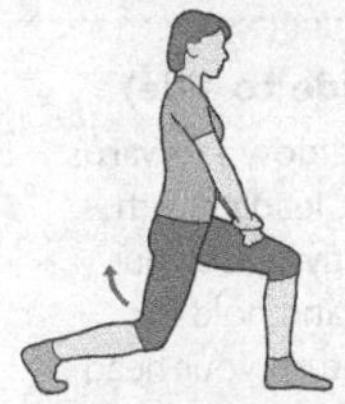

Deep Lunge

Kneel on one knee, the other foot in front. Facing forwards, lift the back knee up. Hold for 5 seconds. Repeat 3times on each side.

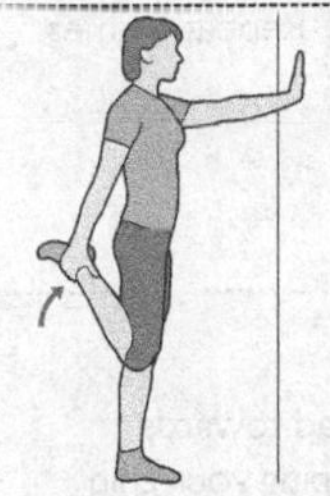

One-leg stand (front)

Holding onto something for support if needed, bend one leg up behind you. Hold for 5 seconds. Repeat 3 times on each side.

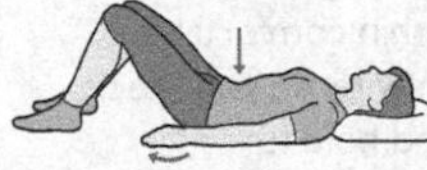

Pelvic tilt

Lie down with your knees bent. Tighten your stomach muscles, flattening your back against the floor. Hold for 5 seconds. Repeat 5 times.

Fig 11.3 Exercises for back pain.

Reproduced from Knee Pain 2301/P-BACK/12-9: Arthritis Research UK with kind permission from Versus Arthritis.

Simple exercises

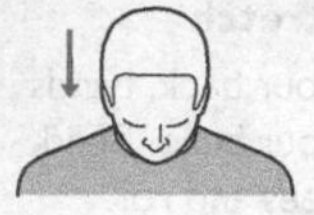

Neck tilt

Tilt your head down to rest your chin on your chest. Gently tense your neck muscles and hold for 5 seconds. Return to a neutral position and repeat 5 times.

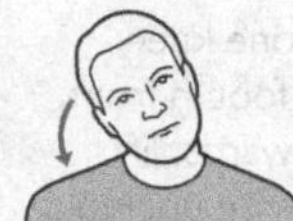

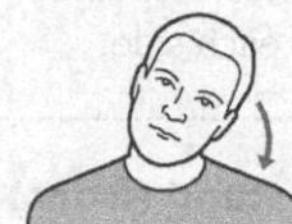

Neck tilt (side to side)

Tilt your head down towards your shoulder, leading with your ear. Gently tense your neck muscles and hold for 5 seconds. Return your head to centre and repeat on the opposite side. Repeat 5 times on each side.

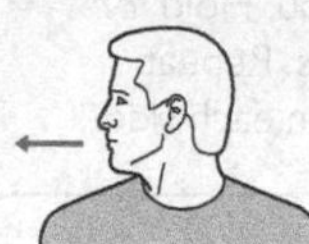

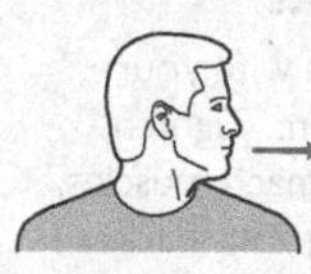

Neck turn

Turn your head towards one side, keeping your chin at the same height and moving within comfortable limits. Gently tense your neck muscles and hold for 5 seconds. Return your head to the centre and repeat on the opposite side. Repeat 5 times on each side.

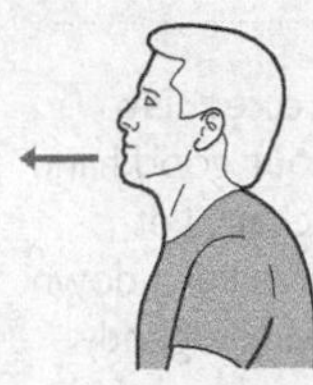

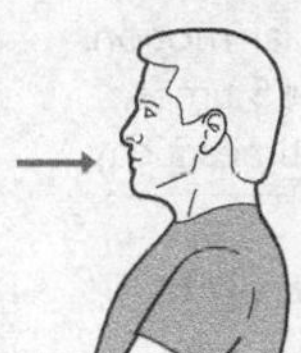

Neck stretch

Keeping the rest of the body straight, push your chin forward so your throat is stretched. Gently tense your neck muscles and hold for 5 seconds. Return your head to the centre and push it backwards, keeping your chin up. Hold for 5 seconds. Repeat 5 times.

Fig 11.4 Exercises for neck pain.

Reproduced from Neck Pain 2305/P-NECK/12-9: Arthritis Research UK with kind permission from Versus Arthritis.

Simple exercises

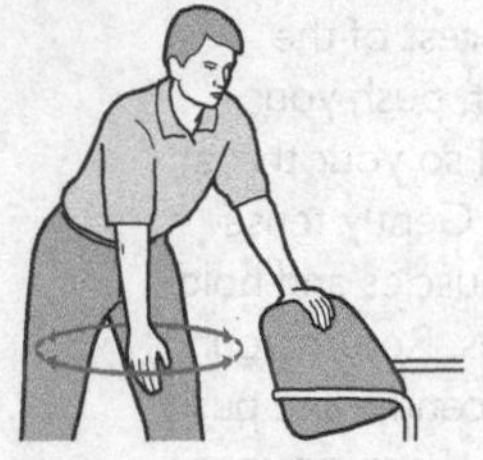

Pendulum exercise
Stand with your good hand resting on a chair. Let your other arm hang down and try to swing it gently backwards and forwards and in a circular motion. Repeat about 5 times. Try this 2–3 times a day.

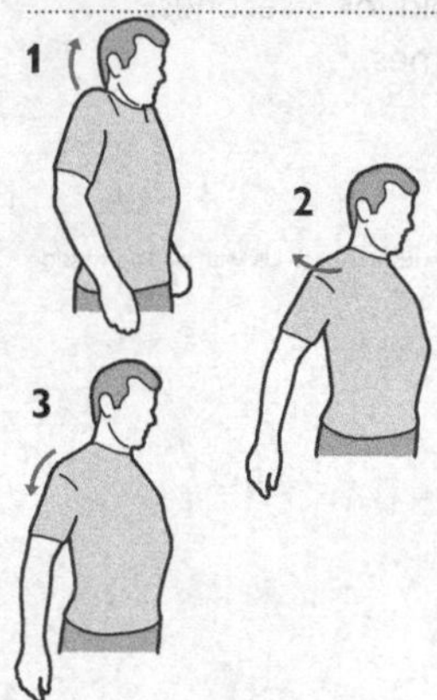

Shoulder stretch
Stand and raise your shoulders. Hold for 5 seconds. Squeeze your shoulder blades back and together and hold for 5 seconds. Pull your shoulder blades downward and hold for 5 seconds. Relax and repeat 10 times.

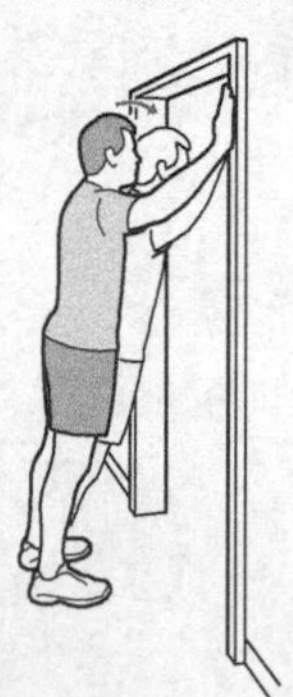

Door lean
Stand in a doorway with both arms on the wall slightly above your head. Slowly lean forward until you feel a stretch in the front of your shoulders. Hold for 15–30 seconds. Repeat 3 times. This exercise isn't suitable if you have a sholuder impingement.

Fig 11.5 Exercises for shoulder pain.

Reproduced from Shoulder Pain 2306/P-SHOU/12-9: Arthritis Research UK with kind permission from Versus Arthritis.

Social and voluntary sector

In the UK, historically health, social care, and voluntary sector provision all worked separately with little in the way of a strategic approach to provision of funding and numerous barriers to achieving a flexible approach to the provision of services for those in need. Excellent services were provided by a number of organizations although many were forced to work in silos (financially or organizationally). The provision of healthcare should encompass all spectrums of health and Illness. In the future, it is advocated that care will be improved by providing a system-wide transformation built upon genuine local partnerships between:

- NHS.
- 1° care services.
- Local authorities.
- Voluntary and social enterprise organizations.
- Other statutory agencies.
- User and carer communities.

The provision of a whole-systems approach for a community will be achieved using local Service Level Agreements (SLAs)[1] ensuring an agreed allocation of budgets based upon collaboration with all organizations. The strategies are developed in the context of national policies but are based upon community-based health needs assessments for each region. This will enable greater interdependence between work, health, and well-being in the context of the needs of the individual, including:

- Their wish to live independently:
  - Encourage independent living, e.g. for older people, those with a chronic condition, disabled, or mental health problems.
- Staying healthy and recovering from illness.
- Exercising and maintaining control of their lives.
- Sustaining family communities.
- Equal citizenship—economically and socially.
- Optimizing their quality of life.
- Retaining their dignity and respect.

A wide spectrum of policies and services need to identify the strategy to ensure each community has the services that are required through all stages of health and illness:

- Public health policies, e.g. infection control and falls prevention.
- Hospital care including strategies to ensure effective discharge management.
- Intermediate care.
- Management of LTCs.
- Packages of care that consider health and nurse care needs.
- Community equipment services.
- Informational resources—that have universal use and value for all members of the population.
- Carer support including public and patient involvement,[2] e.g. recognizing the expertise of the carer and the role in healthcare provision.
- Systems to manage poor performance/complaints of care provided.

Social services

A number of services are provided under the auspices of social services. Many of these focus specifically on those who need additional support including:

- The fail/older person.
- Those with physical, sensory, or learning disabilities.
- Those with mental health problems.

Support provided is extensive and can include:

- Care homes and care services at home.
- 'Meals on wheels'.
- Equipment and adaptations.
- Day care services.
- Social worker support and advice (children/adult needs):
  - Disability services.
  - Support for vulnerable children and their families.

Voluntary sector

There are many voluntary or social enterprise organizations that have provided essential and much valued services, often developed as a result of shortfalls in the provision of services funded by the NHS or local social services. These services are often provided by volunteers directly to patient groups or within a specific community. Examples include:

- Library services in hospitals.
- EPP—social enterprise.
- 'Meet and greet' volunteers in hospital and medical centres.
- Social support and information sharing for individuals with LTCs, e.g. RA.
- Alzheimer's Society helpline, research, and support.
- Assist—impartial advice and support for the disabled.
- Carers UK helping carers recognize their needs.
- The DLF provides information and advice on disability equipment and ways of managing disability.
- The Samaritans provides a range of completely confidential services for those who are suicidal or experiencing emotional distress.
- Educational and training opportunities activities for those with medical conditions—available from a range of voluntary sector organizations.

Many of the voluntary sector organizations provide websites, literature, telephone advice line support, and local meetings/activities.

Nurses should ensure that they have a good understanding of services available within the community and proactively voice new ways of working that will encompass all social and voluntary organizations.

Social prescribing, a way of linking patients in 1° care with sources of support within the community to help improve their health and well-being[3] is increasingly encouraged as part of a non-pharmacological intervention provision in the NHS. Accordingly, the DH, NHS England, and Public Health England are working with voluntary, community, and social enterprise (VCSE) organizations through the Health and Wellbeing Fund to promote equality, address health inequalities, and support the well-being of people, families and communities.[4]

References

1. NHS Health at Work Network. Service Level Agreement (SLA). https://www.nhshealthatwork.co.uk/commissioningohservices.asp
2. INVOLVE. What is public involvement in research? http://www.invo.org.uk/find-out-more/what-is-public-involvement-in-research-2/
3. Bickerdike L, Booth A, Wilson PM, et al. (2017). Social prescribing: less rhetoric and more reality. A systematic review of the evidence. *BMJ Open* 7:e013384.
4. Department of Health and Social Care and Public Health England. Health and Wellbeing Fund 2017–2018. https://www.gov.uk/government/publications/health-and-wellbeing-fund-2017-to-2018-application-form

Further reading

Care Services Improvement Partnership (2007). *Integration for Social Enterprise.* London: Care Services Improvement Partnership.

Department of Health (2007). *Putting People First: A Shared Vision and Commitment to the Transformation of Adult Social Care.* London: DH.

Department of Health (2010). *Prioritising Need in the Context of "Putting People First": A Whole System Approach to Eligibility for Social Care—Guidance on Eligibility Criteria for Adult Social Care, England 2010.* London: The Stationery Office.

Department of Health (2011). *Fairer Care Funding: The Report of the Commission on Funding of Care and Support* (Dilnot Commission). London: DH

Department of Health (2012). *Caring for our Future: Reforming Care and Support.* London: The Stationery Office.

Department of Health (2013). *Adult Social Care: Choice Framework.* London: DH.

Law Commission (2011). *Adult Social Care.* London: The Stationery Office.

NICE (2013). Patient and public involvement policy. https://www.nice.org.uk/media/default/About/NICE-Communities/Public-involvement/Patient-and-public-involvement-policy/Patient-and-public-involvement-policy-November-2013.pdf

Chapter 12

Ward-based care and referral to the multidisciplinary team

Ward-based care: overview

As >20% of the UK population have to cope with a MSC at any one time, it will be inevitable that nurses in all care settings will come across individuals with a MSC. The costs of MSCs are felt by the individual and society as they have the potential to affect work-related capacity and the use of healthcare resources. It is ∴ highly likely that you will encounter such patients during your work on the ward. The benefits of understanding MSCs and providing nursing expertise will be in aiding the patient's physical and mental rehabilitation while working as part of a MDT. Equally, ensuring you are aware of drug therapies used in MSCs may reduce the risk related to polypharmacy

The common MSCs include:

- OA.
- Osteoporosis.
- Trauma and soft tissue injury, e.g. rotator cuff rupture in the shoulder, meniscal tear in the knee, and road traffic collisions causing fractures.
- Inflammatory joint conditions such as RA, PsA, AS, and CTDs. These conditions have systemic and long-term effects.

➲ Also see 'Classifying joint disease', Chapter 1, pp. 7–9; ➲ 'Orthopaedic management', Chapter 7, pp. 249–285.

New models of care such as triage, rapid assessment, and proactive reviews of patients with MSC, coupled with the advent of new targeted drug therapies, have accelerated changes in the work of rheumatology services. In Europe, rheumatology care is predominantly an outpatient and day case-based specialty and is delivered by a MDT. Yet despite all these developments, MSCs have a major impact on the individual, affecting not only function and quality of life but with some long-term inflammatory conditions the disease can result in additional systemic effects on major bodily systems such as the heart, lungs, skin, and kidney and cause deformity and damage to joints. Dedicated rheumatology inpatient beds are in short supply and in many circumstances, patients are admitted according to the organ involvement (e.g. respiratory or cardiology wards). Hospital admissions may be required for:

- Management of an exacerbation of the disease (flare) and rehabilitation.
- Underlying co-morbidities as a result of the systemic effects of the disease, e.g. cardiovascular disease.
- Toxicity/adverse events of treatment, e.g. MTX pneumonitis/infection.
- Blood and imaging investigations.
- Assessment by other medical specialists and members of the MDT.
- Planned surgical procedures.
- Day case treatments.

Key points for nurses to consider in ward-based care

- Symptom control needs:
  - Patients with IJD experience EMS.
  - Pain and analgesia needs.
- Functional needs of the patient in relation to the environment, e.g. chair raisers, tap turners, or other assistive devices.

- Patients may have problems with independent activities, particularly postoperatively, as they may be unable to lift themselves up, get on and off a bedpan, or reach for a drink, unlike the more mobile patients.
- Knowledge of drug therapies commonly prescribed, monitoring, and potential side effects.
- Referral points and when and how to access specialist or MDT support.

➲ Also see 'Orthopaedic care', Chapter 7, pp. 249–284; ➲ 'Pharmacological management', Chapter 16, pp. 445–503; ➲ 'Symptom control', p. 307; ➲ 'Multidisciplinary referrals', Chapter 12, pp. 392–393.

General care issues

When a patient is admitted to hospital it is an ideal opportunity to look holistically at all aspects of their care, using a problem-solving approach to achieve optimum disease control. The patient's rehabilitation plans and discharge should be effectively assessed to ensure a prompt and effective discharge that considers the patient's needs and supports ongoing management plans.

Assessment of ADLs

- The nurse makes a full assessment to include past medical history; current drug therapies and previous drug history; reason for admission and level of disease activity; and social history encompassing living conditions, social support, work, and leisure pursuits.
- Physical assessment of joints and skin.
- Mobility status and use of walking aids and, if required, availability of toilet and chair raisers, tap turners, etc. on the ward.
- Pain status to identify the patient's methods of coping with pain.
- Psychological status to identify the patient's coping methods and current concerns.

Investigations

- A range of tests will be required from blood tests, imaging, urine, faeces, sputum, synovial fluid, and skin biopsy.
- The nurse can ensure, if personally responsible for the collection of samples, that these are obtained and sent with appropriate documentation as soon as possible.
- The nurse can obtain the results, so they are available for review, and explain the meaning of the results to the patient.

Pain management

- The patient's pain should be reviewed regularly using a validated pain measurement tool such as a 10 cm VAS or pain diary to collect information on the nature, severity, and frequency of pain. This facilitates modification of analgesia and evaluation to achieve optimum pain control. It also allows tailoring of care based upon levels of pain.
- Where patient self-administration of medication is possible and appropriate, patients should be supported to perform this. Timing of medications is important to patients who have self-managed their conditions for many years.
- Care should be taken to establish how the patient wants to be lifted as inappropriate lifting can cause significant pain.
- Assess the frequency of bowel movements as analgesia cause constipation.
- Periods of quiet time should be incorporated into the patient's care plan to facilitate a balance of rest and relaxation.
- Observe the patient's sleep pattern to ensure that pain is not disturbing sleep.

Psychological support

Patients cope better psychologically when their pain is recognized, and support is provided in controlling the symptoms. The nurse needs to talk and listen to the patient regarding all aspects of care, especially when decisions about changes to treatment and management have taken place. This can help to clarify salient points, alleviate anxiety, and allow the patient's views to be taken into account.

Rehabilitation and discharge planning

- Immediately following the patient's initial assessment, a plan for discharge should be prepared. This will allow for all social issues that might prevent a timely discharge from hospital to be addressed.
- Early referral to relevant MDT members is needed for assessment, programme of rehabilitation, and guidance on discharge needs.

➲ See 'Multidisciplinary referrals', Chapter 12, pp. 392–393.

Hygiene and toileting

- Care must be taken to provide privacy and dignity wherever possible while respecting the person's wish for independence, particularly for toileting and hygiene needs. This can be a specific problem for those with damaged joints or those experiencing a flare.
- It is good practice to ask the patient what they can do for themselves and what they require help with. Patients experience EMS so it is preferable to allow this to ease off, and immersion in a bath or shower later in the morning can help significantly ↑ independence.

Tissue viability

- Patients often have paper-thin fragile skin (often steroid related) and this, coupled with ↓ mobility, leads to a higher objective measurement of pressure sore risk. Be aware of vulnerable areas such as elbows and heels.
- Tissue viability can be improved by regularly inspecting the skin to detect potential breakdown and by keeping the skin moisturized. Good diet and fluid intake should be encouraged. Injury from sharp objects such as rings and watches should be avoided. Pressure should be regularly relieved by moving and mobilizing the patient and by using pressure-relieving devices.
- Many drug therapies can give rise to rashes. These should be reported promptly and managed to avoid tissue damage.
- Report signs of abnormal bruising, bleeding, or discoloration of digits.

➲ Also see 'Primary systemic vasculitis', Chapter 5, pp. 165–167.

Diet

- Assess normal dietary intake and preferences.
- Refer to the dietician if the patient has become emaciated prior to their admission, for advice regarding a build-up diet, and also seek advice for patients who would benefit from losing weight.
- Ask and support the patient if assistance is required with feeding, e.g. cutting up meat and getting the tops off containers. Equally, referral to an OT may be able to facilitate greater independence using aids and devices (such as dressing aids or special cutlery).
- Don't overfill water jugs and ensure that they are accessible.

➲ See 'Joint protection', Chapter 19, pp. 584–585.

Further reading

Dougherty L, Lister S (eds) (2015). *The Royal Marsden Manual of Clinical Nursing Procedures*, 9th edn. Chichester: Wiley-Blackwell.

Risks related to inpatient care

Patients with long-term musculoskeletal/functional limitations are prone to falling

- Recurrent inflammation leads to loss of muscle bulk and stretching of tendons, ligaments, and the capsule that support joints.
- Osteoporosis is induced by the inflammatory process, immobility, and long-term use of steroids. Falls often result in fracture of the humerus, wrist, thoracic spine, pelvis, or femur.
- Steroid use thins the skin and falls often result in soft tissue injury, such as full-tissue skin tears and chronic ulceration.
- Patients may be on a combination of several drugs thereby ↑ the likelihood of drug interactions and confusion so ↑ the risk of falling.
- Falls and significant injury greatly ↑ the risk of premature death, loss of confidence, and mobility leading to greater disability.
- Careful assessment and support to mobilize patients must be considered, e.g. the use of a walking aid might be appropriate in order to reduce the risk of falling and injury or onward referral to a falls clinic.
- Provide a safe, clutter-free environment and ensure the nurse call button is accessible.

Infection

- Immunosuppressant drugs such as MTX, biological agents, and steroids are commonly prescribed. In some circumstances, bone marrow suppression may make the patient more susceptible to infections, sometimes fatally.
- Unusual infections such as TB, osteomyelitis, and septic arthritis can occur.
- Infection can accelerate very quickly. Concomitant steroid therapy can mask the onset of infection and the patient can become rapidly overwhelmed.
- Regular monitoring of patients' general well-being, temperature, and vital signs are paramount in early detection and treatment of infection.
- If infection occurs, they may need a combination of aggressive antibiotic therapy.
- Ideally, immunosuppressed patients should be isolated from other patients with infection.
- Effective hand washing and disinfecting procedures are crucial to avoid cross infection from one patient to another.

Points to consider in drug therapies

Disease-modifying drugs need to be taken on a regular basis. If a patient fails to continue their DMARD for several weeks, it is highly likely that they will relapse.

- On occasions, drug treatment can be accidentally discontinued, e.g. patients routinely stop their DMARD for surgical procedures such as hip replacement and there is a failure to inform the patient that the drug should be recommenced. An ideal way to counteract this difficulty is to ensure that the DMARD is prescribed in their medication to take home on discharge.

- Discharge from hospital can be a risk to the patient as they are often lost to follow-up or receive no monitoring.
- Following hospital admission, patients may relapse very quickly and therefore it is good practice to ensure that the patient receives a review in the clinic within 6 weeks.
- Monitoring arrangements should be confirmed before discharge. GPs may be unable to provide monitoring and it will be necessary to arrange for a follow-up appointment with the rheumatology nurse specialist.
- It is helpful to ensure that monitoring blood tests are taken and checked prior to the patient discharge—optimizing the interval before they have to return to the hospital or their GP.
- Often patients will be on subcutaneous MTX. If the patient or carer is unable to inject then a nurse competent in administration of cytotoxic drugs should be identified to administer this medication.
- Patients who hold shared care monitoring booklets should have information updated and returned to the patient prior to discharge.

Points to consider for patients attending as a day case

Day case patients attend usually for a short period ∴ all relevant information needs to be conveyed about the treatment to be given and actions to be taken at home, especially when an invasive procedure has been administered such as carpal tunnel release, injection, or infusion treatment.

Multidisciplinary team referrals

Referrals to the MDT will be required at times when patients are admitted with a MSC. The rheumatology nurse specialist is often in a key position to coordinate MDT referrals and can therefore advise ward-based nurses on the most appropriate referral for the patient.

Rheumatology nurse specialist

- Acts as an expert resource for ward and teams managing patients with complex, long-term MSCs.
- Can, in many cases, undertake an assessment of disease activity in relation to the MSC.
- Educates patients about the disease and treatment, and facilitates development of coping skills.
- Provides nurse-led clinics for review and tight control of the patient's disease activity.
- Offers telephone support for patients, carers, and HCPs.
- Coordinates referrals to the MDT.

Physiotherapist

- Teaches patients exercise regimens to build muscle strength and maintain a full range of movements in joints.
- Provides targeted treatment to joints or muscle groups, e.g. for frozen shoulder, and some give joint injections.
- Offers other treatments such as acupuncture and TENS.
- Manages hydrotherapy, OA, and back pain classes and falls clinics.
- Provide musculoskeletal triage services working as extended scope PTs.

Occupational therapist

- Educates patients on joint protection, e.g. using assistive devices such as a helping hand or kettle tipper, and energy conservation by planning and pacing daily activities.
- Supplies and fits custom-make hand and finger splints.
- Assesses patients in the home or workplace, advising on the organization of the environment to enable tasks to be performed more easily.
- Provides wheelchair assessments.

➔ Also see 'Equipment aids and devices', Chapter 11, pp. 361–363.

Podiatrist

- Assesses the function of the lower limb in order to make orthotic appliances such as a metatarsal support to redistribute loading, reduce pain, and facilitate mobility.
- Educates on foot care.
- Provides joint injections to the lower limb and performs minor surgery under local anaesthetic, such as tenotomy and excision of metatarsal heads.

Orthotist

Measures and provides a wide range of orthotic appliances such as insoles, bespoke footwear, knee braces, hand splints, and cervical collars. Works in conjunction with the podiatrist on provision of lower limb appliances.

Dietician

- Provides expert advice on specific dietary needs in the context of a condition, e.g. calcium and vitamin D intake for those at risk of osteoporosis.
- Provides education on a healthy diet and important food groups to be included in reducing and weight-gain diets.
- Advises and supports patients on the use of dietary supplements and exclusion diets.

Clinical psychologist/health psychologist

- Assesses the impact of the condition to help resolve personal and emotional issues and aid in the development of effective coping. One such strategy is CBT, which enables patients to alter their thinking and gain control.
- If a qualified prescriber, may also advise on the use of antidepressant and pain management drugs.

Pharmacist

- Educates patients on drug treatments, checks the safety of drugs prescribed, supports patients entering drug trials, and provides drug information and support to prescribers.
- Reviews polypharmacy and identifies potential drug interactions/side effects.
- Medicines management for discharge from hospital.

Social worker

Advises on social issues of self-care, respite care, housing, aids, adaptations, and benefits.

Medical referrals

A specialist opinion is often required about the systemic effects of arthritis. In complex cases, the patient might be referred to any of the following specialties: renal, hepatology, respiratory, cardiology, neurology, dermatology, haematology, urology, ophthalmology, rehabilitation, and pain team.

Surgical referrals

Surgical opinions are often required, including from vascular, plastics, hand, foot, arthroplasty, and spinal surgeons.

➲ See Chapter 15, 'Pharmacological management: pain relief', pp. 429–444.

Self-management and monitoring of drug therapy

It is recognized that patients must be central to their own care and involved in decisions made about their management so they can adjust to and live with their long-term MSC. This approach also enables the patient to navigate their way through the healthcare system, make shared decisions about how their condition is managed, improve their concordance with treatment, utilize health resources appropriately, and enjoy improved health outcome and quality of life. Patients are increasingly being recognized as consumers and are being consulted on redesign and delivery of services.

Self-management

The patient can only develop and maintain their self-management skills if they are:

- Informed about the importance of their involvement and the role they are to play.
- Given access to full, transparent, and unbiased information about their condition, prognosis, treatment interventions, and the service that they can expect to receive.
- Given consistent advice from all health professional groups.
- Able to build a rapport with their HCPs.
- Offered a range of treatment options over which they feel they have a choice.
- Good practice is to provide the patient with a copy of the clinic letters so they are aware of the next steps in their treatment plan and coordinate with other HCPs.
- Given helpline support and can gain rapid access for reassessment.
- Given prompt support from point of diagnosis that continues throughout their care pathway.
- Provided with access to support groups in the voluntary sector.
- Provided access to nurse-led clinics for review and tight control of disease activity.
- Offered telephone support for patients, carers, and HCPs.
- Provided with access to members of the MDT.

➲ Also see 'Self-management', Chapter 10, pp. 343–344; ➲ 'Patient education', Chapter 10, pp. 336–338.

Patient education

- Is a set of spontaneous or planned activities aimed at facilitating the acquisition of knowledge, self-management skills, coping, improvement in mood, pain control, and health behaviour.
- Can be on a one-to-one basis by the bedside, in clinic, over the telephone, or using digital technology. A classroom approach to patient education groups has fallen out of favour in Europe, with a greater emphasis on one-to-one sessions. (➲ See Chapter 10, 'Holistic and patient-centred care', pp. 329–350.)
- Can take place alongside the patient's carer.
- Can be in the form of a leaflet, booklet, or online module, especially to back up a verbal discussion.

Patient pathway

- Increasingly, patients are entering pathways of care that coordinate care across acute and 1° care settings and time interventions to improve health outcomes.
- Regardless of the aim of care pathways, patients with arthritis face constant uncertainty and unplanned exacerbations are an ongoing factor in their lives. The nature of the disease is of remission and relapse and it is important for patients to know what the next steps in their pathway will be. This helps to alleviate anxiety, enabling them to plan, mentally prepare, and recognize that options have not run out

Monitoring of drug therapy

DMARDs can result in a range of minor to extremely severe side effects so monitoring is vital. The side effects and frequency of monitoring vary for each drug based upon national guidelines.[1] The term 'monitoring' is not just about identifying side effects but also about monitoring the patient's well-being, disease activity, and response to treatment.

- Patients need to be taught how to self-monitor and about the action they must take should a side effect occur.
- Monitoring usually takes place in the rheumatology clinic and GP surgery, but it might also need to be done on the ward/rheumatology day case unit initially if the patient has commenced a new DMARD in hospital.
- A general principle is to monitor FBC and liver and renal function tests initially and based upon national DMARD guidelines (2–4-weekly may be required) for most drugs. This helps to identify trends in blood results, indicating development of immunosuppression, anaemia, and liver and renal abnormalities.
- Blood tests to measure levels of inflammation such as ESR and CRP help to gauge the level of disease activity alongside a physical examination of the patient.
- Urine tests and blood pressure monitoring are required for some drugs as they can cause proteinuria and hypertension.
- Assess the patient and ask about symptoms of mucositis, stomatitis, herpes simplex, rashes, infection, dyspnoea, nausea, vomiting, diarrhoea, hair loss, bruising and bleeding, and anything new or unusual about their health.
- Seek advice over any monitoring concerns from an expert rheumatology practitioner.

➲ Also see 'Pharmacological management', Chapter 16, pp. 445–503.

Reference

1. Ledingham J, Gullick N, Irving K, et al. (2017). BSR and BHPR guidelines for the prescription and monitoring of non-biologic disease-modifying anti rheumatic drugs. *Rheumatology* 56:865–8.

Patient-held record (shared care card)

If patients are being treated with DMARDs, they will require regular blood tests to monitor efficacy and potential side effects/toxicity of treatment. It is considered good practice to provide those prescribed DMARDs with their own patient-held monitoring booklet although evaluating the benefits of patient-held records still requires further research. Anecdotally, patients value holding their own monitoring booklet and it enables them to be more informed about their blood results and more actively engaged with their treatment and management.

➔ See Chapter 16, 'Pharmacological management: pain relief', Chapter 15, pp. 429–444.

Whenever a patient receives care, either as a day case or inpatient they would bring along their patient-held monitoring record. It is a record that belongs to the patient and should be returned to them (Fig. 12.1). It is important to ensure relevant blood tests or treatments are recorded in this document, as well as relevant information e.g. DAS score/injection of Depo-Medrone®.

This information will be helpful to the specialist team reviewing the patient at the next clinic appointment but, most importantly, will continue the principles of:

- Self-management and patient knowledge about blood monitoring and trends in blood results.
- Reducing potential risk related to treatments and changes in blood results.
- Providing an important aide memoir for the patient of treatments received, e.g. treatment, dose, and date administered.
- Reinforces to the patient the value of close monitoring of their treatment and response to treatment.

CURRENT BIOLOGIC:

DMARD:

PREVIOUS DMARDs	DATE STOPPED	IN COMBINATION WITH
PREVIOUS BIOLOGIC:		

DATE					
HB					
WCC					
NEUTROPHILS					
PLATELETS					
MCV					
ALT					
ALK PHOS					
ESR/CRP					
VIS					
B/P					
URINE HAQ SCORE					
DOSE CHANGES					
DAS					
COMMENTS					

Fig. 12.1 Example of a shared care monitoring booklet.

The patient-held blood monitoring booklet:

- Details the baseline and sequential monitoring blood results, drugs, and dose titration; important instructions for patients; and rheumatology department contact numbers.
- Enables identification of worrying trends and action to be taken.
- Facilitates information exchange and communication between care settings.
- Gives the patient information to provide to any healthcare worker and shows evidence of improvement and deterioration.
- Patients need to be educated about the details that are recorded.

➲ See 'Blood tests and investigations', Chapter 17, pp. 505–535.

Further reading

British Society of Rheumatology (2015). *The State of Play in UK Rheumatology: Insights into Service Pressures and Solutions*. London: BSR.

Sartain SA, Stressing S, Prieto J (2014). Patients' views on the effectiveness of patient-held records: a systematic review and thematic synthesis of qualitative studies. *Health Expect* 18:2666–77.

Chapter 13

Rapid access and emergency issues

Infections in musculoskeletal conditions

Introduction

An infection can cause an individual to present with symptoms that lead a clinician to consider a diagnosis of some form of arthritis. In some circumstances, the joint pain is driven by an acute infective episode that will not result in a diagnosis of a long-term rheumatological condition. The most serious example is septic arthritis. This is discussed in detail later in this chapter (➲ see 'Septic arthritis', Chapter 13, pp. 404–407).

This section will discuss infection occurring in patients with a pre-existing rheumatological condition. For these patients the first point of contact will often be the specialist nurse in a rheumatology department or a member of the 1° care team. It is essential to be aware of the potential risks of infection in this patient group in order to have clarity about a differential diagnosis, the next steps in management, or urgent referral to the rheumatologist.[1]

Infection risk due to rheumatological disease

Patients with rheumatological disease have an ↑ risk of infection, independent of treatment. This is due to tissue damage, organ dysfunction, and the immunomodulatory effects of the disease itself. The risk is higher with more active, aggressive disease.

- RhA has at least twice the risk of infection than the general population. Most common are pneumonia and soft tissue infection.
- Other arthritic diseases (e.g. PsA, AS, and ReA) have much lower risks.
- CTDs and systemic vasculitis have substantial risks of infection with a high mortality.
- SLE patients are at high risk, with infection being the second most common cause of death in the first 5 years after diagnosis.
- ANCA-associated vasculitis—in the first year after diagnosis, infection remains the most common cause of death.

Infection risk due to treatment

Almost all forms of DMARDs including corticosteroids in higher doses have the potential to ↑ the risk of infection. Note: gold, D-penicillamine, and hydroxychloroquine have no ↑ risk. Immunosuppression is also associated with:

- Unusual (opportunistic) organisms causing infection.
- Reactivation of latent infection, e.g. *Mycobacterium tuberculosis*, herpes zoster, and hepatitis viruses.
- Masking of usual signs and symptoms of infection making assessment difficult.
- Unusual presentations of infection e.g. disseminated forms of TB.
- Bacterial infections remain the most frequent problem and can develop rapidly.
- The pattern of infection varies between the different immunosuppressive agents, e.g. an ↑ risk of TB is seen with most bDMARDs but not rituximab. ➲ See Chapter 16 for information on individual drugs, pp. 445–503.

Nursing care issues in management

- The nurse in 1° care or rapid access clinics must be vigilant for the signs of infection. Always consider the patient's underlying diagnosis, the current activity of their disease, and their treatment. The history should include the details of the acute illness, any co-morbidities, and other risk factors such as travel and occupation.
- Examination must include the vital signs of temperature, heart rate, respiratory rate, and blood pressure and focus on any symptomatic areas. If there is diagnostic doubt or any worrying features in the history or screening examination, then a full general examination should be done looking for unsuspected sources of infection, rashes, or other abnormal signs. Patients treated with biologics, especially anti-TNFα, may be apyrexial despite infection.
- With this information, a decision must be made to manage the condition, request further investigations, or seek a medical opinion. The threshold should be lower in high-risk patients.
- Investigations will usually include FBC, CRP/ESR, U&Es, LFTs, and blood cultures. Other specimens for culture and serology will depend on the individual case. Chest radiography may be useful even if there are no respiratory symptoms.
- No test is 100% reliable, e.g. in the SLE patient with infection, the rise in CRP may be much reduced. Clinical judgement is vital. If in doubt, discuss or refer.
- Inflammatory complications of rheumatic diseases can mimic an infective process. Note: when in doubt, manage as an infection initially.
- Corticosteroids must not be stopped in an infection. Corticosteroids may need to be ↑ temporarily or given intravenously.
- DMARDs will usually be stopped until the infection has resolved.

Review

Monitor signs and symptoms of fever, ESR, CRP, and WBC count. Assess the patient thoroughly to ensure resolution of symptoms. It is essential to monitor and review clinical progress and investigations.

Social and psychological impact of infections

Patients will be anxious about the risk of infection, fearful about withholding their immunotherapy, and the consequences to their condition generally as well as risk of disease flares. It is imperative, ∴ to ensure patients are adequately informed. Information should be provided about investigations and treatment plans, together with general advice and support to improve outcomes and concordance.

Further reading

Clunie GPR, Wilkinson N, Nikiphorou E, Jadon D (eds) (2018). *Oxford Handbook of Rheumatology*, 4th edn. Oxford: Oxford University Press.

Accessing key management information in caring for those with musculoskeletal infections

- Communicate with rheumatology team. Use a rheumatology nurse specialist helpline as the first point of contact.
- Liaise with the rheumatology team to access monitoring protocols and advice regarding trends/abnormal values and when to stop treatment.

Points to note

- Concerns exist regarding the ↑ risk of TB with biological therapies. Biologics are used in the treatment of RA, PsA, AS, and some forms of vasculitis and mixed CTD. Patients should carry a biologics alert card is receiving a bDMARD (Fig. 13.1).
- Signs and symptoms of pneumonitis (which can be related to MTX), such as SOB, cough, and fever, must not be confused with infection. Patients require prompt investigation (HRCT lungs and PFTs) and stop MTX immediately.
- Surgery: cDMARDs can be continued during surgery unless a specific risk of infection is identified. Advice on bDMARDs varies based upon:
  - The mechanisms of action of the bDMARD.
  - The SPC and whether it remains a black triangle drug.
  - The half-life of the drug.
  - The risk and benefits related to the individual's disease control and general health.

➔ Also see 'Septic arthritis', Chapter 13, pp. 404–407; ➔ Chapter 16, 'Pharmacological management: disease-modifying drugs', pp. 445–503.

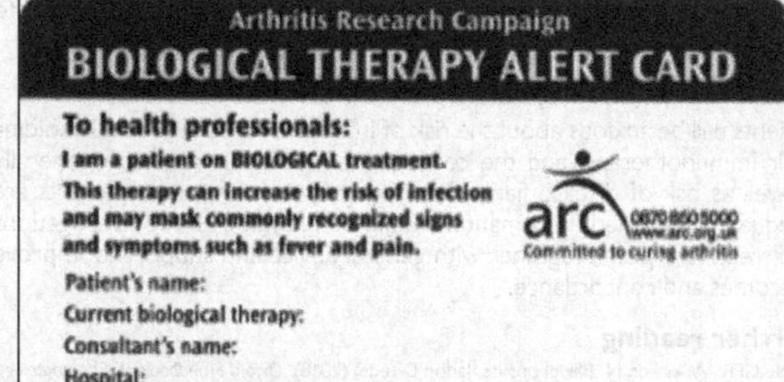
Arthritis Research Campaign

BIOLOGICAL THERAPY ALERT CARD

To health professionals:

I am a patient on BIOLOGICAL treatment.

This therapy can increase the risk of infection and may mask commonly recognized signs and symptoms such as fever and pain.

Patient's name:

Current biological therapy:

Consultant's name:

Hospital:

Hospital phone no:

Arthritis Research Campaign, Copeman House, St. Mary's Gate, Chesterfield, Derbyshire S41 7TD

Fig. 13.1 Example of a biologic alert card.

Reproduced with kind permission from the Arthritis Research Council.

Further reading

NICE website for interactive pathways guidance on all rheumatological conditions: https://pathways.nice.org.uk/Search?q=Rheumatology&pwbu=

Royal College of Nursing (2017). Assessing, management and monitoring biologic therapies for inflammatory arthritis. https://www.rcn.org.uk/professional-development/publications/pdf-005579

Septic arthritis

Septic arthritis

The sudden or subacute development of a hot, swollen joint should always raise the suspicion of a bacterial infection in the joint. Septic arthritis is a medical emergency requiring urgent and expert assessment if the substantial risk of death and long-term morbidity is to be minimized. The four key principles of management are:

- Prompt diagnosis.
- Early antibiotics.
- Adequate drainage.
- Close monitoring to confirm successful treatment.

See Box 13.1 for an overview of septic arthritis and Table 13.1 and ➲ 'Septic arthritis: other infective agents and septic bursitis', Chapter 13, pp. 404–407, for further details on the diagnosis and management. There is a differential diagnosis, most commonly crystal arthropathy. Unless a non-infective diagnosis can be made with confidence, an emergency referral to 2° care should be made. If diagnostic doubt remains, treat for septic arthritis until proven otherwise.

Nursing care issues in septic arthritis

For advanced practitioners undertaking IA joint injection clinics, it is imperative that they are aware of the risk of a case of septic arthritis being referred into the clinic as gout or a 'flare' of the arthritis.

Nurses have a key role in achieving the four principles of management of septic arthritis set out earlier.

In the acute phase, pain control is important and will require monitoring and adjustment. The affected joint will be rested and weight-bearing not permitted until the inflammation and pain settle. Mobilization should then be encouraged. Refer to inpatient physiotherapy to support mobilization, and passive and active exercise, once the acute phase has resolved.

Patients can feel extremely unwell and anxious. Successful pain relief and ensuring that the patient is fully informed about the treatment and management approach will help alleviate anxiety.

Box 13.1 Septic arthritis: overview

Risk factors for septic arthritis (examples)

- Pre-existing joint disease, particularly RA, joint replacement.
- Older age, diabetes mellitus, chronic renal failure, or alcoholism.
- Immunosuppression (e.g. AIDs, hypogammaglobinaemia).
- Skin damage (e.g. cutaneous ulcers, recent IA injection, penetrating injury, or IV drug user).

Presentation

- Hot, swollen, tender joint. Usually large joint, especially knee.
- Fever, but absence of fever does **not** exclude diagnosis.
- Short history, typically <2 weeks.

Diagnostic considerations

- Differential diagnoses, e.g. crystal arthritis (gout, pseudogout), monoarthritis in IJD, trauma, and haemarthrosis.
- If a prosthetic joint, refer to orthopaedic surgeon.
- In the absence of fever but with a high clinical suspicion, treat as septic arthritis.

Likely organisms

- *Staphylococcus aureus, S. epidermidis* in prosthetic joint, and streptococci.
- Gonococcus in sexually active young and Gram negative in elderly people.

Investigations

- Joint aspiration to dryness and send for Gram stain and culture before antibiotics.
- Blood cultures, WBC, CRP or ESR, U&Es, and LFTs.
- If a potential infective source identified, take swabs.
- Echocardiogram and cardiac opinion if IV drug user, ?endocarditis.

Treatment

- Antibiotics are given IV for 2 weeks, or until improvement and then orally for 4 weeks.
- An IV penicillin to cover *S. aureus* while awaiting culture results, e.g. IV flucloxacillin 2 g four times daily.
- If penicillin allergic, clindamycin may be an appropriate choice.
- High risk—elderly, frail, urinary tract infection, add IV cephalosporin, e.g. cefuroxime 1.5 g three times daily.
- MRSA risk—IV cephalosporin and IV vancomycin.

  ► Seek guidance for local antibiotic therapy prescribing policy.

Monitoring

- Daily clinical examination plus FBC, U&E, and CRP/ESR initially.
- Repeat aspiration if effusion reaccumulates.

Table 13.1 Other infective agents causing arthritis

Class	Examples	Disorder and features
Bacteria	*Mycobacterium tuberculosis*	Spinal TB—destruction of vertebral disc and adjacent bodies. Monoarthritis, commonly large joint
Bacteria	Group A streptococci	Rheumatic fever. Delayed autoimmune response with arthritis, carditis and valve damage, chorea
Spirochete	*Borrelia burgdorferi*	Lyme disease transmitted by ticks
Virus	Parvovirus B19 HIV	Slapped cheek syndrome Polyarthralgia, various patterns
Tropical virus	Chikungunya	Mosquito borne, often epidemic, may be persistent arthritis

Further reading

Clunie G, Wilkinson N, Nikiphoru E, Jadon D (eds) (2018). *Oxford Handbook of Rheumatology*, 4th edn. Oxford: Oxford University Press.

Field M, Mathews C, Field M, et al. (2006). BSR and BHPR, BOA, RGCP and BSAC Guidelines for management of the hot swollen joint in adults. *Rheumatology (Oxford)* 45:1039–41. [Guidelines reviewed 2017 and left unchanged.]

Watts RA, Conaghan PG, Denton C, et al. (eds) (2013). Section 9: Infection in rheumatic disease. In: *Oxford Textbook of Rheumatology*, 4th edn, online update 2018. Oxford: Oxford University Press.

Septic arthritis: other infective agents and septic bursitis

A range of infectious agents can cause arthritis via a direct infective mechanism or indirectly (through organism-specific or immunological mechanisms). The clinical course may be slower than septic arthritis and multiple joint involvement is commoner. In viral infections, pain may be marked even in the absence of abnormality on examination of the joints. Diseases (e.g. HIV) or treatments (e.g. anti-TNFα or glucocorticosteroids) which cause marked immunosuppression can leave the patient vulnerable to unusual pathogens. Immunosuppression may also modify the presentation making diagnosis difficult.

Septic bursitis

The two most common sites are the olecranon and pre-patellar bursae. They are managed with serial aspirations and oral antibiotics. However, if there is no response, IV antibiotics should be used.

Further reading

Clunie G, Wilkinson N, Nikiphoru E, Jadon D (eds) (2018). *Oxford Handbook of Rheumatology*, 4th edn. Oxford: Oxford University Press.

Field M, Mathews C, Field M, et al. (2006). BSR and BHPR, BOA, RGCP and BSAC Guidelines for management of the hot swollen joint in adults. *Rheumatology (Oxford)* 45:1039–41. [Guidelines reviewed 2017 and left unchanged.]

Watts RA, Conaghan PG, Denton C, et al. (eds) (2013). Section 9: Infection in rheumatic disease. In: *Oxford Textbook of Rheumatology*, 4th edn, online update 2018. Oxford: Oxford University Press.

Rapid access and emergency complications

This section advises the practitioner on clinical issues that require prompt, early specialist medical opinion.

Drug toxicity

Drug-induced pneumonitis (e.g. MTX)

MTX pneumonitis, generally thought to be the result of a sensitivity reaction, occurs within the first 6 months of commencing the drug. If suspected, MTX should be stopped immediately and an urgent specialist referral made. This complication can progress rapidly and may be fatal if not detected and treated early.

Presentation

- Sudden dry cough.
- SOB.

On examination

- Sometimes fever.
- May have fine crackles on auscultation.

Investigation

- FBC—eosinophilia.
- PFTs.
- HRCT of the lungs.

Treatment

- Prednisolone at high dose, 60 mg/day.

▶ Drug-induced pneumonitis can present with a number of medications.

Overdose of MTX

In the case of an accidental overdose potentially causing acute toxicity, treat with folinic acid 15 mg every 6 hours for 24 hours and monitor LFTs, U&Es, and FBC. The pharmacist can provide guidance on management.

Leflunomide toxicity

In the case of severe toxicity affecting LFTs and skin, stop leflunomide and administer washout procedure, colestyramine 8 g administered three times a day usually for 11 days. Alternatively, 50 g of activated, powdered charcoal may be administered four times a day. Monitor LFTs.

Respiratory complications

Lung disease and respiratory complications are a common complication of RA. This may be part of the disease process or due to the toxicity of the medication prescribed. Seek guidance from the rheumatology team, especially if taking biologic therapies.

Rheumatoid lung disease

Rheumatoid lung disease is manifested as interstitial lung disease or restrictive lung disease. The single most important advice to patients is to give up and stop smoking.

Differentials

- Lung disease related to drug toxicity.
- Infection.
- Other coexisting medical conditions.

For investigations, chest examination, and treatment, a lung biopsy may be required—see ➲ 'MTX pneumonitis', Chapter 16, pp. 466–468 and Chapter 17, pp. 515–517.

Pneumonitis

This basically translates to inflammation of the lung tissue and chronic inflammation can lead to irreversible scarring known as pulmonary fibrosis. For presentation, chest examination, and management—see ➲ 'MTX pneumonitis, Chapter 17, pp. 515–517.

Respiratory infections

Chest infections may be acute or chronic (e.g. those seen with COPD) and are usually bacterial. Pleurisy, however, is different as this is an infection of the lining of the lung rather than the airways.

Causes of chest infection in patients with RA

- Immune system response ↓ due to immunosuppressive therapy.

Presentation

- Chesty cough.
- Discoloured sputum (yellow/green).
- SOB.
- Chest pain.

On examination

- Fever.
- Coarse crackles on auscultation.

Investigations

- ESR and CRP.
- Sputum specimen for culture and sensitivity.
- Chest X-ray.
- HRCT of the lungs may be required.

Treatment

- Antibiotics.
- Analgesia.
- Fluids.
- Oxygen.
- Advise patients to stop smoking and a review of therapy may be required.

Further reading

BNF: 🔗 https://bnf.nice.org.uk/

Pulmonary hypertension

Introduction

Pulmonary hypertension (PH) is a serious, often fatal, complication of a number of CTDs. It is particularly common in scleroderma and accounts for at least one-third of early deaths, either alone or with interstitial lung disease. PH is also seen in SLE, mixed CTD, and RA although the prevalence is much lower than in scleroderma.

PH is defined as an elevated mean pulmonary artery pressure of >25 mmHg at rest. In health, the pressures in the pulmonary artery and the right heart chambers are very low which explains why the walls of these chambers are much thinner than in the left heart. When PH develops, the right heart is put under strain and will compensate by hypertrophy, but as the disease progresses, right heart failure occurs.

Pathogenesis and classification of PH

PH in CTDs develops because of progressive narrowing of the finer branches of the pulmonary arteries within the lungs. This ↑ the resistance to blood flow through the lungs. This subtype of PH is called pulmonary arterial hypertension (PAH), and is group 1 of the WHO classification of PH. Other causes of PH are more common. These include PH due to left heart disease (group 2 in the classification), due to lung disease ± chronic hypoxaemia (group 3), and due to pulmonary emboli blocking larger pulmonary arteries (group 4).

Diagnosis and treatment

The onset of PAH is typically insidious with breathlessness and fatigue. When severe, right heart failure develops with peripheral oedema and ascites. Exercise-related syncope is a symptom of very advanced disease. Examination is usually unhelpful in the early stages and routine clinic investigations including ECG, chest X-ray, and spirometry may be normal at presentation. An estimate of pulmonary artery pressure can be obtained by echocardiogram but can be misleading. Definitive diagnosis needs a right heart catheter study performed in a centre expert in the assessment of PH. Early diagnosis is important before irreversible narrowing of the small pulmonary arteries occurs. The key is a high index of suspicion in patients at risk, particularly scleroderma, and referral to an expert centre if in doubt.

Once the diagnosis of PAH in a CTD patient is made, treatment will include:

- Explanation of the diagnosis and continuing support.
- Consideration of more intensive management of underlying CTD.
- Management of complications such as right heart failure and hypoxaemia.
- Specific therapies for PAH (e.g. vasodilators, endothelin receptor antagonists).

This is a complex and evolving field. In the UK, eight hospitals have been designated as PH centres. Suspected cases of PAH will be referred to one of these centres or to a more local 'satellite' clinic which collaborates with a PH centre. The prognosis for PAH is improving but it remains a challenge with a substantial mortality.

Breathlessness

Breathlessness is a relatively common problem seen in patients with rheumatological disease. It is worth having a framework to enable you to undertake a good clinical history and make a management plan.

Framework

Breathlessness could be due to:

- A cardiac or respiratory complication of the condition.
- Lung disease related to drug toxicity.
- Pulmonary infection as a result of immunosuppression, e.g. pneumonia.
- A co-morbidity, e.g. asthma, COPD, or heart failure.

►► The most important thing to rule out immediately is infection.

An initial assessment of severity

- Vital signs—temperature, pulse rate, respiration rate, blood pressure, and breathing pattern.
- Oxygen saturation.
- ↓ in exercise tolerance from the patient's usual level.
- Evidence of other system involvement, e.g. hypotension, ankle oedema, and poor urine output.

History of acute event

- Duration of breathlessness.
- Pattern of symptoms—worsening rapidly, episodic?
- Symptoms to suggest infections—fever, chills, night sweats, or productive purulent sputum.
- Direct questioning for features of respiratory and cardiac disease.
- Recent immobility or major surgery, and other risk factors for PE.

Drug history

- On immunosuppressant?
- On drugs that cause lung toxicity?
- ► Many drugs can cause pulmonary complications, e.g. SAS and MTX pneumonitis.

Coexisting disease

- Smoking history.
- Cardiovascular disease, e.g. hypotension/hypertension, ischaemic heart disease.
- Respiratory disease, e.g. asthma, COPD.
- Ask the patient: 'Does the problem present in a similar way to previous exacerbations?'

➲ For underlying conditions, e.g. hypertension or asthma, refer to appropriate treatment guidelines.

Observations and investigations

- Temperature, pulse rate, respiratory rate, blood pressure, and calculation of early warning score if acutely ill.
- Oxygen saturation and, if asthmatic, peak flow.

- Bloods—FBC, CRP, and U&E, as a minimum.
- Chest X-ray and ECG.
- If patient reports purulent sputum—specimen for culture (to identify organism).
- Consider blood culture if features suggesting infection.

At the end of this process you will have an idea of the following

- Is the symptom complex suggestive of an infective, a respiratory, or a cardiac cause?
- Worsening of coexisting disease—manage according to treatment for underlying condition.
- Is this a new problem requiring a medical assessment?
- Severity and pace of change of breathlessness.

❶ If following assessment the patient appears severely ill, or there is a rapid deterioration, or if infection is likely—seek urgent medical advice.

❶ If a patient is taking a bDMARD they may not present with classical signs of infection.

➲ Also see 'Pharmacological management', Chapter 16, pp. 445–503; ➲ 'Assessing the patient', Chapter 8, pp. 290–291; ➲ 'Rapid access and emergency issues', Chapter 13, pp. 408–409.

Further reading

British Lung Foundation: ℬ https://www.blf.org.uk

British Thoracic Society: ℬ https://www.brit-thoracic.org.uk

Galie N, et al (2016). ESC/ERS Guidelines for the diagnosis and treatment of pulmonary hypertension. *European Heart Journal* 37:67–119 doi:10.1093/eurheartj/ehv317. https://www.blf.org.uk/support-for-you/pulmonary-hypertension

Shaw M, Collins BF, Ho LA, Raghu G (2015). Rheumatoid arthritis-associated lung disease. *Eur Respir Rev* 24:1–16.

Frequently asked questions

What if an infection does not settle?

The diagnosis should be reviewed, and the patient reassessed. Medical advice should be sought for those with polypharmacy or complex disease presentations. If patients are being treated with biologic therapies, it is essential that they get an urgent medical opinion.

When should a GP/community nurse refer to 2° care?

Firstly, seek advice by telephone or email initially. Urgently refer any patient with suspected septic arthritis, or systemic infection, to 2° care or emergency services. If patients appear systemically unwell and the disease activity ↑, specialist advice should be sought to guide management. More recently, there is a good range of communication available with specialist teams including telephone consultations and rapid email referral clinics. If in doubt or there is difficulty in accessing a member of the team, contact the specialist nursing team.

Do DMARDs, steroids, or biologics mask infection?

Yes, some of these drugs may mask infection showing a normal WBC count and lack of fever. Patients who are on these therapies are immunosuppressed and have an ↑ risk of infections, so a high index of suspicion should be maintained. Good clinical acumen and patient reports should aid consideration but refer/seek 2° if in doubt.

How can I tell the difference between a chesty cold and drug-induced pneumonitis?

This can be very difficult even for the specialist nurses receiving reports over the phone from the patient about a 'cold' or 'cough', especially during winter months. If a patient is prescribed a drug recognized to cause pneumonitis (e.g. MTX or gold therapy), you need to seek medical advice if there is any doubt. The cough can come on suddenly or gradually, will be unproductive, and may or may not be accompanied by breathlessness. Additional questions to exclude a cold may be helpful (e.g. have they had a runny nose and sore throat?). However, if there is any doubt whatsoever, medical advice should be sought and the patient should be advised to withhold treatment.

Fertility, pregnancy, and relationships

Fertility and conception

Sexual and reproductive health issues are important considerations in patients with rheumatic disease that are frequently overlooked in clinical consultations. For HCPs, the challenges are those of maintaining disease control with the patient's desire to become a parent. For patients parenting a child, decisions are even more complex, particularly when drug regimens are needed for life and may impact fertility, conception, and pregnancy decisions. Furthermore, certain treatments may have adverse effects upon pregnancy. Therefore, patients need careful counselling and support. Specialist guidance should be provided on:

- Contraceptive advice that is appropriate for the underlying disease.
- Long-term strategy on family planning, e.g. treatments may ↓ fertility (e.g. storage of eggs or sperm prior to starting treatment).
- Preconception counselling regarding the ideal timing of pregnancy in relation to disease activity/manifestations and for those with antiphospholipid antibodies (aPL) (↑ risk adverse pregnancy outcomes) or anti-Ro and anti-La antibodies (↑ risk of congenital heart block and delivering babies with neonatal skin rash).
- Clinical decisions on maintaining disease control and well-being (± medication) while attempting to conceive and during pregnancy.

As many inflammatory rheumatic diseases predominately affect ♀ of child-bearing age, discussions often focus on ♀ regarding pregnancy issues but ♂ with an inflammatory rheumatic disease who may be fathering a child must also be counselled and advised. The welfare of the mother and unborn child must be considered as certain treatments may adversely affect pregnancy. All patients on drug therapies with the potential to affect the unborn child must have:

- Appropriate information and advice about the treatment prescribed.
- Contraceptive advice tailored to the individual and underlying disease.

The most significant conditions that face these challenges include:

- RA, APS, primary systemic vasculitis (PSV) (➔ Chapter 5, p. 165).
- SLE, especially those with APS (➔ Chapter 5, p. 132).
- Scleroderma, also called systemic sclerosis, especially those diagnosed with pulmonary hypertension or ♂ with erectile dysfunction.
- Sjögren's syndrome in those with antibodies to anti-Ro and anti-La (➔ see 'Sjögren's syndrome', Chapter 5, pp. 142–146).
- Marfan's syndrome—pregnancy carries an ↑ risk of aortic and cardiac problems.

Fertility and contraceptive advice

Family size is reduced among patients with rheumatic disease for many reasons including impaired sexual function, pregnancy loss, and personal choice.

- Evidence suggests ↓ fertility when disease is poorly controlled or when there are additional disease complications (e.g. lupus nephritis may be associated with amenorrhea).
- Proposed links between aPL and infertility remain unproven.
- Specialist support may be required to select a contraceptive (e.g. hand function difficulties fitting contraceptive diaphragm/use of intrauterine coil).

- Consideration of the type of sex hormone used is important for lupus patients with aPL or associated with APS—contraceptive should be progesterone only (there is an ↑ risk of blood clots with combined oestrogen-containing types of contraceptive pill).
- Ovulation induction and *in vitro* fertilization can be safely used in patients with SLE with stable/inactive disease but certain ↑ risks (fetal and maternal) have been identified including:
  - Ovarian hyperstimulation.
  - Thrombosis, particularly in patients with positive aPL.
- Medication reviews prior to conception and when breastfeeding:
  - Most antirheumatic drugs do not impair fertility. The main exceptions are cyclophosphamide that has gonadotoxic effects on ♂ and ♀ fertility and SAS in ♂ causing reduced sperm count (reversible on cessation). Although MTX has been linked with ♂ reduced sperm count, current guidelines do not require ♂ to stop SAS or MTX prior to conception.
  - MTX and SAS deplete folate—provide folate therapy.
  - ♂ with erectile dysfunction may require specialist advice.

➲ See also Chapter 16, 'Pharmacological management: disease-modifying drugs', pp. 445–503.

Drug therapies: fertility and safety issues

- Preconception treatment plans should be carefully considered in consultation with the patient and clinician. Conception should be planned at a time of disease quiescence of 3–6 months on stable medication. Longer periods of 6–12 months may be advised in cases of severe internal organ involvement and/or drug change. It is important to stratify drug therapies to safely maintain disease control during conception and pregnancy as loss of disease control on stopping treatment can harm mother and unborn child.
- Many conditions are treated with cytotoxic therapies that must be avoided during pregnancy (e.g. MTX, MMF), due to ↑ risks related to first-trimester exposure, e.g. congenital abnormalities.
- Some drug therapies that may be continued during pregnancy (based on risk/benefit discussions) include:
  - Hydroxychloroquine (HCQ) sulphate.
  - SAS, AZA, and ciclosporin.
- High-dose corticosteroids may safely be used to treat disease flares in pregnancy.
- Avoid prolonged systemic treatment unless risks to the patient are higher than those to the unborn child.
- Pulsed therapies may be considered for some patients.
- Ensure adequate vitamin D treatment.
- Cyclophosphamide continued with acute multisystem episodes. Associated with ovarian failure but dependent on:
  - Age of ♀ at start of treatment (the younger the patient, the ↓ risk).
  - Cumulative dose and route of administration—IV probably safer than oral.
- Avoid NSAIDs at third trimester—after 32 weeks of gestation (risks of premature closure of ductus arteriosus and oligohydramnios).

- Increasing preliminary observational data on pregnancies while treated with new bDMARDs (particularly anti-TNF drugs—adalimumab, etanercept, and infliximab) are reassuring. In fact, certolizumab pegol, a PEGylated form of anti-TNF drug with minimal rates of placental and breastmilk transfer, is now licensed by the European Medicines Agency. Current British and European guidance gives detailed recommendations on the potential use of these and other biologic drugs in pregnancy. Importantly, if a biologic drug is given in the third trimester of pregnancy then live vaccines should not be given to the infant until 7 months of age.

Key point

There are improved outcomes for mother and unborn child if conception and the prenatal phase are achieved while disease activity is quiescent.

Further reading

Andreoli L, Bertsias GK, Agmon-Levin N, et al. (2017). EULAR recommendations for women's health and the management of family planning, assisted reproduction, pregnancy and menopause in patients with systemic lupus erythematosus and/or antiphospholipid syndrome. *Ann Rheum Dis* 76:476–85.

Flint J, Panchal S, Hurrell A, et al. (2016). BSR and BHPR guideline on prescribing drugs in pregnancy and breastfeeding—part I: standard and biologic disease modifying anti-rheumatic drugs and corticosteroids. *Rheumatology (Oxford)* 55:1693–7.

Flint J, Panchal S, Hurrell A, et al. (2016). BSR and BHPR guideline on prescribing drugs in pregnancy and breastfeeding—part II: analgesics and other drugs used in rheumatology practice. *Rheumatology (Oxford)* 55:1698–702.

Götestam Skorpen C, Hoeltzenbein M, Tincani A, et al. (2016). The EULAR points to consider for the use of antirheumatic drugs before pregnancy and during pregnancy and lactation. *Ann Rheum Dis* 75:795–810.

Pregnancy and long-term conditions

Many inflammatory rheumatic diseases are systemic, with the potential for significant internal organ involvement and requirement for long-term medications to control the disease, principally:

- RA.
- Spondyloarthropathies, e.g. AS.
- SLE.
- PSV.
- Scleroderma/systemic sclerosis.
- APS.

There are therefore important issues for patients (♂ and ♀) to consider before planning for a family (➔ see 'Fertility and conception', pp. 416–417).

Pregnancy

About 2–3% of *all* pregnancies in the normal population result in major congenital anomalies and the frequency of minor (cosmetic) anomalies are much higher. Early fetal development is the most vulnerable time of gestation in relation to malformations and drug toxicity issues; ∴ essential prerequisites for all patients should be:

- Initial drug counselling when starting treatment with cytotoxic or DMARDs in relation to risks and benefits of treatment and consequences of conception while on treatment.
- Preconception counselling for all patients receiving treatments for LTCs of child-bearing potential.
- The aim of care will be to achieve remission or at least maintain optimum disease control during the pregnancy but with the minimal drug toxicity/risk of teratogenicity. Specialist support required to manage complex pregnancies includes rheumatology and obstetric teams and, depending upon the condition and organ involvement, other specialist teams. Careful monitoring of the patient and unborn child is required. For some conditions, there are additional risks to the mother during pregnancy (e.g. SLE) and in others, evidence of management and outcomes is limited (e.g. PSV). High disease activity in SLE, APS, and systemic sclerosis at conception and prenatal phases appear to be linked with worst outcomes for the mother and unborn child.

AS and RA

- AS—limited data, low chance of remission during pregnancy. Mechanical problems may relate to sacroiliitis.
- RA—remission during pregnancy (~50%).
- RA—↑ risk of premature birth, low birth weight, and pre-eclampsia.
- RA—frequently relapse of disease 3–4 months postpartum requiring specialist support to establish disease control.

Systemic sclerosis: limited evidence but some reports suggest:

- ↑ frequency in pre-term births and small full-term infants but frequency miscarriage and neonatal survival no different from controls.

- Contraindications to pregnancy include pulmonary hypertension and uncontrolled hypertension. Diffuse scleroderma—wait until disease is stable.
- Evaluation of cardiac and pulmonary function may be required.
- Reflux oesophagitis and cardiopulmonary decompensation may develop but Raynaud's phenomenon likely to improve.

SLE

- Pregnancy in SLE associated with renal disease leads to ↑ risk of poor outcomes. Close monitoring necessary.
- Low C3, C4 levels, and/or high anti-double-stranded DNA levels ↑ risk flare SLE in pregnancy and pregnancy loss.
- Maternal anti-Ro and anti-La antibodies associated with 0.7–2% risk of congenital heart block. If first child delivered with congenital heart block, subsequent pregnancies are at ↑ risk of congenital heart block.
- SLE patients with high-risk aPL profile (persistent moderate to high aPL titres, LA positivity or multiple aPL positivity) or patients with APS will need:
  - Anticoagulant therapy—aspirin and low-molecular-weight heparin should replace pre-existing warfarin in pregnancy and up to 6 weeks postpartum.
  - Obstetric monitoring and obstetric-led birth.
  - HCQ is recommended preconceptually and in all SLE pregnancies.
- To reduce the risk of pre-eclampsia, low-dose aspirin is recommended in all SLE pregnancies.
- Active disease may be treated with HCQ, AZA, ciclosporin, tacrolimus, or glucocorticoids.
- MMF should be stopped prepregnancy and switched to AZA.

PSV

- ↑ risk of thromboembolic events during pregnancy—treatment as for SLE.
- Pregnancy in Takayasu arteritis—limited evidence outlines:
  - Severe hypertension and/or pre-eclampsia most common maternal complications in ~40%.
  - Low birth weight and intrauterine growth restriction most frequent fetal complications in 20%.
  - If Takayasu arteritis with abdominal aorta involvement—↑ risk to mother and unborn child.
  - Despite ↑ complications, pregnancy outcomes favourable in most cases.
- Pregnancies rare in GPA (older age group, rare disease). Very limited evidence shows patients with active disease at conception or disease onset during pregnancy are at high risk of maternal complications and death.
- Pregnancy in EGPA—despite affecting ♀ of child-bearing potential, data on pregnancy are extremely limited.
- May require corticosteroids and AZA to maintain disease control during pregnancy. Immunoglobulin treatment may also be given during pregnancy.

- Pregnancy in polyarteritis nodosa rare (older age group). Very limited evidence. Patients who conceive during remission have favourable outcome.
- Those diagnosed late in pregnancy appear to have high rates of maternal death.
- Pregnancy in MPA—extremely rare case reports. Use same management principles as for GPA.

➲ See 'Fertility and conception', pp. 416–417.
➲ Also see Chapter 10, 'Holistic and patient-centred care', pp. 329–350; ➲ Chapter 16, Pharmacological management: disease-modifying drugs', pp. 445–503.

Key point

Disease control is essential for good maternal and fetal outcomes. Establish disease control during ante- and postpartum care and provide support to mother and family in caring for infant.

Further reading

Andreoli L, Bertsias GK, Agmon-Levin N, et al. (2017). EULAR recommendations for women's health and the management of family planning, assisted reproduction, pregnancy and menopause in patients with systemic lupus erythematosus and/or antiphospholipid syndrome. *Ann Rheum Dis* 76:476–85.

Ching Soh MC, Nelson-Piercy C (2015). High-risk pregnancy and the rheumatologist. *Rheumatology (Oxford)* 54:572.

Gatto M, Iaccarino L, Canova M, et al. (2012). Pregnancy and vasculitis: a systemic review of the literature. *Autoimmun Rev* 11:A447.

Breastfeeding and medications

There are multiple health benefits to mother and baby from breastfeeding. Studies on the excretion of any drugs into breastmilk are rare and very few antirheumatic drugs have been studied. Breast milk is an emulsion containing water, lipids, carbohydrates, minerals, and proteins. Only the unbound fraction of a drug is transferred into breast milk by passive diffusion to reach equilibrium from blood. Drugs can also be transferred into breast milk by carrier-mediated transport.

Concentrations of drug in breast milk may be affected by the following:

- Non-ionized and lipophilic agents with a low molecular weight are most likely to be transferred into breast milk.
- Highly protein-bound drugs or agents with high molecular weight are unlikely to cross extensively into breast milk.
- Term neonate, older or partially breastfed babies are usually at low risk for side effects of drugs in breast milk.
- The molecular weight and dose and dosage intervals of the medication.
- The drug's half-life will affect how long the drug is found in the breast milk.

The changes seen during pregnancy (e.g. ↑ in body weight, body fat, GI absorption, and enhanced hepatic metabolism) will also affect drug absorption and metabolism. These changes have little impact on the drug therapies prescribed for rheumatic diseases or for the mother but may be important when having to consider drug dosages passed on via breast milk to an infant.

The amount of drug excreted in breast milk can be reduced by considering the timing of breastfeeds and medications (e.g. ensuring that oral drugs are taken just before breastfeeding where there will be insufficient time for drugs to concentrate in breast milk).

There is limited information on the risks to the breastfed child while the mother is taking medication.

- Drugs that can safely be used during breastfeeding include NSAIDs and paracetamol, corticosteroids, HCQ, SAS, and AZA
- Due to limited data, patients should be advised to avoid breastfeeding while on antirheumatic drugs such as MTX, leflunomide, and MMF. MTX levels excreted in breast milk are said to be <10% of those in plasma; however, as little is known of the harmful and cumulative effects on the developing child, MTX should be avoided if breastfeeding.

For more detailed information regarding the risks of medications while pregnant or breastfeeding refer to the BSR and EULAR recommendations referenced previously and the online LactMed database—🔗 https://toxnet.nlm.nih.gov/newtoxnet/lactmed.htm.

Sexuality

Sexual problems are very common for patients. However, offering emotional support and practical solutions can radically improve the patient's quality of life.

Identify possible causes

Physical causes consider:

- Joint pain.
- Joint stiffness.
- Fatigue.
- ↓ or altered sensation or poor blood circulation causing erectile or orgasmic dysfunction; dry vagina causing dyspareunia.
- Medications triggering loss of libido, erectile dysfunction, or anorgasmia.

Psychological factors

Psychological factors play an important role in perceived:

- Feelings of unattractiveness or poor body image.
- Low esteem affecting libido.
- Helplessness lowering desire and affecting performance.

Relationship

Illness and ensuing dependency may cause guilt, resentment, withdrawal by partner, and couple conflict.

Offer emotional support

Be aware …

that sex may be an important part of an individual's life independent of illness, age, or marital status.

Subtly mention the problem …

in the right environment try to take the initiative so the patient doesn't have to. You can make this less of a big issue by normalizing: 'Is arthritis affecting your sexuality in any way?'

Normalize …

explain that the problem is common and acceptable. Consider using examples such as this: 'Many patients with your condition find it's difficult to make love'.

Create emotional space …

support by allowing patients to express anxiety, guilt, and anger. Consider open questions such as 'Do you want to talk about how you feel?'

Empower …

so patient feels more hopeful and in control. Offer statements such as 'There's lots you can do to improve things'.

Offer general solutions

- Examine the list of medications and treatment plans; identify any medications that may be the source of sexual problems.
- Discuss with the patient possible support such as painkillers or erectile dysfunction medication.

- Encourage the patient to be physically affectionate with their partner, to offset the lack of sexual contact.
- Suggest options such as relationship-building strategies, such as better communication. If necessary, suggest seeking additional support.

Get patient to use sex-specific solutions

Identifying times of day when pain level is lower:

- Suggest resting before and after sex to lower fatigue.
- Encourage them to ensure the room is well heated to avoid getting cold during sex.
- Before sex, easing pain with hot bath, massage, or painkillers.
- Raising libido through erotic magazines or DVDs.
- Applying lubricant to offset vaginal dryness.
- Shortening foreplay if pain or stiffness builds.
- Using sex toys such as vibrators.
- Choosing more pain-free techniques—oral or hand sex may be easier than intercourse.
- Experimenting to find more comfortable sexual positions; ➔ the following 'Further reading' section includes suggestions for online publications.

Further reading

Arthritis Foundation (life-stages/relationships): https://www.arthritis.org

National Rheumatoid Arthritis Society (https://www.nras.org.uk) has some interesting and useful pieces about sexuality and RA, including 'Emotions, relationships and sexuality' (2013) https://www.nras.org.uk/emotions-relationships-and-sexuality-booklet

Regard (an organization for gay men and lesbians): http://www.regard.org.uk

Relate (for problems that require specific support/advice on relationships suggest seeking additional support from Relate): https://www.relate.org.uk

Scleroderma Foundation (2015). Sexuality and scleroderma. https://www.scleroderma.org

Versus Arthritis (formed in 2018 from a merger of Arthritis Research UK and Arthritis Care), advice on sex relationships and arthritis: M https://www.versusarthritis.org/; Feelings matter: emotional wellbeing and arthritis (2016) M https://www.arthritiscare.org.uk/assets/000/001/842/Emotional_wellbeing_2017_update_original.pdf?1509538654

Self-esteem and effect on relationships

Self-esteem is a person's own appraisal of their worth and combines personal beliefs ('I can manage to undertake normal work activities') and emotions ('My disease makes me feel like a second-class citizen'). Individuals with a LTC can face numerous challenges to their self-esteem and these effects can impact their personal relationships.

- The disease itself may be perceived by some members of the lay public in negative ways (e.g. AIDS) or be perceived as principally an old age condition, despite the person being relatively young and possibly with no outward signs of disease (e.g. SLE).
- Society perceives sexuality as belonging to the young, fit, and healthy—adding to the burden the patient may perceive about their disease.
- The patient may feel a sense of shame about their condition, e.g. perceiving themselves as inferior in society or feeling guilty because of the adjustments that have to be made as a result of their condition and effect on their significant others.

The consequences of the conditions may disrupt perceptions of self by:

- The variable nature of the condition—leading to a poor sense of 'control' over life and ability to plan and manage daily activities.
- Disrupt life with frequent reminders of the chronic disease status—e.g. numerous outpatient appointments, frequent blood tests, drug regimens, or a disease that excludes activities or social participation, e.g. consumption of alcohol, sporting activities, or dietary restrictions.
- Changes that occur to body image, e.g. joint changes seen in the hands of those with RA or obvious skin rashes in PsA or SLE.
- Facial changes that may occur as a result of GPA or butterfly rash seen in SLE.

The condition may significantly ↑ reliance on others, e.g.:

- Inability to complete tasks such as dressing, personal hygiene, or preparing a meal.
- Changes that result in role reversals in relationships, e.g. 'traditional' roles undertaken by a ♀ in a relationship may have to be undertaken by her ♂ partner (e.g. hanging the washing on the line); for a ♂, the loss of key roles may affect their long-standing perceived position as breadwinner or 'protector'.
- Loss of work participation may affect financial standing and security, ↑ the sense of loss that comes with changes to their perceived role in society or ability to manage/control family income.
- Changes may affect the individual's perception of attractiveness and belief in their appeal sexually. This will affect sexual relationships with their partner, for example.
- Partners who also provide a role as carer may find it hard to revert then to sexual partner.
- Changes in body image may make the person nervous of making the first sexual approaches—fearing they are no longer attractive.
- Individuals may find it difficult to communicate their anxieties and challenges with their partner.
- Patients may worry about being seen unclothed.

- Pain and fatigue from the disease may also have a negative impact on the wish to be touched.

Social participation

Evidence suggests that those with a LTC who have a good level of social support (in the form of satisfactory relationships and financial infrastructures) have a high level of perceived self-efficacy and have improved outcomes. Individuals should be supported in coming to terms with their condition and negotiating their healthcare needs. When self-esteem is low, it can be difficult for patients to effectively negotiate without an advocate.

The role of the nurse in enhancing self-esteem

- Patients will, over time, need differing levels of support and may take time to feel able to discuss issues related to relationships. Enhancing the therapeutic relationships and encouraging a holistic and patient-centred approach to care should encourage practitioner/patient communication.
- The partner or close family/friends supporting someone with a LTC may often go unrecognized or unsupported and need to be considered in the context of the patient's self-esteem and ability to participate actively in society.

Nurses should:

- Provide an opportunity for the patient (and, if the patient consents, the partner) to be able to discuss issues of concern.
- Provide an environment conducive to discussing such personal issues.
- Be comfortable and receptive to discussing relationship issues.
- Normalize the problem. Provide reassurance and appropriate information to enable the patient to recognize their problems are not unique and support is available to them.
- Enable the patient to achieve personal goals in improving self-esteem:
  - Set goals, e.g. taking up a small, part-time, voluntary post.
  - Refer to OT for aids and devices for independent living, e.g. kitchen equipment or aids to enable ease of dressing.
- Advise on ways that they can participate and network where appropriate with organizations or support groups that will allow the patient access to other patients with similar experiences.
  - EPPs or voluntary network groups such as the NRAS.
- Where appropriate, provide contact details for organizations such as marriage guidance for those with specific relationships problems

➔ Also see 'Sexuality', pp. 423–424.

Further reading

National Rheumatoid Arthritis Society (2013). Emotions, relationships and sexuality. https://www.nras.org.uk/emotions-relationships-and-sexuality-booklet

Versus Arthritis (advice on sex, relationships, and arthritis): https://www.versusarthritis.org/

Part III

Nursing care issues

Treatment, nursing management, and tools

Pharmacological management: Pain relief

Pretreatment and review: prescribing issues

Pretreatment assessment

Pain is a complex experience influenced by physical, psychological and social factors. The presenting complaint of pain may also be linked to other factors that may heighten or precipitate the sensations of pain. These include:

- Prior experience of pain and ability to control symptoms.
- Intensity, frequency, and duration of pain.
- Low mood and anxiety.
- Beliefs, behaviours, and cultural factors that may affect pain or perceptions of pain and controlling pain.
- Social factors such as dissatisfaction at work or family difficulties.

Pretreatment assessment of risk and benefit of prescribing analgesia

An assessment should include:

- General health status and evaluation of co-morbidities or prior illness, and surgical treatments.
- Current prescribed medications and potential drug interactions.
- Drug history in relation to drug allergies, adverse events, or treatment side effects.
- The presenting history, duration of presenting complaint, and causal factors to pain, e.g. ↑ inflammatory activity.

Following this assessment, the nurse should have sufficient information to know about:

- Prior treatments and potential drug interactions/adverse events.
- The patient's previous experience of different analgesia or pain-relieving strategies and benefits gained.
- Cautions and contraindications to consider, e.g. prior history of GI blood or steroid psychosis.
- The nature of symptoms, e.g. duration/intensity of pain, with an assessment of the level of pain experienced by the patient, e.g. use of a VAS.

A purely pharmacological approach to pain management may fail to adequately control pain and prescribers should explore the following with the patient:

- The individual's knowledge of pain and how pain relief works, e.g. to achieve effective pain control, regular dosing may be required rather than waiting for the pain to become unbearable before taking medications.
- Other non-pharmacological approaches that may be an adjunct to prescribed medications.
- An assessment of current pain scores, and the patient's needs and expectations of symptom control.
- A planned review process to examine changes in pain scores and benefits of prescribed pain relief.

➲ Also see 'Assessing pain', Chapter 9, pp. 310–312.

The review process

If the patient is to have confidence in achieving effective pain relief, they should be offered a review appointment with a specified time frame for their current drug regimen. A prescribing plan must include a review process. This will build a safety framework to ensure a thorough assessment of the treatment prescribed and subsequent prescribing plans—e.g. can an effective treatment such as paracetamol be added to their repeat prescriptions?

A number of analgesics may be considered safe and effective over a short period of time but may not be appropriate to consider as part of a long-term strategy.

Patient information

- Patients should receive information on the treatments they are prescribed, including potential risks and benefits of treatment in the context of their health condition.
- Monitoring or clinical attendance responsibilities as part of the prescribing plan.
- Access to support and advice including:
  - Written information on the underlying condition and treatment.
  - Additional information resources such as web-based self-help groups, and health and well-being activities in the community.
  - Patient self-help/support groups.

Ensure patients who have a LTC requiring access to regular pain relief are aware of:

- If prescribed pain relief to have for such episodes, how they should 'step up' or re-start analgesia (and non-pharmacological options) to manage symptoms.
- Guidance on when to 'step down' treatment and how to document changes in their self-medication if required.
- Advice on what to do if initial symptom control fails and they need to seek additional support. If it is likely they will require specialist support/advice—who they contact and contact details.

For those with self-limiting conditions who would not be expected to require follow-up (e.g. referral for joint injection for OA of the knee), guidance should be provided on what to do if the condition fails to resolve as planned, and what to do if they experience side effects from their treatment.

➲ Also see 'Chronic non-inflammatory pain', Chapter 6, pp. 185–199; ➲ 'Symptom control: pain relief', Chapter 9, pp. 315–316; ➲ 'Assessment of pain: red and yellow flags', pp. 313–314; ➲ 'Depression and fatigue', pp. 317–318; ➲ 'Intra-articular injections', Chapter 18, pp. 541–543.

Further reading

British Medical Association (2017). *Chronic Pain: Supporting Safe Prescribing of Analgesia*. London: BMA.
NICE (2016). Multi-morbidity: clinical assessment and management (NG56). https://www.nice.org.uk/guidance/ng56

The analgesic ladder: step one

Introduction

Pain is defined as an unpleasant feeling which may be associated with actual or potential tissue damage and which may have physical, emotional, and social components. Before prescribing analgesia it is useful to identify whether the patient's pain has one or more of four components:

- Mechanical nociceptive.
- Inflammatory nociceptive.
- Neuropathic—pain related to lesions/dysfunction of the peripheral nervous system.
- Psychological component driving the pain.

► Nociception is a neurophysiological term and refers to specific activity in nerve pathways.

➜ Also see 'Assessing pain', Chapter 9, pp. 310–311; ➜ 'Symptom control: assessing pain', chapter 9, pp. 315–316; ➜ 'Assessment tools', Chapter 20, pp. 595–612; ➜ 'Chronic non-inflammatory pain', Chapter 6, pp. 185–198.

Chronic pain syndromes: assessing pain

The analgesic ladder as defined by the WHO for nociceptive pain outlines a step-up approach starting with a non-opioid, moving to a weak opioid, and then a strong opioid (Box 15.1).

Discuss taking analgesia with the patient and include information on potential side effects and benefits. A common problem is that patients frequently fail to take regular analgesia and then wait until the pain has become unbearable. This can result in the patient gaining minimal benefit from analgesia as heightened pain perceptions render the analgesia ineffective or they have to wait for a further 20–30 min for the drug's therapeutic benefits to be achieved. Regular analgesia may be effective but in some cases the patient's analgesia may be ineffective (or side effects may warrant a change) and they will need to move up the analgesic ladder. Responses to analgesia vary and some patients may experience ↑ side effects of a medication, e.g. drowsiness/constipation.

Box 15.1 Analgesic ladder

Step 1

Non-opioid: paracetamol.

Step 2

Weak opioid: codeine.

Step 3

Strong opioid: tramadol, morphine, oxycodone, fentanyl, or buprenorphine.

NB In the original analgesia ladder tramadol was cited at step 2, but due to the reclassification of tramadol as a controlled drug, it is appropriate to place it at step 3.

Example: step one

Paracetamol (acetaminophen)

- Tablets (500 mg); soluble tablets (500 mg); oral suspension (120 mg/5 mL; 250 mg/5 mL); suppositories (250 mg, 500 mg) in a dosage of 0.5–1.0 g every 4–6 hours, with a max dose of 4 g (8 × 500 mg tablets/day).
- This is the first-line treatment for acute and chronic musculoskeletal pain. The mechanism of action is thought to be inhibition of prostaglandins in the brain resulting in an ↑ pain threshold.

Side effects: medication overuse headache.
Relative cautions: liver disease and severe renal impairment.
Contraindications: known hypersensitivity to paracetamol.

Further reading

Clunie GPR, Wilkinson N, Nikiphorou E, Jadon D (eds) (2018). *Oxford Handbook of Rheumatology*, 4th edn. Oxford: Oxford University Press.
WHO. Analgesic pain ladder for adults. https://www.who.int/cancer/palliative/painladder/en/

The analgesic ladder: step two

Example 1: step two

Codeine tablets (15 mg, 30 mg, 60 mg), syrup (25 mg/5 mL)

- Codeine is metabolized in the body by an enzyme process called demethylation to morphine, with 10% of the compound converted to morphine. This process stimulates the opioid (mu and k) receptors in the CNS and causes *inhibition* of the spinal and central processing pain sensation.
- The amount of codeine in combined preparations varies. It is important to be aware of the different dosages and combinations available and try and match them according to the control of pain and side effects the patients is experiencing.
- Codeine may be combined with paracetamol in the form of co-codamol.
- Dosages vary between both codeine and paracetamol as outlined:
  - 8/500 = 8 mg codeine/500 mg paracetamol.
  - 15/500 = 15 mg codeine/500 mg paracetamol.
  - 30/500 = 30 mg codeine/500 mg paracetamol, in a dosage of 30–60 mg every 4–6 hours and a maximum of 240 mg/day.

Side effects

Nausea, vomiting, constipation, dizziness, sweating, dependence, and medication overuse headache.

Cautions

Use as low as possible dose in elderly patients, and patients with hypothyroidism, hypoadrenalism, chronic hepatic disease and renal insufficiency, or asthma. Pregnancy and breastfeeding.

Contraindications

Known hypersensitivity to any of the tablet constituents; respiratory depression, obstructive airways disease, paralytic ileus, head injury, raised intracranial pressure, or acute alcoholism.

Example 2: step three

Tramadol

- Useful when codeine is ineffective or causes constipation. Tramadol may have less respiratory depression.
- Tramadol works from the binding of sigma, kappa, mu opioid receptors, and inhibition of noradrenaline reuptake, and serotonin release.
- Capsules (50 mg), or dispersible tablets (50 mg), or soluble tablets (50 mg), and modified-release tablets (twice-daily regimen): 100 mg, 150 mg, and 200 mg tablets. Dosage is 50–100 mg 4-hourly. Modified release twice-daily preparations initially 50–100 mg twice daily. Maximum dose of 400 mg/day.

Side effects

As with codeine, nausea and vomiting are more common. Abdominal discomfort, hypotension, psychiatric disturbance (hallucinations), or convulsions. Addiction can occur.

Contraindications

Uncontrolled epilepsy, pregnancy, and breastfeeding.

For those patients taking regular 4–6-hourly doses of tramadol, consider a modified-release preparation. If unable to tolerate tramadol, an alternative is Tramacet®. This may have equal potency to tramadol by combining tramadol and paracetamol, with an improved side effect profile.

Pain relief: tricyclics and other antidepressants

Pain is a unique personal experience for the patient and for some people pain is not relieved using non-opioid analgesia and non-pharmacological approaches. Patients who have chronic pain may also experience symptoms of depression or insomnia. The use of an opioid is usually recommended for moderate to severe pain and may not be appropriate for patients with chronic pain. However, another option for chronic unrelieved pain can be the addition of an antidepressant (e.g. tricyclic) which are widely used to treat non-affective symptoms of chronic musculoskeletal pain although currently this is an unlicensed indication (➔ see 'Chronic non-inflammatory pain', p. 186). Refer to the *BNF* for full details and SPC for each drug.

The most effective older tricyclic antidepressants (TCAs) often no longer used to treat depression are used to support pain relief and are thought to work by ↑ levels of chemicals such as noradrenaline.

TCAs

TCAs appear to have a synergistic benefit (when prescribed with a central acting analgesic) for the patient with chronic pain or neuropathic pain unrelieved by traditional pain-relieving approaches. TCAs fall into two broad categories—those that have a sedative effect and those with less sedative effects:

- Sedative effects—amitriptyline, clomipramine, and dosulepin.
- Less sedative effects—imipramine, nortriptyline, and lofepramine.

Evidence suggests they are most effective in conditions such as fibromyalgia to improve sleep quality, pain, and well-being. TCAs used for neuropathic or chronic pain include:

- Amitriptyline (helpful in sleep deprivation): usual dose range 10–50 mg, 2 hours prior to going to bed. Evidence of benefit suggests doses of <50 mg daily.

The TCA dose should be started low and gradually ↑ to achieve effect and limit side effects. Pain relief benefits may take a few months while sleep deprivation may improve within 2 weeks.

Common side effects: dry mouth, blurred vision, low blood pressure, dizziness, and drowsiness.

Cautions

- Arrhythmias and heart block can occur (sudden death has been reported).
- Convulsions—caution in epilepsy.
- Ocular (closed-angle glaucoma) and genitourinary (retention, prostatic hypertrophy).

SSRIs

SSRIs block the uptake of serotonin involved in endogenous pain control but are generally used less for non-affective symptoms. It is important that there is a clear rationale for prescribing a TCA or SSRI, e.g. is it to treat mild depression or for non-affective symptoms? The prescription of antidepressants appears to be ↑ in conditions where there is evidence of an ↑ prevalence of depression:

- Fibromyalgia.
- RA.
- Spondyloarthropathies.
- Low back pain.
- OA.

When using SSRIs, the onset of analgesic effect is usually faster than that expected when used for antidepressant effects and the dose required is usually lower than when treating depression.

SSRIs tend to have fewer side effects than TCAs but appear to be less effective, requiring high dosages. SSRIs used for pain relief include:

- Citalopram 20 mg daily.
- Fluoxetine 20 mg daily.
- Serotonin and noradrenaline re-uptake inhibitors (SNRIs), e.g. venlafaxine and duloxetine, are used for chronic musculoskeletal pain. SNRIs ↑ the amount of specific nerve transmitters in the nervous system reducing pain messages arriving in the brain. They can take several months before they have their full effect.

Common side effects include:

- Nausea, anxiety, and headache.
- Sexual dysfunction.
- Constipation.
- Dry mouth.
- Urinary hesitancy.

Caution

- Elderly patients—regular review and careful monitoring required.
- Glaucoma.
- Cardiac disease.
- Diabetes mellitus.

Antiepileptics—for neuropathic pain

- Gabapentin 300 mg day 1; 300 mg twice daily day 2; 300 mg three times a day day 3; ↑ by 300 mg per day to a maximum dose of 3.6 g daily. Trial for a period of 3–8 weeks.
- Pregabalin 150 mg daily in 2–3 divided doses, ↑ (after 3–7 days) to a maximum of 600 mg if necessary.

Common side effects: dry mouth, dizziness, cognitive impairment, diarrhoea, and nausea.

Caution: avoid during pregnancy and breastfeeding. Avoid abrupt withdrawal.

Pain relief: non-steroidal anti-inflammatory drugs

Introduction

The broad term NSAID will be used to describe both NSAIDs and COX-2 inhibitors unless otherwise stated. NSAIDs can be beneficial for MSCs where there is pain and inflammation (e.g. RA, OA, AS, acute articular and periarticular disorders, cervical spondylitis, acute back pain, and acute gout) or following orthopaedic surgery. NSAIDs should only be prescribed at the lowest effective dose for the shortest duration and considered in the context of an overall pain-relieving approach for conditions that have an inflammatory component. In some circumstances, NSAIDs may form part of a comprehensive pain-relieving approach that includes other forms of analgesia and non-pharmacological approaches.

The mechanism of action is that of inhibiting the release of COX (type 1 and type 2) suppressing the activation of prostaglandins along the pain pathway in the peripheral nervous system. NSAIDs can be broadly classified into two main categories:

- Traditional NSAIDS—may vary in their therapeutic spectrum of inhibiting COX (type 1 and type 2).
- COX-2 inhibitors—preferentially block COX-2, the principal enzyme identified in the production of inflammatory mediators. COX-1 is an essential enzyme for constitutional functions, e.g. gastroprotection, and remains relatively uninhibited by COX-2 therapies.

Traditional or non-selective NSAIDs

- Ibuprofen, 1.2–1.8 g/day in 3–4 divided doses, with a maximum dose of 2.4 g/day.
- Naproxen 500 mg initially for acute pain and 750 mg for acute gout followed by 250 mg every 8 hours until attack passes. For inflammatory arthritides, naproxen 250–500 mg twice a day can be prescribed. Maximum dose for first day 1.25 g.
- Diclofenac at a maximum of 150 mg/day in 2–3 divided doses (as diclofenac has an ↑ risk of cardiovascular events it is not routinely used in the treatment inflammatory arthritis).

COX-2 selective NSAIDs

- Celecoxib—200 mg/day in 1–2 divided doses may be given for OA and elderly patients; 200–400 mg/day in 2 divided doses may be given for RA and AS.
- Etoricoxib—120 mg once daily may be given for acute gout; 60 mg/day maximum may be given for OA; and 90 mg/day maximum for RA.

Side effects

- GI bleed (traditional NSAIDs have a high risk) or dyspepsia.
- Cardiovascular events (stroke or myocardial infarction).
- Side effects related to renal impairment (poor excretion/metabolism).
- Liver impairment (hepatitis and jaundice).
- Exacerbation of asthma.

Other documented side effects include:
Nausea, vomiting, abdominal pain, flatulence, diarrhoea, peptic ulcers, perforation, fluid retention, hypertension, aggravating asthma (bronchospasm), and rashes including photosensitivity. Nephrotoxicity—including interstitial nephritis, nephrotic syndrome, and renal failure.

Cautions with all NSAIDs

Proceed cautiously using NSAIDs in elderly patients and when patients have cardiovascular, renal, and hepatic problems; patients with a history of heart failure, hypertension, asthma; and patients with history of GI problems such as ulcerative colitis and Crohn's disease. Currently evidence suggests that all NSAIDs (non-selective or selective COX-2 inhibitors) can ↑ blood pressure by 3–5 mmHg, ↑ risk of stroke, angina, and heart failure. Avoid NSAIDs in patients who have ischaemic heart and/or cerebrovascular disease.

Contraindications with NSAIDs

NSAIDS are not suitable for patients with a known sensitivity, active peptic ulcer disease, GI bleeding or perforation due to NSAIDs, patients with severe liver, renal, cardiac failure, and patients with ischaemic heart, cardiovascular, or peripheral vascular disease. Patients in last trimester of pregnancy.

For latest guidance refer to:

- The *BNF* and the latest Committee on Safety of Medicines advice.
- NICE.
- The European Medicines Agency on prescribing NSAIDs.
- Product SPC for each drug.

Topical NSAIDs

Topical NSAIDs demonstrate benefits in relieving pain particularly in treating discreet areas or for small to moderate-sized joints (e.g. OA of the base of thumb or knee pain) or for acute musculoskeletal injuries, such as epicondylitis, tendonitis, and tenosynovitis. Creams or gels should have the prescribed amount applied to the affected area—two to four times daily. As long as the patient takes the prescribed dose and dosing regimens, only small amounts of the drug are systemically absorbed.

Possible side effects
Mild to moderate local irritation, erythema, pruritus and dermatitis, and photosensitive skin reaction. Rarely, minor GI side effects such as nausea, dyspepsia, abdominal pain, and dyspnoea.

Further reading

NICE (2015, updated 2018). Non-steroidal anti-inflammatory drugs (KTT13). ℘ https://www.nice.org.uk/advice/ktt13

NICE (2018). Clinical knowledge summaries: NSAIDs—prescribing issues. ℘ https://cks.nice.org.uk/nsaids-prescribing-issues

Gastric cytoprotection

Introduction

GI disorders are a common complaint for many individuals—heartburn, epigastric pain, gastro-oesophageal reflux disease, and GI bleeds. GI symptoms can present as a result of:

- Drug interactions, e.g.:
  - Aspirin and corticosteroids.
  - Nausea and GI symptoms from DMARD therapies.
- Individual patient risk factors including:
  - Previous GI disorders including dyspepsia, or peptic ulceration.
  - Lifestyle factors including high alcohol intake, smoking history, obesity, and poor dietary habits.
- Predisposing factors such as *Helicobacter pylori* status.

Treatment of GI disorders

Treatment of GI disorders must be considered in the context of the underlying pathology but the treatment options include:

- Antacids, compound alginates, or indigestion preparations.
- Antispasmodics and drugs affecting gut motility (used for non-ulcer dyspepsia).
- Ulcer healing drugs (H2-receptor antagonists and PPIs).
- Treatment of *H. pylori* infections.

GI bleeding

A GI bleed is defined as bleeding in the oesophagus, stomach, or duodenum characterized by fresh bleeding or 'coffee-ground' bleeding.

NSAIDs inhibit prostaglandins and ↓ mucous production. Protecting patients from risks related to GI bleeding or ulceration must be considered in the context of prescribing for MSCs. PPIs are routinely prescribed to prevent the risk of GI bleeds related to treatment with NSAIDs. GI bleeds can be related to:

- Varicose bleeding or tear of the stomach due to excess vomiting—Mallory–Weiss tear.
- Drug-induced.
- Polyps and inflammatory diseases.
- Cancer.
- NSAIDs.

Prevention of NSAID-induced GI bleeding

Traditional NSAIDs should be prescribed at the lowest effective dose for the shortest possible duration. Patients who require pain relief should be assessed to find the most appropriate treatment. Cardiovascular and GI risks should also be assessed to ensure eligibility for either a traditional NSAID or a COX-2 inhibitor:

- PPIs are the most effective treatment to be co-prescribed with a traditional NSAID.
- Patients who have no cardiovascular risk factors but identified risks related to GI bleeds should be considered for a COX-2 inhibitor.

PPIs

PPIs act by inhibiting gastric acid secretion by blocking the enzyme secreting system (proton pump) of the gastric parietal cells. The ↓ gastric acidity means that the gut is less effective at preventing bacterial infections such as *Campylobacter* or *Clostridium difficile*.

PPIs are prescribed for:

- Short-term benefit for treatment of gastric and duodenal ulcers and are used as part of the eradication therapy for *H. pylori* in combination with antibacterial therapy.
- Prevention and treatment of ulcers associated with NSAIDs.
- Control of excessive gastric acid secretions.

Cautions

- Liver disease.
- Breastfeeding.
- May mask symptoms of gastric cancer.

Side effects

- Nausea, vomiting, and abdominal pain including flatulence and diarrhoea.
- Headaches and dizziness.

H2-receptor antagonists

The histamine H2-receptor is blocked and as a result gastric acid secretion is reduced. Examples of H2-receptor antagonists include ranitidine and famotidine.

H2-receptor antagonists are prescribed to:

- Heal gastric and duodenal ulcers.
- Relieve symptoms of gastro-oesophageal reflux disease.
- Treat NSAID-associated ulcers.

Cautions

- Renal impairment.
- Pregnancy and breastfeeding.
- May mask symptoms of gastric cancer.

Side effects

- Diarrhoea and abdominal discomfort.
- Headaches and dizziness.
- Changes in LFTs (rarely liver damage).

Further reading

NICE (2014). Gastro-oesophageal reflux disease and dyspepsia in adults: investigations and management (CG184). https://www.nice.org.uk/guidance/cg184

NICE (2014, updated 2017). Osteoarthritis: care and management (G177). https://www.nice.org.uk/guidance/cg177

NICE (2018). Rheumatoid arthritis in adults: management (NG100). https://www.nice.org.uk/guidance/ng100

Topical therapies

Topical therapies are sometimes used as an adjunct to other pain-relieving strategies for acute or chronic pain although the evidence supporting their use currently remains limited. They may also be used for those who are intolerant to oral analgesics. The rationale for topical therapies is that by applying topically, the systemic effects will be reduced. Rubefacient is a term that may be applied to such topical agents, however terminology does differ and clarification may be needed to ensure whether NSAIDs are considered part of this category or not.

A systematic review to explore quality, validity, and effect size of topical non-steroidal anti-inflammatory therapies has shown a modest short-term benefit (2 weeks) in pain relief for conditions such as acute sprains and OA. Topical therapies used as analgesics for MSC include:

- Rubefacients containing salicylates or capsaicin.
- NSAIDs, e.g. diclofenac, ibuprofen, and piroxicam.
- Local anaesthetics (e.g. lidocaine)—chiefly used for post-herpetic neuralgia or where allodynia is prominent.

Rubefacients

Rubefacients include a wide range of different chemicals. The broad term of rubefacients frequently includes salicylates (that are pharmacologically similar to non-steroidal anti-inflammatory agents) and compounds such as capsaicin which is said to work by acting as a counter-irritant, reducing musculoskeletal pain by acting as distraction to the pain by producing an irritation to the skin. Counter-irritation is said to result in a pleasant sensation that relieves discomfort experienced in muscles and tendons, altering/offsetting the sensations of pain in the sensory nerve endings. Further research is needed to demonstrate their efficacy in acute injuries or chronic conditions.

Salicylates

Topical salicylates have shown mixed results in acute and chronic pain. Limited evidence suggests that efficacy is demonstrated in acute pain at 7 days although poor to moderate efficacy is seen in chronic pain at 14 days.

Capsaicin

Capsaicin is extracted from chili peppers and is a naturally occurring alkaloid. It appears to affect the sensory nerve endings. Available in strengths of 0.075% (post-herpetic neuralgia) or 0.025% (for OA) and are usually applied three to four times a day.

NSAIDs

The use of topical NSAIDs remains controversial particularly in the UK where the Prescription Pricing Authority data suggest they make up 10% of the total cost of analgesics and NSAID prescribing. NSAIDs need to be able to penetrate the skin and be actively absorbed in high concentrations so that they can actively inhibit COX enzymes before producing pain relief. Evidence suggests that topical therapies have a much lower systemic dose accounting for the reduction in side effects but also potentially the sustained therapeutic benefit (plasma concentration at 1–2 hours declines rapidly).

Issues to consider in the use of topical therapies

- Acute conditions (e.g. joint strains, sprains) are likely to gain the most benefit from topical NSAIDs.
- Chronic MSCs may benefit from topical therapies in the short term (number needed to treat = 5 although evidence is weak).
- Differing terminology used to describe different topical therapies.
- Variations in concentrations of the topical agent being prescribed.
- Topical therapies may be more a more expensive option than oral analgesia.
- A number of preparations can be purchased by the patient over the counter; some contain NSAIDs and/or counter-irritants.
- Although evidence is limited and further research is needed, topical therapies as an adjunct to other treatment modalities may enhance the patient's perception of empowerment/self-efficacy in managing the condition.
- Therapeutic effect of topical NSAIDS relies upon skin integrity and vasculature.

Advice to give the patient

- General information on the use of pain-relieving strategies and how to step-up or step-down management based upon pain assessment.
- Provide detailed information on the risks and benefits of treatment centred upon individual treatment choices, based upon a patient-centred assessment.
- Topical therapies must not be applied to broken or infected skin.
- They may experience a transient burning sensation.
- Ensure they wash their hands immediately after applying the treatment.
- Patients with a known allergy to aspirin or NSAIDs should avoid topical therapies (e.g. asthmatics).
- Adverse events include:
    - Number needed to harm = 2.5.
    - >50% of patients experience local adverse event (burning sensation).
    - Photosensitivity is rare (1–2 cases per 10,000 patients) with topical NSAIDs.

➲ Also see 'Symptom control', Chapter 9, pp. 315–320.

Further reading

Derry S, Matthews PRL, Wiffen PJ, Moore RA (2014). Salicylate-containing rubefacients for acute and chronic musculoskeletal pain in adults. *Cochrane Database Syst Rev* 11:CD007403.

Derry S, Moore R, Gaskell H, et al. (2015). Topical NSAIDs for acute musculoskeletal pain in adults. *Cochrane Database Syst Rev* 6:CD007402.

Frequently asked questions

Is analgesia addictive?

In some cases, the use of opiates has led to their abuse and dependence but only when used on a regular basis in an inappropriate way. Used appropriately in the context of severe pain this is not a concern.

What is meant by medication overuse headache?

Headaches can occur when analgesic levels trough, e.g. the patient wakes with a morning headache. It is thought that sustained analgesia use can cause pain signalling mechanisms to become more sensitive.

Who are the most at-risk group of patients for GI complications?

The highest risk group are those who are >65 years, also using medications likely to ↑ GI side effects, e.g. anticoagulants, corticosteroids; or with serious co-morbidity; or those with a prior history of peptic ulcer ± complication, who may require prolonged use of or the maximum recommended doses of NSAIDs.

What is the best advice to give those most at risk?

Use the lowest effective dose for the shortest duration. Review the pain-relieving benefits and other supporting strategies regularly. Encourage the patient to report any gastric symptoms and to take their medication with food. A traditional NSAID prescribed with gastroprotection (usually a PPI) may be considered if they have no contraindications (e.g. prior GI risks). If prior previous peptic ulceration (and there are no cardiovascular contraindications), a COX-2 inhibitor can be prescribed together with a PPI. Encourage a pharmacological and non-pharmacological approach to pain management and encourage the patient to use self-management strategies such as the use of cold packs, rest and relaxation, and joint protection.

Which NSAID would be the most effective?

NSAIDs have a highly variable effect between patients so it is vital to find one that suits the individual, allow up to 4 weeks of taking the NSAID on a regular basis for the full anti-inflammatory effect. It is important to allow an adequate trial and evaluate the benefits to the patient by reviewing the level of pain relief achieved. Scoring pain may be helpful, such as a simple VAS or rating pain from 1 to 10. It may be necessary to have a short trial of a few NSAIDs before finding the one that provides the maximum benefit to the patient.

Chapter 16

Pharmacological management: Disease-modifying drugs

Pharmacological management: pretreatment assessment

Nurses play an important role in preparing patients before starting a new treatment. A thorough screening process should encourage concordance and reduce risks related to poor knowledge of drug therapies or anxieties about what to do if side effects are experienced.

The level of screening may vary according to the therapy being prescribed (e.g. being prescribed a short course of paracetamol for knee pain in an otherwise healthy patient will differ from a patient who has diabetes and primary systemic vasculitides who is being prescribed cyclophosphamide). All screening should consider:

- A patient-centred approach.
- A thorough medical assessment and baseline clinical examination.

A patient-centred approach

Patients may be anxious about the treatment prescribed or adjusting psychologically to a diagnosis or change in disease state. The patient should be actively encouraged to participate and ask questions and discuss any of their personal anxieties/goals. Screening often incorporates education about the disease and the drug therapies prescribed (➲ see 'Blood tests and investigation', Chapter 17, pp. 505–534; ➲ 'Patient consent and shared decision making', Chapter 10, pp. 332–335).

An assessment of medical history and baseline clinical history

The nurse should ensure they undertake a review of the medical record and specific risk factors related to the proposed drug therapy and combine this with a consultation that reviews:

- General health status, previous medical and surgical history, and co-morbidities. Assess rate, strength, and rhythm of pulse, and blood pressure.
- Baseline height and weight.
- Age, smoking status, and alcohol consumption.
- Family history—including any linked to genetic predispositions.
- Previous drug history, previous allergic reactions, and side effects.
- Current prescribed medication and over-the-counter treatments (including complementary therapies). Consider polypharmacy risks.
- Lifestyle or social issues that may affect risks to treatment, monitoring, or concordance:
  - Discuss fertility and contraceptive use.
- National guidelines now advocate viral hepatic screening prior to use for all DMARDs.

General baseline assessments

There may also be assessments that are essential prior to commencing treatment to assess eligibility criteria for treatment (e.g. risk of osteoporosis). Initial pretreatment assessments and time-specific reviews of disease control may be essential for adherence to NICE guidance.

- NICE set out individual information based upon the drug therapy and the disease being treated. See specific conditions to identify assessments required. For example:
  - CG146: 'Osteoporosis: assessing the risk of fragility fractures'.
  - NG100: 'Rheumatoid arthritis in adults: management'.
  - NG65: 'Spondyloarthritis in over 16's: diagnosis and management'.
- Update of EULAR recommendations for the treatment of systemic sclerosis:
  - European League Against Rheumatism (EULAR) recommendations for the management of psoriatic arthritis with pharmacological therapies: 2015 update.

Further reading

BNF for drug information: http://www.bnf.nice.org.uk

NICE (2014). Cardiovascular disease: risk assessment and reduction including lipid modification (CG181). https://www.nice.org.uk/guidance/cg181

NICE guidelines: http://www.nice.org.uk

Baseline assessments: body systems

The body systems should be reviewed as part of the nursing pre-assessment process. These include:

- **Immune status**—consider general information but also:
  - Corticosteroids, and all prior or current DMARD therapies—review immunization status of TB history, hepatitis and HIV risks, and chickenpox.
  - Immunizations may be required prior to starting treatment, e.g. administration of live vaccines.
- **Screen for infections** or risk related to re-emergence of latent infections, e.g. TB or serious underlying infections (e.g. prior septic arthroplasty where joint remains *in situ*).
- Cardiovascular:
  - Cardiac risk factor, e.g. high-density lipoprotein/↑ blood pressure. Hypertension and lipid levels may need specific review before commencing a therapy (e.g. ciclosporin).
  - Underlying cardiovascular disease. Some therapies (e.g. bDMARDs) refer to the NYHA classification criteria to exclude those at risk of developing side effects.
  - In some cases, a pretreatment electrocardiograph may be required.
- Gastrointestinal:
  - Prior history of gastrointestinal bleed, dyspepsia, or predisposing factors that ↑ risks (e.g. aspirin/steroid).
  - Gastric symptoms prior to starting a bisphosphonate for osteoporosis.
  - Risk factors may determine choice of NSAID and addition of PPI.
- Haematological:
  - FBC, U&Es including creatinine, LFTs, CRP, ESR, and PV—prior results and baseline assessments. Inflammatory markers (e.g. ESR or CRP) for baseline composite scores (e.g. DAS 28).
  - Pre-screening results must be scrutinized to ensure safety of commencing treatment—refer to protocols/guidelines or seek advice for abnormal results.
- Hepatic:
  - LFTs will be considered with all blood tests and should be considered in the context of predisposing risk factors, underlying disease, or lifestyle factors (e.g. alcohol consumption). Dermatologists sometimes request a pre-screening test to assess hepatic status—procollagen III (PIIINP); however, this test is affected by active bone remodelling or joint inflammation and ∴ is less useful in rheumatology.
- Neurological:
  - Identification of any neurological conditions or family history (e.g. demyelinating disease) should be documented. Biologic therapies may precipitate exacerbation of demyelinating disease.
- Renal:
  - Good renal function is essential for excretion of many therapies. Poor function may ↑ risk of toxicities. Drugs may exclude treatment if there is renal impairment.
  - Urinalysis (e.g. screen for infections or urinary proteins).

- Respiratory:
  - Interstitial lung disease, prior pulmonary TB, or poor respiratory function should be reviewed with the prescribing physician.
  - Chest X-ray or PFTs may be necessary prior to starting MTX or biologic therapy.
- Skin: examine for signs of bacterial or fungal infections, or the presence of rashes, lesions, or vasculitis changes.

➲ See Chapter 8 for more details on assessing the patient. p. 289.

Further reading

Holroyd CR, Seth R, Bukhari M, et al. (2019). The British Society for Rheumatology biologic DMARD safety guidelines in inflammatory arthritis. *Rheumatology (Oxford)* 58:220–6.

Ledingham J, Gullick N, Irving K, et al. (2017). BSR and BHPR guideline for the prescription and monitoring of non-biologic disease-modifying anti-rheumatic drugs. *Rheumatology* 56:865–8.

Screening before treatment: documentation and decisions

The screening process combined with good documented evidence of pre-treatment health status and exclusion of risk factors is an essential component to nursing support in drug therapies.

In addition to the actual screening process, documentation should include:

- Evidence that the patient has been provided with written and verbal information about the treatment and has had an opportunity to explore all questions/anxieties about the treatment.
- Information including outcomes from a patient-centred consultation, documented in the notes (➲ see 'Nursing issues and the patient-centred approach', Chapter 10, pp. 332–334).
- The patient has reviewed the information, understands their responsibilities in undertaking regular blood monitoring and concordance with treatment, and that they consent to treatment.
- The patient has been provided with a patient-held monitoring booklet/record or passport that informs them of:
  - The treatment they are prescribed, dose, timing. and duration of treatment.
  - Their recent test results.
  - When they will be seen again.
  - Side effects of treatment and what to do should they develop, e.g. treatment and telephone advice line at the hospital.
  - Individual issues or risk factors identified in the assessment or as a result of the consultation.
  - What they should expect in the next few weeks of treatment and what to do if something untoward happens.

Decisions to be made when screening patients

Nurses should have the knowledge and skills to be able to screen patients, interpret the results, and recognize when to seek guidance from the prescribing clinician following the screening process. The screening process may reveal:

- Previously missed cautions or contraindications to the proposed treatment:
  - Co-prescribing factors that may enhance or reduce the proposed drug dosage or route of administration.
  - Co-morbidities that may be affected by the proposed treatment, e.g. exacerbation of demyelinating disease.
- Pre-screening tests may reveal factors that require further investigation, e.g. previous history of untreated TB or impaired renal function.
- The patient may decline treatment and alternative treatment may need to be offered.
- General health status may have declined or changed since referral and require intervention or review, e.g. recent infection.

Tools to support screening clinics

- Specific nurse-led drug screening/monitoring protocols and guidelines.
- Regional or national screening guidelines.
- Treatment protocols for specific drug therapies.
- Regional or national treatment monitoring guidelines.
- NICE guidelines to screen for adherence to guidance.
- Drug SPC: http://www.medicines.org.uk.
- The *BNF*: http://www.bnf.org.

Additional resources

- NICE clinical knowledge summaries: https://cks.nice.org.uk/clinicalspeciality#?speciality=Musculoskeletal.
- Medical Health Products Regulatory Agency: http://www.mhra.gov.uk.
- National Patient Safety Agency: https://improvement.nhs.uk/resources/learning-from-patient-safety-incidents/.

Further reading

Clunie GPR, Wilkinson N, Nikiphorou E, Jadon D (eds) (2018). *Oxford Handbook of Rheumatology*, 4th edn. Oxford: Oxford University Press.

Ledingham J, Gullick N, Irving K, et al. (2017). BSR and BHPR guideline for the prescription and monitoring of non-biologic disease-modifying anti-rheumatic drugs. *Rheumatology* 56:865–8.

Disease-modifying antirheumatic drugs

A number of MSCs have an underlying inflammatory component and many of these are as a result of an autoimmune process. There has been significant progress in the last 25years in understanding the key cell-to-cell interactions in the autoimmune pathway. This has meant that many new therapies have been developed, targeting the body's specific cell-to-cell interactions responsible for driving inflammatory autoimmune conditions, and their mechanism of action is better understood, unlike the older traditional DMARDs. Ultimately, the aim is to suppress the disease and stop the resulting damage that occurs (e.g. tissue or organ damage, synovial proliferation, joint erosions, and long-term disability).

Treatment options for inflammatory autoimmune-driven conditions include a range of therapies, but the main focus should be on achieving rapid and proactive management to ensure disease control/suppression.

- Symptom relief—analgesia and NSAIDs.
- Symptom relief and modification of inflammatory component—corticosteroid therapies.
- Disease modification—cDMARDs, e.g.:
  - Azathioprine (AZA)
  - Ciclosporin.
  - d- penicillamine and sodium aurothiomalate (Myocrisin—intramuscular gold).
  - Hydroxychloroquine.
  - Leflunomide.
  - Methotrexate (MTX).
  - Mycophenolate.
  - Sulfasalazine (SAS).
  - Tacrolimus.
- Disease modification—bDMARDs, e.g.:
  - Adalimumab—Humira® and biosimilars including Halimatoz®, Hefiya®, Hyrimoz®, Amgevita®, Solymbi®, Cyltezo®, and Imraldi®.
  - Etanercept—Enbrel®, Benapali®, and Erelzi®.
  - Infliximab—Remicade®, Remsina®, and Inflectra®.
  - Rituximab—MabThera® and Truxima®.
  - Abatacept—Orencia®.
  - Certolizumab pegol®.
  - Tocilizumab—RoActemra®.
  - Sarliumab -Kevzara®.
  - Ustekinumab—Stelara®.
  - Secukinumab—Cosentyx®.
  - Ixekizumab—Talz®

➲ Also see 'Biological disease-modifying drug therapies', pp. 485–495.

Licensed and unlicensed use of DMARDs

DMARDs are used in the treatment of a number of conditions not all of which are prescribed under their licensed indications. These include:

- AS.
- CTDs:
  - Behçet's disease.
  - Vasculitides.
- Felty syndrome.
- Inflammatory myopathies such as dermatomyositis and polymyositis.
- Pemphigus vulgaris.
- PMR.
- Polyarteritis.
- PsA.
- RA.
- Scleroderma.
- Systemic and discoid lupus erythematosus.

DMARDs are immunological modifiers and require regular monitoring for adverse events and efficacy. They usually take a number of weeks before benefits are achieved and can cause unpleasant side effects, particularly in the early phases of treatment. They vary in efficacy for the range of treatments outlined and toxicity profiles.

➔ See 'Key points and top tips in reviewing blood results', Chapter 17, pp. 515–516.

For detailed licensed indications of each medication and clinical case scenarios exploring management issues of individual DMARDs, see https://cks.nice.org.uk/dmards.

Further reading

Ledingham J, Gullick N, Irving K, et al. (2017). BSR and BHPR guideline for the prescription and monitoring of non-biologic disease-modifying anti-rheumatic drugs. *Rheumatology* 56:865–8.

Conventional disease-modifying antirheumatic drugs

Introduction

cDMARDs have been used in the treatment of inflammatory forms of joint disease for >60 years. These DMARD therapies traditionally evolved in an ad hoc way with a limited understanding of the mechanisms of action; however, in the last decade there has been a more targeted approach with drugs designed to interact and alter the autoimmune response at cellular level (e.g. the pathway of TNFα). The bDMARDs followed more recently by tsDMARDs have transformed the management of patients with inflammatory arthritides.

However, both cDMARDs and bDMARDs inhibit the immunological response to an inflammatory process. cDMARDs and bDMARDs require care before prescribing.

cDMARD monitoring guidelines published by the British Society for Rheumatology and the British Health Professionals in Rheumatology provide a strong guidance for health professionals in the UK. These guidelines are supported by local authority guidelines to ensure effective and safe screening and monitoring of patients receiving cDMARDs.

The process of preparing and managing a patient should include:

- An assessment of the disease activity using recognized diagnostic and treatment criteria.
- Screening of the patient for underlying infections prior to treatment.
- A general health screen to ensure normal function:
  - Haematology and biochemistry (liver and renal).
  - Renal function—normal renal function (or may require dose reductions). See Table 16.1.
  - Respiratory—in some cases detailed respiratory function tests.
  - Cardiac status.
  - Other co-morbidities—e.g. demyelinating disease and diabetes.
- Some DMARDs may require additional screening tests:
  - AZA—thiopurine methyl transferase status.
  - Ciclosporin—lipid profiles.
  - bDMARDs and tsDMARDs—screening for TB status as well as the others listed.
- Some DMARD dosages are calculated based upon weight. Best practice recommends height, weight, and blood pressure measurements prior to starting DMARDs.

Combination therapy with traditional DMARDs

It is common practice for combination therapy to be used to achieve proactive and targeted management of the condition. There is strong evidence particularly in the inflammatory arthritides (e.g. RA) to support aggressive treatment regimens. Combination therapies use two or three DMARD therapies together—e.g. MTX, SAS, and hydroxychloroquine. The combination therapies appear to have no additional risks in relation to toxicity when prescribed together. When patients are on triple therapy regimens, base the blood monitoring requirements on the DMARD requiring the most frequent monitoring.

Table 16.1 Summary of monitoring requirements

Drug	Laboratory monitoring	Other monitoring
Apremilast	No routine laboratory monitoring	None
AZA	Standard monitoring schedule[a]	None
Ciclosporin	Extend monthly monitoring longer term[b]	BP and glucose at each monitoring visit
Gold	Standard monitoring schedule[a]	Urinalysis for blood and protein prior to each dose
HCQ	No routine laboratory monitoring	Annual eye assessment (ideally including optical coherence tomography) if continued for >5 years
LEF	Standard monitoring schedule[a]	BP and weight at each monitoring visit
Mepacrine	No routine laboratory monitoring	None
MTX	Standard monitoring schedule[a]	None
MTX and LEF combined	Extend monthly monitoring longer term[b]	None
Minocycline	No routine laboratory monitoring	None
Mycophenolate	Standard monitoring schedule[a]	None
SSZ	Standard monitoring schedule for 12 months then no routine monitoring needed	None
Tacrolimus	Extend monthly monitoring longer term[b]	BP and glucose at each monitoring visit

BP, blood pressure; HCQ, hydroxychloroquine; LEF, leflunomide; MTX, methotrexate; SSZ, sulfasalazine.

[a] Standard monitoring as per recommendations I and II for DMARD blood monitoring schedule when starting or adding a new DMARD.

[b] Patients who have been stable for 12 months can be considered for reduced frequency monitoring on an individual patient basis.

Reprinted from Ledingham J, Gullick N, *et al.* (2017) "BSR and BHPR guideline for the prescription and monitoring of non-biologic disease-modifying anti-rheumatic drugs" *Rheumatology* 56(6):865–868, with permission from Oxford University Press.

Further reading

➲ Detailed information on specific DMARDs can be found elsewhere in this chapter under specific drug therapies.

➲ Also see Chapter 10, p. 329; ➲ 'The nurse specialist role, Chapter 21, pp. 613–615.

For detailed licensed indications of each medication and clinical case scenarios exploring management issues of individual DMARDs, see ☞ https://cks.nice.org.uk/dmards

Ledingham J, Gullick N, Irving K, et al. (2017). BSR and BHPR guideline for the prescription and monitoring of non-biologic disease-modifying anti-rheumatic drugs. *Rheumatology* 56:865–8.

Azathioprine and ciclosporin

AZA and ciclosporin were originally developed to prevent rejection of organ transplants but are now also used as traditional DMARDs to control the underlying immunological inflammatory response. They suppress the inflammatory processes and as a result, inhibit progression of damaging joint and tissue destruction.

AZA and ciclosporin general management

- Pre-screening required for both therapies: haematological, pregnancy, and immunological status (➔ see 'Screening prior to DMARD treatment', p. 450).
- Before commencing AZA, baseline thiopurine methyltransferase status must be checked. ➔ See 'Key factors in nursing management of patients taking AZA', p. 457.
- Regular blood monitoring required (plus blood pressure for ciclosporin):
  - FBC including WCC.
  - LFTs.
  - U&Es (including K^+), creatinine for ciclosporin.
  - Blood glucose monitoring for ciclosporin.
- Vigilance for evidence of skin rashes, bruising or mucocutaneous ulcers.

⚠ Note: a trend in blood results is as important as absolute values.

Note: weight needs to be monitored regularly as the AZA dose is calculated on body weight.

➔ Also see Chapter 17, p. 505.

Patients treated with AZA and ciclosporin should be advised:

- It will take up to 3 months before they feel the benefit of treatment although they may feel a benefit earlier.
- They may experience side effects during this time and these should abate. Side effects include:
  - Nausea, loss of appetite (occur in ~23% of patients on AZA).
  - Itching, rashes, or mouth ulcers.
  - Muscle aches.
- Monitoring for any side effects include tests to check bloods, liver function, and renal function.
- To not alter the dose they are prescribed.
- Report promptly any infections they experience (occur in ~9% of patients on AZA) **or** any signs of myelosuppression (e.g. bruising or bleeding).
- They must not get pregnant while on treatment (use an effective method of contraception).
- Blood monitoring regimens are important and will help identify problems.
- They should not have any live vaccines while on treatment.
- Herbal or complementary therapies—advise the doctor or nurse of any being taken as there may be interactions.
- If side effects become a problem or if they are uncertain about their treatment, seek advice as there is always something that can be done to help with side effects.

Key factors in nursing management of patients taking AZA

AZA is an immune-modulating drug that inhibits DNA synthesis, inhibiting cell replication. It is a pro-drug metabolized by the liver, 30% is protein bound, and 45% is excreted in urine with the remainder metabolized by 6-methylmercaptopurine (6MMP).

An inability to metabolize AZA due to an enzyme deficiency means some patients are vulnerable to serious adverse events. The deficiency of thiopurine methyltransferase is classified as:

- Homozygous state—AZA should be avoided and can be fatal (within 6 weeks).
- Heterozygous state—may be subject to delayed bone marrow toxicity (symptoms may not be evident until 6 months after starting treatment).
- ❶ Screening of thiopurine methyltransferase does not exclude the risk of myelosuppression, ∴ monitoring is essential.

Dose of oral azathioprine

A typical dose is usually 1 mg/kg/day, ↑ after 4–6 weeks to 2–3 mg/kg/day.

⚠ Drug interactions may ↑ the risk of toxicity, e.g. if there is co-prescription of allopurinol, the dose of AZA should be **cut to 25% of original dose.**

Key factors in nursing management of patients taking ciclosporin

Ciclosporin has an immunosuppressive action on proinflammatory cytokines by inhibiting responses by T cells. Observe for potential side effects which can include:

- Impairment of renal function.
- ↑ in lipids (reversible).
- Observe serum: ↑ creatinine may necessitate dose reductions.
- Limited evidence in the elderly.
- ⚠ Significant drug interactions, e.g. pharmacodynamics with co-prescriptions:
  - NSAIDs may adversely affect renal function.
  - Hepatotoxicity potential with NSAIDs.
  - Nifedipine use with caution.
  - Avoid colchicine and potassium-sparing diuretics.
- ⚠ Patient self-administered:
  - Interactions with St John's wort (↓ ciclosporin effectiveness).
  - Grapefruit (flesh and juice) must be avoided for 1 hour prior to taking ciclosporin as it ↓ bioavailability.
- ► Note blood trends or unexplained bruising (with or without sore throat)—withhold treatment and seek medical advice.

Dose of oral ciclosporin

Treatment is normally started as two divided doses of 2.5 mg/kg/day and gradually ↑ after 2–4-week interval by 25 mg each, ↑ until clinically effective (maximum dose of 4 mg/kg/day). Maintenance dose usually effective at 2.5–3.2 mg/kg/day (titrate according to tolerance and efficacy).

Further reading

AZA and ciclosporin: refer to the SPC for licensed indications and the BNF for prescribing information.

Ledingham J, Gullick N, Irving K, et al. (2017). BSR and BHPR guideline for the prescription and monitoring of non-biologic disease-modifying anti-rheumatic drugs. *Rheumatology* 56:865–8.

NICE (2018). Case scenarios of each DMARD: https://cks.nice.org.uk/dmards

Patient information leaflets on all drug therapies are available from Versus Arthritis: https://www.versusarthritis.org

D-penicillamine and sodium aurothiomalate (Myocrisin®—intramuscular gold)

General management

D-penicillamine and sodium aurothiomalate (Myocrisin®) are the older generation of DMARD therapies and are rarely prescribed in the UK today. This is partly due to the effectiveness of other cDMARDs (e.g. MTX) but also the additional risk from D-penicillamine and Myocrisin® (gold) of life-threatening rash or anaphylactic reaction.

Both drugs require:

- Pre-screening: haematological, pregnancy, and immunological status.
- Regular blood monitoring:
  - ~50% of RA patients experience an adverse event in the first 6 months of treatment.
  - 25% will discontinue treatment.
- Regular urinalysis for Myocrisin® before each dose. Both drugs have the potential to cause renal impairment and are excreted in the urine.
- For prescribing information and rare adverse events refer to SPC and *BNF* for prescribing information.

⚠ A trend in blood results is as important as absolute values.

➲ Also see Chapter 17, p. 505; ➲ 'Screening prior to DMARD treatment', p. 450.

Patients treated with D-penicillamine and sodium aurothiomalate (IM gold) should be advised:

- It may take 3–6 months before they feel the benefit of treatment although they may feel a benefit earlier.
- To not alter the dose they are prescribed.
- They may experience minor side effects during this time and these should abate. Side effects include:
  - Nausea, loss of appetite (taking medication before bed may reduce nausea).
  - Abnormal taste sensations with D-penicillamine (should resolve spontaneously).
- They should not have any live vaccines while on treatment.
- They should advise the doctor or nurse if taking herbal or complementary therapies—as they may interaction with the medication.
- They must not get pregnant while on treatment (use an effective method of contraception).
- That medical staff monitor for side effects related to bloods, liver, and kidneys and blood monitoring regimens are important and will help identify problems.
- If side effects become a problem or if they are uncertain about their treatment, seek advice as there is always something that can be done to help with side effects.

- ❗ However, some side effects must not be ignored and should be reported promptly:
  - Itching, rashes, or mouth ulcers (do not ignore rashes—even those that appear late in treatment—they can be serious).
  - Abnormal bruising or severe sore throat.
- Report promptly any infections they experience.

Key factors in the management of penicillamine and IM gold

► Note blood trends or unexplained bruising (with or without sore throat)—withhold treatment and seek medical advice.

Dose of oral D-penicillamine

A typical dose in two divided doses: 125–250 mg/day, ↑ by 125 mg every 4 weeks to 500 mg/day. The dose may be ↑ to 750 mg/day if response is not achieved in 3 months. Patients should be advised:

- Milk, antacids, zinc supplements, or iron tablets must be administered at least 2 hours after taking D-penicillamine as they interfere with drug absorption.
- Haematological side effects include neutropenia, thrombocytopenia, and aplastic anaemias—rapid or gradual changes in the blood picture may be seen.
- Contraindicated in moderate to severe renal impairment.

⚠ Drug interactions include digoxin and antipsychotics. Also consider drugs with concomitant nephrotoxicity (including sodium aurothiomalate).

Note: observe weight and review if there is weight loss—dose is calculated according to weight.

Cautions

⚠ Caution if co-prescribed:

- Aspirin—may exacerbate hepatic dysfunction.
- Phenylbutazone or oxyphenbutazone—hepatic dysfunction.
- Angiotensin-converting enzyme inhibitors due to an ↑ risk of severe anaphylactoid reaction in these patients.

Contraindications

These include severe renal or hepatic impairment, history of blood disorders/marrow aplasia, SLE, significant pulmonary fibrosis, porphyria, and pregnancy or lactation.

⚠ *IM gold*

In the elderly, renal or hepatic impairment (moderate), history of urticaria, eczema, or inflammatory bowel disease. Rare anaphylactic reactions may occur (dizziness, nausea, sweating, and facial flushing) a few minutes after injection. Treat according to policy on anaphylaxis and discontinue treatment.

Dose of sodium aurothiomalate (IM gold)

A test dose of 10 mg sodium aurothiomalate should be administered in the clinic/ward—observe patients for 30 min for any signs of allergic reaction. Injections of 50 mg sodium aurothiomalate should then continue once a week until a significant treatment response is seen.

Review of treatment response

Benefits should be seen at a cumulative dose of at 500 mg although efficacy should be assessed after a cumulative dose of 1 g has been administered. Responders to treatment—↑ the interval between injections to one every 4 weeks (50 mg dose). If no response is seen after cumulative doses of 1 g, consider an alternative DMARD.

➲ See Table 16.1, p. 455, for the blood monitoring regimen.

Further reading

British Society for Rheumatology: ℘ http://www.rheumatology.org.uk

Ledingham J, Gullick N, Irving K, et al. (2017). BSR and BHPR guideline for the prescription and monitoring of non-biologic disease-modifying anti-rheumatic drugs. *Rheumatology* 56:865–8.

NICE (2018). Case scenarios of each DMARD: ℘ https://cks.nice.org.uk/dmards

Patient information leaflets on all drug therapies are available from Versus Arthritis: ℘ https://www.versusarthritis.org

Hydroxychloroquine sulfate

Hydroxychloroquine is principally used as a prophylaxis against malaria although benefits in treating RA and SLE have been demonstrated for many years. Hydroxychloroquine has a lower toxicity profile compared to other DMARDs but also a lower therapeutic benefit and is therefore chiefly confined to treating milder disease or in combination therapy.[1]

General management

- Ophthalmic pre-screening is required for hydroxychloroquine. This should include visual acuity of each eye and an annual review with the optometrist while on treatment for any signs of blurred vision. Eye examination should include optical coherence tomography recommended with 1 year of starting treatment.

Caution

- ↑ risk of retinal toxicity if dose exceeds 6 mg/kg and long-term use over 5 years. Check visual acuity.
- Renal or hepatic impairment. Therapeutic doses may need to be adjusted for those with renal impairment (40% renal excretion).
- Patients with epilepsy—may reduce threshold for convulsions.
- Dose is calculated based on weight—check weight regularly as dose changes may be required.

Contraindications

- Breastfeeding.
- Pre-existing maculopathy.

Drug interactions

These include ↑ plasma concentrations of digoxin, MTX, and ciclosporin. Avoid use with amiodarone, moxifloxacin, mefloquine, and quinine.

Relatively safe in pregnancy—risk:benefit analysis should consider relative potential harm to unborn child against the relative risks of stopping treatment.

Patients treated with hydroxychloroquine should be advised:

- To take hydroxychloroquine with food to avoid gastrointestinal symptoms.
- To avoid antacids within 4 hours of dose.
- Side effects usually resolve with continuation of treatment, but these include:
  - Nausea, diarrhoea, and abdominal discomfort.
  - Blurred vision, irreversible retinal damage, headaches, and dizziness.
  - Skin reactions (rashes, itching). May exacerbate psoriasis.
  - Hair loss.

Dose of hydroxychloroquine sulfate (oral)

A typical regimen would be 200–400 mg daily. Dosage may be reduced to 200 mg daily depending upon clinical response.

➔ Also see 'Screening prior to DMARD treatment', p. 450 and Table 16.1, p. 455.

Reference

1. Royal College of Ophthalmologists (2018). Hydroxychloroquine and chloroquine retinopathy: new screening recommendations. https://www.rcophth.ac.uk/2018/03/rcophth-guideline-hydroxychloroquine-and-chloroquine-retinopathy-new-screening-recommendations-february-2018/

Further reading

Ledingham J, Gullick N, Irving K, et al. (2017). BSR and BHPR guideline for the prescription and monitoring of non-biologic disease-modifying anti-rheumatic drugs. *Rheumatology* 56:865–8.

National Rheumatoid Arthritis Society. Patient organization with information including drug information: http://www.nras.org.uk

NICE (2018). Case scenarios of each DMARD: https://cks.nice.org.uk/dmards

Patient information leaflets on all drug therapies are available from Versus Arthritis: https://www.versusarthritis.org

Leflunomide

Leflunomide is one of the most recently developed cDMARDs. It has an active metabolite that inhibits the human enzyme dihydroorotate dehydrogenase and as a result has antiproliferative activity and arrests lymphocyte activation. It has a long half-life (~2 weeks) and is strongly protein bound. There is no dose adjustment recommended in patients with mild renal insufficiency.

General management

- Pre-screening required for haematological, pregnancy, and immunological status (➔ see 'Screening prior to DMARD treatment', p. 450).
- Allergic responses, toxicities, pregnancy, or severe side effects will require an urgent therapeutic washout.
- Pre-existing anaemia, leucopenia, and/or thrombocytopenia, or patients with impaired function of the bone marrow function are at risk of ↑ haematological disorders.
- Early signs of skin or mucosal reactions raise the suspicion of allergic reaction.
- ► Interstitial lung disease has developed while being treated—observe for cough and dyspnoea and report urgently.

Patients treated with leflunomide should be advised:

- They may experience side effects; this should abate over time. Side effects include:
    - Nausea, loss of appetite, and diarrhoea.
    - Hair loss.
    - Liver impairment—alcohol should be avoided/or limited to within national limits (e.g. 4–8 units per week).
- Side effects can occur which is why medical staff monitor to make sure the bloods, liver, and kidneys are functioning normally. Blood monitoring regimens are important and will help identify problems.
- The benefits of treatment are usually seen between 4 and 6 weeks after starting treatment and may further improve up to 4–6 months.
- Not to alter the dose they are prescribed.
- Report promptly any infections they experience as they may require treatment.
- They must not get pregnant while on treatment (use an effective method of contraception). They should contact their doctor/nurse immediately if they believe they might be pregnant—a therapeutic drug washout may be required.
- They should not have any live vaccines while on treatment.
- Herbal or complementary therapies—advise the doctor or nurse of any being taken as there may be interactions (➔ see 'Ciclosporin', p. 456).
- If side effects become a problem or if they are uncertain about their treatment, seek advice as there is always something that can be done to help with side effects.

Cautions

- Localized or systemic infections including hepatitis B or C.
- History of TB.
- Potential hepatotoxicity/haematotoxic issues related to co-prescription of other drug therapies (e.g. phenytoin, warfarin, or tolbutamide). MTX is listed as a caution although it is often prescribed in combination therapy with leflunomide.
- Note: during a serious infection, leflunomide should be temporarily withheld until the patient has recovered from the infection.

Contraindications

- Severe immunodeficiency.
- Serious infections.
- Liver impairment or moderate to severe renal impairment.
- Hypoproteinaemia.
- Bone marrow impairment, e.g. anaemia or cytopenias.

⚠ Note: a trend in blood results is as important as absolute values.

Key factors in nursing management

► Note blood trends or unexplained bruising (with or without sore throat)—withhold treatment and seek urgent medical advice. Note: toxicity may require washout (➲ see Chapter 17, p. 505).

► ➲ See Table 16.1, p. 455, for the blood monitoring regimen.

❶ If leflunomide is co-prescribed with MTX, extra vigilance is required when monitoring side effects/toxicities.

Dose of leflunomide (oral only)

The licensed indications suggest a loading dose of 100 mg once daily for 3 days (in practice this is no longer prescribed in the UK due to an ↑ incidence of side effects with loading dose). Frequently patients are commenced on a maintenance dose of leflunomide 10–20 mg once daily for RA; for PsA, the dose is 20 mg once daily.

Further reading

For licensed indications, prescribing, and rare adverse events see the SPC and the *BNF*.

Joint Formulary Committee (2019). DMARDs: leflunomide. In: *British National Formulary*, 77th edn. London: British Medical Association and Royal Pharmaceutical Society of Great Britain. https://bnf.nice.org.uk/

Ledingham J, Gullick N, Irving K, et al. (2017). BSR and BHPR guideline for the prescription and monitoring of non-biologic disease-modifying anti-rheumatic drugs. *Rheumatology* 56:865–8.

NICE (2018). Case scenarios of each DMARD: https://cks.nice.org.uk/dmards

Patient information leaflets on all drug therapies are available from Versus Arthritis: https://www.versusarthritis.org

Methotrexate

MTX is the 'gold' standard of traditional disease-modifying drug therapies suppressing disease activity for IJDs. Gastrointestinal and bone marrow toxicities with MTX are significantly ↓ if folic acid is prescribed. MTX is prescribed in oncology and gynaecology to prevent cell replication. MTX inhibits the activity of an enzyme (dihydrofolate reductase) responsible for the synthesis of purines implicated in cell replication (DNA) resulting in a fall of malignant and, it appears, inflammatory cells. MTX is frequently prescribed in combination with other traditional DMARDs (e.g. MTX and SAS) and co-prescribed when patients are treated with a bDMARD. MTX can be administered subcutaneously (better bioavailability).

General management

- Pre-screening required, includes haematological, respiratory function, pregnancy, and immunological status.
- In patients with clinical suspicion of parenchymal lung disease, formal lung function testing and imaging should be performed and may require referral to a respiratory specialist.
- Dermatologists may require an additional pre-screening test to monitor liver status (pro-collagen III levels).
- Regular blood monitoring required—FBC, U&E, and LFTs.
- ► Vigilance for signs of toxicity—these can occur at any time during treatment, e.g. pulmonary pneumonitis (cough, dyspnoea)—if any suspicion, seek urgent medical advice.
- Frail and elderly patients require lower doses. Observe for signs of renal impairment: ↑ risk of toxicity.
- ⚠ Note: a trend in blood results is as important as absolute values.

➲ Also see 'Screening prior to DMARD treatment', p. 450.

Patients treated with MTX should be advised:

- They may experience side effects; this should abate over time. Side effects may be reduced if MTX is taken at night with a full glass of water. Side effects include:
  - Nausea, loss of appetite, diarrhoea, and headaches.
  - Hair loss or skin rashes.
  - Mouth ulcers.
  - Liver impairment—seek medical advice regarding alcohol consumption while on treatment (should be at least less than nationally recommended levels).
  - Rare but important risk of developing respiratory problems—seek medical advice for unexplained cough or dyspnoea.
  - They will also be co-prescribed folic acid 5 mg—dosing regimens vary.
- If side effects become a problem or if they are uncertain about their treatment, seek advice as there is always something that can be done to help with side effects.

- MTX is prescribed **as a once-a-week dose.** They must not alter the dose they are prescribed. If they forget to take a dose:
  - Delay 1–2 days, take dose and return to normal dosing day the following week.
  - >3 days, make a note they have missed the dose and then take their normal dose on their normal dosing day the following week.
- Folic acid is prescribed (usually at a minimal dose of 5 mg weekly). It is important they continue taking it as prescribed.
- Side effects can occur which is why medical staff monitor to make sure the bloods, liver, and kidneys are functioning normally. Blood monitoring regimens are important and will help identify problems.
- Report unexplained bleeding or bruising.
- Treatment can take up to 3 months for benefits to be achieved.
- Report promptly any infections as they may require treatment.
- Conception while receiving treatment must be avoided (use an effective method of contraception). Seek medical advice promptly if pregnancy occurs.
- They should not have any live vaccines while on treatment.
- Herbal or complementary therapies—advise the doctor or nurse of any being taken as there may be interactions.

Cautions

- Localized or systemic infections including hepatitis B or C.
- History of TB.
- Potential hepatotoxicity/haematotoxic issues related to co-prescription of other drug therapies (e.g. phenytoin, probenecid, penicillin, tolbutamide, co-trimoxazole, or trimethoprim).

Contraindications

- Pregnancy or breastfeeding.
- Liver impairment or moderate to severe renal impairment.
- Suspicion of local or systemic infection.
- Hypoproteinaemia.
- Bone marrow impairment, e.g. anaemia or cytopenias.

Key factors in nursing management for patients taking MTX

- MTX is a **once-a-week dose only.** ⚠ Patients must check tablets (dosages of 2.5 mg or 10 mg tablets).[1]
- Folic acid is usually not administered on the day that MTX is taken.
- Side effects and toxicities can occur at any time during treatment.
- ► Note blood trends or unexplained bruising (with or without sore throat)—withhold treatment and seek medical advice.
- If overdosage occurs, seek prompt medical/pharmacist advice to enable chemical washout.
- ❗ If leflunomide is co-prescribed with MTX, extra vigilance is required when monitoring side effects/toxicities.

Drug dose (oral, SC, or IM routes prescribed for MSCs)

These will vary according to age, renal function, and route of administration but doses range from 5 to 25 mg once a week.

➔ Also see Chapter 17, p. 505.

Reference

1. NHS Improvement. Learning from patient safety incidents. https://improvement.nhs.uk/resources/learning-from-patient-safety-incidents/

Further reading

Ledingham J, Gullick N, Irving K, et al. (2017). BSR and BHPR guideline for the prescription and monitoring of non-biologic disease-modifying anti-rheumatic drugs. *Rheumatology* 56:865–8.

NICE (2018). Case scenarios of each DMARD: https://cks.nice.org.uk/dmards

Patient information leaflets on all drug therapies are available from Versus Arthritis: https://www.versusarthritis.org

Mycophenolate mofetil

MMF inhibits the pathway of active metabolites required for the synthesis of DNA. This inhibition results in a reduction in T and B lymphocytes as they are critically dependent for their proliferation on *de novo* synthesis of purines necessary for DNA.

General management

- Pre-screening required.
- MMF does not normally cause major organ toxicity.
- Note: live vaccines should not be administered to patients on MMF.
- ⚠ Note: a trend in blood results is as important as absolute values.

➲ Also see 'Screening prior to DMARD treatment', p. 450.

Cautions

- Suspected lymphoproliferative disorders or unexplained anaemias/ leucopenia and thrombocytopenia.
- Localized or systemic infection.
- Active serious digestive system disease.
- Frail and elderly patients.

Contraindications

- Pregnancy and breastfeeding.
- Localized or systemic infections.
- Should not be co-prescribed with AZA.

Patients treated with mycophenolate should be advised:

- They may experience side effects which are usually related to the dose. Side effects if severe will abate on cessation of treatment but include:
  - Sickness, nausea, loss of appetite, diarrhoea, vomiting, or abdominal pain.
  - Hair loss, skin rashes, and bruising.
  - Mouth ulcers.
  - Urinary—urgent sensation to pass urine.
- It is important to use sun block or sunscreen and avoid exposure to strong sunlight as there is a slight ↑ in skin cancers and lymphoma.
- Symptoms of allergy including wheezing, SOB, swelling of face, lips, or tongue—stop treatment and seek medical advice.
- If side effects become a problem or if they are uncertain about their treatment, seek advice as there is always something that can be done to help with side effects.
- MMF is prescribed as a capsule and should be taken on an empty stomach.
- Side effects can occur which is why medical staff monitor to make sure the bloods, liver, and kidneys are functioning normally. Blood monitoring regimens are important and will help identify problems.
- Report unexplained bleeding or bruising.
- Treatment can take up to 3 months before the benefits are achieved.
- Report promptly any infections they experience as they may require treatment.

- ♂ and ♀ patients need to be aware that conception while receiving treatment must be avoided (use an effective method of contraception). Seek medical advice promptly if a pregnancy occurs.
- They should not have any live vaccines while on treatment.
- Herbal or complementary therapies—advise the doctor or nurse of any being taken as there may be interactions.

Key factors in nursing management

- ▶ Note blood trends or unexplained bruising (with or without sore throat)—withhold treatment and seek medical advice.
  - Severe neutropenias occur in ~0.5% for those receiving the full dose.
- Drug interactions include:
  - Cholestyramine ↓ absorption of MMF by ~40%.
  - Antacids containing aluminium and magnesium hydroxide ↓ absorption of MMF by 33%.
  - Probenecid ↑ plasma concentration of MMF.
  - Note: if patients have renal impairment and are co-prescribed aciclovir with mycophenolate they will have raised concentrations of both aciclovir and mycophenolate.

➔ Also see Chapter 17, p. 505.

Drug dosage (oral or IV routes available)

The typical dose is 500 mg twice a day, gradually ↑ over weeks until the optimum dose is achieved, e.g. if well tolerated this may be ↑ to 1 g twice a day thereafter. Maximum is usually 3 g/day.

Further reading

Ledingham J, Gullick N, Irving K, et al. (2017). BSR and BHPR guideline for the prescription and monitoring of non-biologic disease-modifying anti-rheumatic drugs. *Rheumatology* 56:865–8.

NICE (2018). Case scenarios of each DMARD: ℛ https://cks.nice.org.uk/dmards

Patient information leaflets on all drug therapies are available from Versus Arthritis: ℛ https://www.versusarthritis.org

Sulfasalazine

It appears that SAS may work by inhibiting specific metabolites that have a disease-modifying effect on conditions such as inflammatory bowel disease or IJD. The enteric coated form should be prescribed.

General management

- Pre-screening required for haematological, pregnancy, and immunological status.
- ⚠ Note: a trend in blood results is as important as absolute values.

➲ Also see 'Screening prior to DMARD treatment', pp. 450 and 455; ➲ Table 16.1, p. 455, for the blood monitoring regimen.

Cautions

- Haemolysis may occur for those with glucose-6-phosphate dehydrogenase deficiency.
- Moderate renal impairment—encourage high fluid intake, may cause crystalluria.

Contraindications

- Severe renal impairment.
- Hypersensitivity to sulphonamides/co-trimoxazole.
- Acute intermittent porphyria.
- Pregnancy (a relative contraindication—depending upon risk:benefit analysis of benefit and harms to the patient versus the unborn child).
- Breastfeeding.

Patients treated with SAS should be advised:

- They may experience side effects during this time and these should settle with continuation of treatment. Side effects include:
  - Nausea, loss of appetite, and dyspepsia.
  - Dizziness and headaches.
  - Abnormal LFTs.
  - Itching, skin rashes, or mouth ulcers.
- It may take up to 3 months before they feel the benefit of treatment although they may feel a benefit earlier.
- Side effects that can occur include changes in the bloods, liver, and kidneys—which medical staff will monitor especially for the first year of treatment.
- To not alter the dose they are prescribed.
- Report promptly any infections they experience.
- General advice highlights the importance of not getting pregnant while on treatment and to use an effective method of contraception; however, SAS has been shown to be relatively safe during pregnancy. The doctor will discuss this to ensure a risk:benefit analysis is undertaken to support treatment with SAS during pregnancy.
- Herbal or complementary therapies—advise the doctor or nurse so they can document these and review should there be any interactions.
- SAS may make urine a yellow-orange colour. It may also affect contact lenses, staining them a yellow-orange colour.

- If side effects become a problem or if they are uncertain about their treatment, seek advice as there is always something that can be done to help with side effects.

Key factors in nursing management

- Rarely eosinophilic pneumonitis can occur—dyspnoea, fever, weight loss, ↓ pulmonary function, and changes suggesting infiltration on chest X-ray.
- If iron or antacids are prescribed, avoid/withhold SAS administration until 2 hours has elapsed.
- Usually well tolerated.
- Slow acetylator (a genetic predisposition to be a slow or fast acetylator/metabolizer) of drug may result in drug-induced lupus-like syndrome.
- May impair folate absorption.
- ♂ should be aware of transient and reversible oligospermia.
- In some circumstances, a risk:benefit analysis may mean that some patients remain on treatment while wishing to conceive. It may be appropriate in these patients to have a folic acid supplementation.
- Drug interactions include:
  - AZA may contribute to bone marrow toxicity.
  - Cardiac glycosides may reduce absorption of digoxin.
- ► Note blood trends or unexplained bruising (with or without sore throat)—withhold treatment and seek urgent medical advice.
- ► Rash—withhold treatment and seek urgent medical advice.

➲ Also see Chapter 17, p. 505.

Drug dosage

SAS is usually commenced at a dose of 500 mg once a day for a week, ↑ weekly to gradually ↑ over weeks to a maximum dose of 2–3 g per day.

Further reading

Ledingham J, Gullick N, Irving K, et al. (2017). BSR and BHPR guideline for the prescription and monitoring of non-biologic disease-modifying anti-rheumatic drugs. *Rheumatology* 56:865–8.

NICE (2018). Case scenarios of each DMARD: ℜ https://cks.nice.org.uk/dmards

Patient information leaflets on all drug therapies are available from Versus Arthritis: ℜ https://www.versusarthritis.org

Tacrolimus

Tacrolimus inhibits calcineurin, a key component that enables message transduction in activated T cells and appears in cell cultures to inhibit IL-5 production (a cytokine). It is licensed for immunosuppression in organ transplant surgery but has been used for MSCs.

General management

- Pre-screening required for pregnancy and immunological status.
- Should not be co-prescribed with ciclosporin.
- St John's wort or herbal preparation should not be taken with tacrolimus: ↓ blood concentrations of tacrolimus.
- Grapefruit and pomelo ↑ levels of tacrolimus.
- Should not breastfeed while on treatment.

Dose reduction may be required if blood pressure is raised or there is a deterioration in renal function:

- Monitor for signs of hypertension (treat hypertension).
- Monitor kidney function for signs of ↑ creatinine.
- Evidence suggests potential risk of diabetes—monitor blood glucose.
- If contraception required, non-hormonal methods should be used.

➲ Also see 'Screening prior to DMARD treatment', p. 450.

Cautions

Galactose intolerance.

Contraindications

Sensitivity of tacrolimus.

Note: tacrolimus requires extended monitoring—➲ see Table 16.1, p. 455.

Patients treated with tacrolimus should be advised:

- They may experience side effects which are usually related to the dose. Side effects if severe will abate on cessation of treatment but include:
  - Flu-like symptoms.
  - Diarrhoea, nausea, abdominal pain, dyspepsia, and headaches (occur in >5%).
  - Tremor.
  - Sickness, nausea, loss of appetite, diarrhoea (>5%), vomiting, or abdominal pain.
  - Skin rashes and bruising.
  - Mouth ulcers.
- It is important to use sun block or sunscreen and avoid exposure to strong sunlight as there is a slight ↑ in skin cancers.
- They must not take herbal or complementary therapies while on treatment as there are drug interactions.
- If side effects become a problem or if they are uncertain about their treatment, seek advice as there is always something that can be done to help with side effects.

- Side effects can occur which is why medical staff monitor to make sure the bloods, liver, and kidneys are functioning normally. Blood monitoring regimens are important and will help identify problems.
- Report unexplained bleeding or bruising.
- Treatment can take up to 3 months before the benefits are achieved.
- Report promptly any infections they experience as they may require treatment.
- ♂ and ♀ patients need to be aware that conception while receiving treatment must be avoided (use an effective method of contraception). Seek medical advice promptly if an unplanned pregnancy occurs.
- They should not have any live vaccines while on treatment.

Key factors in nursing management

Tacrolimus is chiefly prescribed for transplant patients. Evidence suggests risks of side effects are lower with RA than in organ transplantation possibly related to lower dosing regimens.

- Monitor blood pressure and renal function/creatinine levels.
- Tacrolimus may be prescribed during pregnancy in some cases—based on a risk:benefit analysis of treatment against no treatment.
- Drug interactions:
  - The dose of tacrolimus may need to be reduced when prescribed with antifungals (e.g. ketoconazole, fluconazole), macrolide antibiotic erythromycin or rifampicin, phenytoin, or HIV protease inhibitors (e.g. ritonavir).
  - Carbamazepine, metamizole, and isoniazid may reduce the action of tacrolimus.
- ⚠ Note: a trend in blood results is as important as absolute values.
- ▶ Note blood trends or unexplained bruising (with or without sore throat)—withhold treatment and seek medical advice.

➲ Also see Chapter 17, p. 505.

Drug dosage

Tacrolimus should be prescribed as a morning, once-daily dose on an empty stomach or 2–3 hours after a meal. A typical dose might be 3 mg/day for RA. The dose should be taken promptly once released from the blister pack. It may take several days before a stable dose is achieved.

Further reading

Ledingham J, Gullick N, Irving K, et al. (2017). BSR and BHPR guideline for the prescription and monitoring of non-biologic disease-modifying anti-rheumatic drugs. *Rheumatology* 56:865–8.

NICE (2018). Case scenarios of each DMARD: https://cks.nice.org.uk/dmards

Patient information leaflets on all drug therapies are available from Versus Arthritis: https://www.versusarthritis.org

Oral targeted synthetic disease-modifying antirheumatic drugs

This section will briefly outline three new licensed oral therapies used in rheumatology.

Apremilast, baricitinib, and tofacitinib are referred to as targeted synthetic disease-modifying antirheumatic drugs (tsDMARDs).

Apremilast

Apremilast is a small molecule that works by inhibiting phosphodiesterase 4 (PDE4) intracellularly. This results in a reduction of proinflammatory cytokines such as TNFα, IL-17, and IL-23 but also increases the expression of anti-inflammatory mediators such as IL-10.

Apremilast is used to treat active:

- Psoriatic arthritis (in combination with a DMARD or alone) for those who have had an inadequate response to prior DMARDs.
- Moderate to severe chronic plaque psoriasis that has not responded to standard treatment or when contraindicated.

General management/screening

- History of psychiatric disorders (see 'Cautions').
- Renal function (reduced dose if estimated glomerular filtration rate) <30 mL/min/1.73 m^2.
- Pregnancy (those with childbearing potential must be advised to use an effective method of contraception during treatment).
- Monitor the patient's weight—see 'Cautions'.
- Check the patient is not being treated with any drugs that are strong cytochrome P450 3A4 enzyme inducers (e.g. rifampicin)—check with the prescribing clinician as this may result in a loss of efficacy.
- Note: no routine laboratory monitoring is required.

Cautions

- Diarrhoea, nausea, and vomiting have been reported in the first few weeks of treatment. Patients >65 years of age may be at higher risk. If there are severe symptoms, treatment may need to be discontinued.
- Patients with rare hereditary galactose intolerance should not be prescribed apremilast (see the *BNF* for further details).
- In **severe** renal impairment, the dose is reduced to 30 mg once daily.
- Risk of psychiatric disorders, e.g. insomnia, depression, and suicidal behaviour have been reported. Risks and benefits of treatment should be carefully assessed if previous episodes of psychiatric disorders. If any worsening of psychiatric symptoms, patient/carers should notify team and stop treatment.
- Underweight patients at the start of treatment should have their body weight monitored regularly. If significant weight loss, refer to prescribing clinician, as they may require discontinuation of treatment.

- If the patient is co-prescribed a cytochrome P450 3A4 enzyme inducer (e.g. rifampicin) or is taking St John's wort there may be a loss of efficacy of apremilast and ∴ is not recommended.
- Pre-assessment should include screening for risk of pregnancy in those with childbearing potential.

Contraindications

- Pregnancy (apremilast is teratogenic in animal studies).
- Nursing mothers should not be prescribed apremilast while breastfeeding.

Drug dosage

Apremilast is taken orally. Treatment starts at a dose of 10 mg daily gradually increasing to 30 mg twice daily after 6 days.

- 10 mg—first day.
- 10 mg (twice daily) morning and evening—second day.
- 10 mg am and 20 mg in the evening—third day.
- 20 mg twice daily—fourth day.
- 20 mg am and 30 mg in the evening—fifth day.
- 30 mg (twice daily)—12 hours apart.

This gradual introduction potentially reduces the risk of potential gastrointestinal side effects. If a dose is missed, the dose should be taken as soon as possible afterwards, then the next dose should be taken at the usual time. If close to the time for the next dose, leave out the forgotten dose and return to the usual regimen the next day.

Patients should be advised:

- Apremilast can be taken with or without food.
- If they experience mild gastrointestinal side effects (including diarrhoea, nausea) in the first 2 weeks, this should resolve after a few weeks. If these are severe and do not resolve or there is significant weight loss, seek advice from the team.
- Other side effects are usually mild and include upper respiratory tract infections and headache.
- In clinical trials, weight loss was observed. In only 0.1% of patients did this require discontinuation of treatment.
- For those with mild previous psychiatric symptoms (e.g. depression), withhold treatment and seek urgent medical advice if they experience changes in behaviour, suicidal ideation, or mood.
- See advice on dosage and missing a dose (as previously described)
- Herbal or complementary therapies—advise team so this can be documented. Do not take St John's wort while being treated with apremilast.

For further information, see: ☞ https://bnf.nice.org.uk/drug/apremilast.html and for psoriasis patient information: ☞ http://www.bad.org.uk.

Baricitinib

Baricitinib and tofacitinib are oral Janus kinase (JAK) inhibitor medications. JAK inhibitors present a new era of treatment for individuals with RA and possibly other forms of inflammatory arthritis in the future. JAK inhibitors are very small intracellular molecules that interrupt the signalling pathway of JAK group of enzymes. By interrupting the JAK signal transducers and activators of transcription (referred to as JAK–STATs signal pathways), the signalling pathway which would normally activate an immune response usually leading to a pro-inflammation response is hindered. There are four JAKs that have been identified in humans and been shown to be of importance: JAK1, -2, and -3 and tyrosine kinase 2 (TYK2).

Baricitinib is a JAK1/JAK2 inhibitor. It is licensed to treat moderate to severe RA either as a monotherapy or combined with MTX for those who have had an inadequate response or intolerant to one or more DMARDs. ➲ See 'Tofacitinib', pp. 478–479.

General management/screening

Routine blood monitoring is required and in particular:

- FBC, LFTs, and glomerular filtration rate twice weekly until stable dose for 6 weeks—and then monthly for 3 months. Further monitoring if there is an ↑ risk of toxicity.
- If dose is ↑—monitor every 2 weeks until stable and then reduce to 6-monthly.
- Lipids at baseline then 12 weeks after commencing treatment. If hyperlipidaemia—treat according to national guidelines. Then monitor periodically.
- TB and viral hepatitis screening are advocated for all bDMARDs.
- Pre-assessment should include screening for risk of pregnancy in those with childbearing potential.

Note: if haematological abnormalities occur (see 'Contraindications'), withhold treatment and seek prescribing clinician's advice. May be restarted when levels return to acceptable values.

Cautions

- Active, chronic, or recurrent infection. Stop treatment and discuss with prescribing clinician if no response to standard therapy.
- Risk of viral reactivation (e.g. herpes zoster). Interrupt treatment until viral infection is resolved.
- If creatinine clearance is <30–60 mL/min—dose adjustment to 2 mg once daily. If creatinine clearance is <30 mL/min—avoid treatment, discuss with prescribing clinician.

Contraindications

- Lymphocyte count <0.5 × 10^9 cells/L or neutrophil count <1 × 10^9/L or haemoglobin <8 g/dL. Treatment should not be commenced.
- Active TB,
- Pregnancy or breastfeeding.
- Avoid in severe hepatic impairment,

Drug dosage

- For adults aged 18–74 years—4 mg once daily.
- For adults 75 years and over—2 mg once daily.

Note: dose reductions may be necessary if there are side effects or a history of infections (refer to the *BNF* or SPC).

Patients should be advised:

- They may experience side effects when they commence treatment, these should settle. If they become severe, they should contact their specialist team for advice.
- They must not become pregnant while on treatment, so an effective method of contraception is essential for women of childbearing potential.
- Side effects include:
    - Gastroenteritis and nausea.
    - Cold sores (herpes simplex) or shingles (herpes zoster) can be reactivated. Withhold treatment and contact your specialist team.
- Blood monitoring regimens are important and will help identify problems.
- Side effects that can occur include changes in the bloods, liver, and kidneys—which medical staff will monitor especially for the first year of treatment. Monitoring of cholesterol—if raised they may require treatment according to national guidelines.
- To not alter the dose they are prescribed.
- Report promptly any infections they experience.

Tofacitinib

Tofacitinib is a JAK1 and JAK3 inhibitor. It is licensed to treat moderate to severe RA and active psoriatic arthritis that have had an inadequate response or are intolerant to one or more DMARDs. Can be prescribed as a monotherapy or in combination with MTX.

General management/screening

Routine blood monitoring is required and in particular:

- FBC, LFTs, and glomerular filtration rate twice weekly until stable dose for 8 weeks—and then monthly for 3 months. Further monitoring if there is an ↑ risk of toxicity.
- If dose is ↑—monitor every 2 weeks until stable and then reduce to 6-monthly.
- Lipids at baseline then 8 weeks after commencing treatment. If hyperlipidaemia—treat according to national guidelines. Then monitor periodically.
- Lymphocyte count <750 cells/mm^3 or neutrophil count <1000 cells/mm^3/or haemoglobin <9 g/dL—treatment should not be commenced.
- TB and viral hepatitis screening are advocated for all bDMARDs.
- Review vaccination history and offer all recommended vaccines, given before starting treatment. Consider prophylactic varicella zoster vaccination.
- Live vaccines should be given preferably 4 weeks before but at least 2 weeks before starting treatment.
- Pre-assessment should include screening for risk of pregnancy in those with childbearing potential.

Note: if haematological abnormalities occur (see 'Contraindications'), withhold treatment and seek prescribing clinician's advice. May be restarted when levels return to acceptable values.

Cautions

- Active infections, including localized infection—stop treatment and discuss with prescribing clinician. Recommence treatment when infection is controlled.
- Risk of viral reactivation (e.g. herpes zoster). Interrupt treatment until viral infection is resolved.
- If creatinine clearance <30–60 mL/min—dose adjustment to 2 mg once daily. If creatinine clearance <30 mL/min—avoid treatment, discuss with prescribing clinician.
- A patient with a risk of gastrointestinal perforation (e.g. diverticulitis). If the patient presents with new-onset abdominal signs and symptoms, they should be evaluated promptly for gastrointestinal perforation.

Contraindications

- Active TB.
- Pregnancy or breastfeeding.
- Avoid in severe hepatic impairment.
- Prescribing drugs with strong cytochrome P450 3A4 inducers such as rifampicin should be avoided and if co-prescribed, the tofacitinib dose should be reduced by half.
- Avoid in patients with rare hereditary galactose intolerance.

Drug dosage

5 mg twice daily. For patients with severe renal impairment or moderate hepatic impairment (see 'Cautions'), reduce dose to 5 mg daily.

Note: dose reductions may be necessary if side effects or history of infections.

For further information, refer to the *BNF* or SPC.

Patients should be advised:

- They may experience side effects when they commence treatment these should settle. If they become severe, contact your specialist team for advice.
- Side effects include:
  - Gastroenteritis, nausea and headache.
  - Respiratory and urinary tract infections.
  - Cold sores (herpes simplex) or shingles (herpes zoster) can be re-activated. Withhold treatment and contact your specialist team.
- Blood monitoring regimens are important and will help identify problems.
- Side effects that can occur include changes in the bloods, liver, and kidneys—which medical staff will monitor especially for the first year of treatment. Monitoring of cholesterol—if raised they may require treatment according to national guidelines.
- Women of childbearing age must not become pregnant while on treatment. An effective method of contraception is essential.
- To not alter their prescribed dose.
- Report promptly any infections they experience.

Note: UK national guidelines[1] published while going to press have advocated that key principles of general monitoring used for bDMARDs should be applied to all new therapies until there is sufficient post-marketing data available, although they do not refer directly to JAK inhibitors. Early evidence of JAKs appears to show that reactivation of varicella zoster virus is the most characteristic infection seen.[2] Further evidence from drug registries and post marketing surveillance will inform specific screening and monitoring guidance for JAK therapies in the future.

References

1. Holroyd CR, Seth R, Bukhari M, et al. (2019). The British Society for Rheumatology biologic DMARD safety guidelines in inflammatory arthritis. *Rheumatology (Oxford)* 58:220–6.
2. Bechman K, Subesinghe S, Norton S, et al. (2019). A systematic review and meta-analysis of infection risk with small molecule JAK inhibitors in rheumatoid arthritis. *Rheumatology* 58:1755–66.

Further reading

NICE (2017). Baricitinib for moderate to severe rheumatoid arthritis (TA466). ☞ https://www.nice.org.uk/guidance/ta466

NICE (2017). Tofacitinib for moderate to severe rheumatoid arthritis (TA480). ☞ https://www.nice.org.uk/guidance/ta480

NICE (2018). Case scenarios of each DMARD: ☞ https://cks.nice.org.uk/dmards

Corticosteroids: overview

The precise mechanism of corticosteroids and how they suppress inflammation is presently unknown. The body's naturally occurring corticosteroid hormones are produced and sustained by a complex feedback cycle involving the hypothalamus and adrenal glands. Corticosteroids consist of androgenic, glucocorticoids, and mineralocorticoids.

Corticosteroids such as oral prednisolone may be used in the treatment of RA, PMR, GCA, vasculitis, polymyositis, and SLE for disease suppression. Different preparations of steroids and routes of administration include local injections used in MSCs such as soft tissue injuries and sports injuries, IV infusions, and IM injections of preparations such as Depo-Medrone® (➔ see 'Corticosteroids: preparations and routes of administration', p. 483).

The most commonly used treatments for MSCs are:

- 💣 Oral prednisolone—the relative benefits and harms of oral prednisolone use in low doses as part of routine management is contentious. However, oral prednisolone is commonly used in the management of PMR.
- IM, IV, or IA methylprednisolone, hydrocortisone, or triamcinolone acetonide.

When treating with corticosteroids it is important to:

- Use the lowest possible dose for the shortest duration to minimize the risk of side effects, particularly osteoporosis. For this reason, parenteral corticosteroids are often used instead of oral corticosteroids.
- During times of physical stress (health-related crisis, e.g. infection), ↑ corticosteroids may be needed. Regular corticosteroids may suppress the appropriate response.
- If patients have been treated with oral corticosteroids (>3 weeks), adrenal suppression occurs ∴ corticosteroids must not be stopped abruptly; collapse or death from adrenal insufficiency can occur.

❗ Stopping oral corticosteroids abruptly can result in adrenal insufficiency.

❗ Corticosteroids may need to be ↑ at times of additional stress to maintain the same level of steroid effect.

Side effects

- Gastrointestinal—dyspepsia, peptic ulceration, nausea.
- Musculoskeletal—proximal myopathy, osteoporosis, avascular necrosis.
- Endocrine—adrenal suppression, weight gain, ↑ appetite.
- Ophthalmic—glaucoma, corneal or scleral thinning.
- Neuropsychiatric effects—euphoria, depression, psychosis.
- Other effects—bruising, striae, impaired healing, skin atrophy.

Contraindication

Any evidence of systemic infection.

Cautions

- Hypertension, congestive heart failure, liver failure, renal insufficiency, diabetes mellitus, or osteoporosis. In addition, caution should be used if any prior history of severe affective disorders (particularly if a previous history of steroid-induced psychoses), epilepsy or seizure disorders, or peptic ulceration.
- ❶ A previous history of TB or X-ray changes characteristic of TB may be at ↑ risk of re-emergence of latent TB.
- ❶ Corticosteroids suppress inflammatory responses, ↑ the susceptibility to infections. Normal signs of infections may be masked in patients taking prednisolone.
- ❶ Ensure patients are aware that chickenpox, although normally a minor illness, may be fatal in immunosuppressed patients. If in contact during the infective phase, they should seek medical advice promptly.

Nursing management and patient advice

- A full assessment of the patient should be made to clarify their immune status, e.g. history of prior exposure to chickenpox or herpes zoster:
  - If no prior exposure, patients should be advised to seek urgent medical attention if they come in close contact with an infected person. Passive immunization with varicella zoster immunoglobulin can be administered within 10 days of exposure.
  - All patients who have received corticosteroids for >3 months or have completed a course of steroid treatment within the past 3 months should be considered at risk.
  - If chickenpox is diagnosed, the prednisolone dose may need to be ↑.
  - Patients should also be advised to avoid exposure to measles if possible and if necessary to seek immediate medical assistance should exposure occur.
- If it is possible that corticosteroid treatment will extend to a period of 3 months or more (irrespective of dose), then the guidance on preventing corticosteroid-induced osteoporosis should be followed.

Further reading

For detailed guidance refer to http://www.nice.org.uk for specific conditions, e.g.: NICE (2018). Rheumatoid arthritis in adults: management (NG100). https://www.nice.org.uk/guidance/ng100

Also refer to https://bnf.nice.org.uk/ for further information on glucocorticosteroids.

Jacobs WG, Spies CM, Bijlsma WJ, Tuttgereit F (2013, updated 2018). Glucocorticoids. In: Watts RA, Conaghan PG, Denton C, et al. (eds). *Oxford Textbook of Rheumatology*, 4th edn, pp. 607–18. Oxford: Oxford University Press. https://oxfordmedicine.com/view/10.1093/med/9780199642489.001.0001/med-9780199642489-chapter-79

Corticosteroids: preparations and routes of administration

The adrenal cortex and the secretion of steroids in the body have two main functions:

- They allow or manage the normal resting state or actions of hormones that allow normal function.
- Steroids produced in the body are also used at times of stress/fear or need for a rapid response such as 'fear or flight' as a result of a threat or danger.

The adrenal cortex releases several steroid hormones including:

- Androgens—secrete oestrogen and testosterone—peripherally converted (sex hormones).
- Mineralocorticoids—manage the water and mineral balances of the body (e.g. aldosterone).
- Glucocorticoids—have an effect on metabolic, anti-inflammatory responses, levels of awareness, and sleep patterns (hydrocortisone and cortisone).

The use of glucocorticoids can have an effect on normal circadian rhythm (normal wakefulness and sleep patterns).

Glucocorticoids are the key 'steroid' of interest in treating inflammation by reducing signs and symptoms of an inflammatory condition. Steroids are not curative and when stopped may result in a return or exacerbation of the symptoms/condition.

Corticosteroids vary in:

- The potency.
- The preparations and routes of administration:
  - Oral.
  - Topical/eye drops/creams.
  - IA/IM/IV.
  - Inhaled.
  - Rectal.

Cautions

Long-term treatment—there is a need to consider the adverse effects of treatment against the risks of continued use.

Oral prednisolone

- Prednisolone is chiefly a glucocorticoid in activity and is the drug of choice for oral therapy.
- Usually starting at doses of between 10 and 20 mg daily up to 60 mg daily in severe disease (such as GCA or acute polymyositis).

IA or soft tissue routes

IA methylprednisolone (Depo-Medrone®) or triamcinolone (Kenalog®) is indicated for local inflammation of joints and soft tissues. Hydrocortisone is used for superficial soft tissue injections (e.g. for lateral epicondylitis) to minimize the risk of skin atrophy.

- Usual doses—40 mg for medium-sized joints and 10–20 mg for small joints or tendons.

IM route

- IM methylprednisolone (Depo-Medrone®) is used to treat symptoms related to exacerbations of inflammatory arthritis or to provide some symptom control while starting, changing, or escalating disease-modifying therapy.
- Licensed indication is for 40–80 mg but doses are sometimes administered up to 120 mg based on individual patient assessment.

IV infusion

- Methylprednisolone (Solu-Medrone®) can be administered as an IV infusion to treat exacerbations of inflammatory conditions.
- Dose usually up to maximum of 1 g.

Side effects of steroids

Excessive and/or prolonged glucocorticoids results in Cushing's syndrome:

- Moon face.
- Buffalo hump.
- Hypertension.
- Cataracts.
- Avascular necrosis of femoral head/osteoporosis.
- Thinning of skin.
- Bruising.
- Muscle wasting.
- Poor wound healing.
- Tendency to hyperglycaemia.
- ↑ appetite/↑ abdominal fat/obesity.
- ↑ susceptibility to infection.
- Hirsutism.

Further reading

Buckley L, Guyatt G, Fink HA, et al. (2017). 2017 American College of Rheumatology guideline for the prevention and treatment of glucocorticoid-induced osteoporosis. *Arthritis Rheumatol* 69:1521–37.

Duru N, van der Goes MC, Jacobs JW, et al. (2013). EULAR evidence-based and consensus-based recommendations on the management of medium to high-dose glucocorticoid therapy in rheumatic diseases. *Ann Rheum Dis* 72:1905–13.

New disease-modifying drugs: biologic therapies

In the last 10 years, new drug therapies developed to treat many immune-mediated LTCs have had a significant impact on patient outcomes and healthcare resources. These drugs are referred to as 'biologics' because they were developed using biological engineering. Research identified a number of important components to autoimmune diseases and the cell-to-cell interactions involved in the inflammatory responses and sustained attacks upon the individual's tissues with the resulting destruction of specific tissues (autoimmune disease). There is now a greater understanding of the cell-to-cell interactions along the inflammatory pathways as well as clarity about the acquired (adaptive) and active (innate) immunity which are not so clearly delineated as previously thought, with more of an overlap between acquired and active immunity than previously believed.

The biologics 'targeted' approach mimics the body's normal communication processes and introduces treatments that can block these pathways. A specific example is the development of monoclonal antibodies that can communicate and capture or block important inflammatory messengers (cytokines) before they lock in to a receptor and activate an inflammatory response. In the case of IJDs, specific cytokines have been identified that play a pivotal role in the inflammatory pathway. One of the first conditions to benefit from biologic therapies was RA. Other IJDs have increasingly benefited from this research and evidence continues to grow in a wide range of autoimmune-driven conditions.

Disease-modifying drugs

Three categories

- Conventional (or traditional) DMARDs (cDMARDs).
- Biologic DMARDs (bDMARDs).
- Targeted synthetic DMARDs (tsDMARDs).

The cDMARDs, particularly MTX, have been effective to some degree in suppressing the disease in some IJDs. However, evidence (in RA) has demonstrated that radiological damage continues despite treatment, resulting in loss of function and disability. cDMARDs can be effective for a significant proportion of patients in a disease group (e.g. RA), but for a small group the disease is erosive and progressive and traditional drug therapies fail to suppress the disease.

cDMARD therapies vary in their efficacy, toxicity, and length of time that they are effective. During the course of a person's disease, they can easily have exhausted all traditional therapeutic options yet still have active destructive disease with the resulting symptoms of pain, fatigue, and systemic damage. cDMARDs are significantly cheaper than the cost of newer therapies (e.g. the newest of the cDMARDs, leflunomide, costs <£100 per annum (without any administration or monitoring costs)).

The first generation of bDMARDs uses complex and expensive procedures that involve biologically engineering monoclonal antibodies. As a result, many of these therapies can cost between £8000 and £10,000 per annum, on average per patient (£11,400–£14,200) (➲ see 'Disease-modifying antirheumatic drugs', pp. 452–455).

At the time of publication, the cost of biosimilars for etanercept, infliximab, and rituximab is up to half of the originator drug cost although this may vary from country to country.

Benefits of bDMARDs (evidence in RA)

Patients with aggressive and erosive disease have a range of biologic therapeutic options that can demonstrate:

- Evidence to suggest that bDMARDs can halt and in some cases retard radiographic progression.
- Reduction in the sustained effect of inflammatory mechanisms on endothelial tissues and ↓ risks of cardiovascular disease.
- Large observational studies which have to date demonstrated the overall safety of anti-TNFα.
- Patients treated early with bDMARDs have shown significant benefits with greater disease control, minimal joint damage, and reduction in symptoms (pain and fatigue).

Risks of bDMARDs

- Biologics require a thorough assessment and screening process to reduce risks related to treatment.
- There are clear eligibility criteria for commencing and staying on treatment.

➲ Also see 'Anti-tumour necrosis factor alpha: overview'; refer to individual therapies for specific information on each drug, e.g. ➲ 'Rituximab', p. 496; ➲ 'Abatacept', p. 488; ➲ 'Certolizumab pegol', p. 489; ➲ 'Infections in musculoskeletal conditions', Chapter 13, p. 400.

Examples of bDMARD therapies

The term 'biologic' therapy is a general term used to describe technology that biologically manipulates antibodies to enable them to be used as treatments. The composition of each therapy varies depending upon how the antibodies were developed, and the component parts that make up the antibody design (e.g. fixed and variable chains). The biologic therapies developed for MSCs include:

- Abatacept—fully human fusion protein which selectively modulates the activation of T cells.
- Adalimumab—a human monoclonal antibody which binds to inactive (tissue bound) and biologically active (soluble) TNFα.
- Anakinra—a recombinant form of human antibody. IL-1 receptor agonist (IL-1ra): blocks receptors for IL-1 by actively competing with IL-1 receptors.
- Belimumab is a fully humanized monoclonal antibody directed against soluble B lymphocyte stimulator (BLyS).
- Certolizumab pegol is a recombinant, humanized antibody Fab' fragment against TNFα expressed in *Escherichia coli* and conjugated to polyethylene glycol (PEG).

- Etanercept—a fully human p75 TNF receptor (fusion protein): binds to soluble active TNFα and lymphotoxin A (TNFβ).
- Golimumab is a human IgG1κ monoclonal antibody.
- Infliximab—a chimeric (mouse + human) monoclonal antibody: binds with transmembrane (tissue bound) and biologically active (soluble) TNFα.
- Ixekizumab—a human monoclonal antibody that inhibits the release of proinflammatory cytokines as a result of binding to IL-17A.
- Rituximab—a chimeric (mouse + human) monoclonal antibody binds to extra cellular domain of CD-20 B cells.
- Sarilumab is a human monoclonal antibody selective for the IL-6 receptor.
- Secukinumab is a recombinant fully human monoclonal antibody selective for IL-17A.
- Tocilizumab is a humanized IgG1 monoclonal antibody against the human IL-6 receptor.
- Ustekinumab is a fully human IgG1κ monoclonal antibody to IL-12/23.

Further reading

Ryan S, Oliver S, Brownfield A (2007). *Drug Therapy in Rheumatology Nursing*. Chichester: John Wiley and Sons.

Treatment with biologic therapies: key points

- This topic sets out the current licensed indications for biologic therapies for MSCs.
- Further in-depth information should be sought from the SPC or drug information sheets of each therapy, NICE, and the *BNF* (➔ see 'Further reading', p. 492).

Abatacept licensed MSC indications (IV infusion and subcutaneous administration)

IV licensed for RA co-prescribed with MTX, for PsA alone or in combination with MTX, and in polyarticular JIA in combination with MTX.

Subcutaneously licensed for RA co-prescribed with MTX, for PsA alone, or in combination with MTX.

- IV prescribing is dose dependent on weight: <60 kg, 500 mg; >60 kg and <100 kg, 750 mg; or >100 kg, 1000 mg). Treatment 0-, 2-, then 4-weekly.
- Subcutaneous prescribing 125 mg weekly.

Key treatment considerations include:

- Infusion reactions <1%. Other nursing care issues—at present consider as for other biologic therapies until further clinical experience develops.
- Similar issues to other infusions. Early evidence suggests similar nursing care issues to other biologics until clinical evidence available.
- For subcutaneous administration as for adalimumab but no blood monitoring recommended in SPC. If on MTX, blood monitoring will be required.

➔ Also see 'Abatacept', p. 555.

Adalimumab licensed MSC indications (subcutaneous administration)

Licensed indications for AS and non-radiographic axial spondyloarthritis, PsA, RA, and polyarticular JIA (➔ see Chapter 4, 'Inflammatory joint diseases', pp. 61–126).

- Prescribing dose for musculoskeletal indications of 40 mg once a fortnight.
- Can be administered as a monotherapy when intolerant to MTX.

Key treatment considerations include:

- Mild to moderate injection site reactions—common >10%.
- Risk of emergence of latent infection—including TB.
- Risk of exacerbations of demyelinating diseases—review history.
- Contraindicated in those with moderate to severe heart failure.
- Contraindicated in those with active infections including TB.
- Reactivation of hepatitis B.
- Combination therapy with MTX—unless intolerant of MTX.
- Blood monitoring required if on MTX monthly.
- Avoid live vaccines.

➲ Also see 'Adalimumab', pp. 485–488 and pp. 493–495.

Anakinra licensed MSC indications (subcutaneous administration)

Licensed indication for Still's disease (children and adults):

- Prescribing dose in Still's disease of 100 mg once daily in patients >50 kg; in those weighing <50 kg the starting dose is 1–2 mg/kg/day. Must be prescribed in combination with MTX in RA—a once-a-week dose.
- Should not be co-prescribed with an anti-TNFα therapy.

Key treatment considerations include:

- Neutropenia.
- Similar issues to anti-TNFα therapies although should not be prescribed for those with impaired renal function.
- Note: not recommended by NICE.

Belimumab licensed MSC indications (IV infusion)

Licensed indications as an add-on treatment for active autoantibody-positive SLE in adults who are receiving standard therapy.

- Prescribing dose for SLE is 10 mg/kg on days 0, 14, and 28, and at 4-week intervals thereafter.
- Pretreatment with an antihistamine, with or without an antipyretic.

Key treatment considerations include:

- Hypersensitivity and infusion-related reactions in 0.9% of patients up to several hours after the infusion. The risk is greatest after the first two infusions and therefore patients should remain under clinical supervision for several hours after at least the first two infusions.
- Access to specialist infusion clinics–with resuscitation facilities.

➲ Also see 'Belimumab', pp. 559–561.

Certolizumab pegol licensed MSC indications (subcutaneous administration)

Licensed indications for AS and non-radiographic axial spondyloarthritis, PsA, and RA.

- Prescribing dose of 400 mg as a loading dose at 0, 2, and 4 weeks.
- Maintenance dose in RA 200 mg every 2 weeks (can go to 400 mg every 4 weeks once clinical response is confirmed.
- Maintenance dose in axial spondyloarthritis 200 mg every 2 weeks or 400 mg every 4 weeks.
- Maintenance dose in PsA 200 mg every 2 weeks (can go to 400 mg every 4 weeks once clinical response is confirmed.
- In RA and PsA can be administered as a monotherapy when intolerant to MTX.

Key treatment considerations include:

- As for adalimumab but no blood monitoring recommended in SPC. If on MTX, blood monitoring will be required.

➲ Also see Chapter 16, pp. 455 and 466.

Etanercept licensed MSC indications (subcutaneous administration)

Licensed indications for RA, polyarticular and enthesitis-related JIA, PsA, and AS.

- Prescribing dose 25 mg twice weekly or 50 mg weekly.
- Combination therapy with MTX for RA—unless intolerant of MTX.

Key treatment considerations include:

- As for adalimumab but no blood monitoring recommended in SPC. If on MTX, blood monitoring will be required.

➲ Also see 'Etanercept', pp. 488 and 490.

Golimumab licensed MSC indications (subcutaneous administration)

Licensed indications for AS and non-radiographic axial spondyloarthritis, PsA, and RA.

- Prescribing dose of 50 mg once a month on the same date each month, in patients >100 kg of body weight, ↑ to 100 mg once a month if clinical response is not adequate.
- In RA should be given concomitantly with MTX.

Key treatment considerations include:

- As for adalimumab but no blood monitoring recommended in SPC. If on MTX, blood monitoring will be required.

➲ Also see 'Golimumab', pp. 490–493.

Infliximab licensed MSC indications (IV infusion)

Licensed indications for RA, AS, and PsA. Prescribing dose varies according to indication from 3 mg/kg to 5 mg/kg of body weight.

- Musculoskeletal dosing regimen: 0, 2, 6 weeks then 6–8-weekly thereafter (depending upon indication).
- For RA, it must be co-prescribed with MTX; for PsA, it should be administered with MTX unless intolerant or contraindicated.

Key treatment considerations include:

- Infusion-related reactions—within minutes or hours following infusion (~2% in research evidence vs 9% in placebo). <1% develop severe infusion reactions—rarely necessary to discontinue treatment.
- Blood monitoring for MTX.
- As for adalimumab and etanercept.
- Access to specialist infusion clinics—with resuscitation facilities.

➲ Also see 'Infliximab', p. 567.

Rituximab licensed MSC indications (IV infusion)

Licensed indications for RA and ANCA-associated vasculitis.

- Prescribing dose for RA is 1000 mg infusion (day 1 and day 15) with MTX (once-a-week dose).
- Pretreatment of paracetamol 1000 mg, methylprednisolone 100 mg, and chlorphenamine 10 mg IV.

Key treatment considerations include:

- Allow timings to administer pretreatment infusions (60 min before rituximab).
- Withhold antihypertensive therapies for 12 hours prior to infusion.
- Infusion-related reactions—rituximab 36% vs 30% placebo. Mainly mild to moderate. Infusion reactions in RA are significantly lower in rate and severity to those seen in NHL.
- Access to specialist infusion clinics–with resuscitation facilities.

➲ Also see 'Rituximab', p. 574.

Secukinumab licensed MSC indications (subcutaneous administration)

Licensed indications for AS and PsA.

- Prescribing dose for AS and PsA (without moderate to severe plaque psoriasis) of 150 mg at weeks 0, 1, 2, 3, and 4 then monthly. In PsA with moderate to severe plaque psoriasis, 300 mg at above-mentioned intervals.
- In PsA alone or in combination with MTX.

Key treatment considerations include:

- As for adalimumab but no blood monitoring recommended in SPC. If on MTX, blood monitoring will be required.

➲ Also see 'Secukinumab', pp. 485–487.

Tocilizumab licensed MSC indications (IV infusion and subcutaneous administration)

IV licensed for RA and in polyarticular JIA, in combination with MTX unless unable to tolerate or if continued MTX treatment is inappropriate.

SC licensed for RA co-prescribed with MTX (unless unable to tolerate) and for giant cell arteritis in combination with tapering glucocorticoids.

- IV prescribing dose dependent on weight: 8 mg/kg once every 4 weeks (maximum dose 800 mg per infusion in patients >100 kg of body weight) Dose adjustment if abnormal liver enzyme abnormalities and/or low absolute neutrophil count (see SPC for full details or BSR/BHPR guidelines). In JIA, the dose in patients >2 years of age is 8 mg/kg once every 4 weeks in patients weighing ≥30 kg; or 10 mg/kg once every 4 weeks in patients weighing <30 kg.
- SC prescribing of 162 mg weekly.

Key treatment considerations include:

- Infusion reactions <1%. Other nursing care issues—at present consider as for other biologic therapies until further clinical experience develops.
- Similar issues to other infusions. Early evidence suggests similar nursing care issues to other biologics until clinical evidence available.
- Caution in diverticulitis.
- Dose reduction if liver enzyme test abnormalities and/or low absolute neutrophil count as recommended in SPC and BSR guidance. If on MTX, blood monitoring will be required.
- Check serum lipids at 3 months, treat if abnormal; repeat at clinician's discretion.

➲ Also see 'Tocilizumab', p. 578.

Further reading

BNF: https://bnf.nice.org.uk/

BSR: https://www.rheumatology.org.uk

Holroyd CR, Seth R, Bukhari M, et al. (2019). The British Society for Rheumatology biologic DMARD safety guidelines in inflammatory arthritis. *Rheumatology (Oxford)* 58:220–6.

NICE: https://www.nice.org.uk

Royal College of Nursing (2017). *Assessing, Managing and Monitoring Biologic Therapies for Inflammatory Arthritis*, 4th edn. London: RCN.

Summaries of Product Characteristics: http://www.medicines.org.uk

Anti-tumour necrosis factor alpha: overview

TNFα is an important proinflammatory cytokine (chemical messenger) implicated in MSCs such as RA and other IJDs. TNFα is considered to be the pivotal cytokine that starts the process of an inflammatory cascade within the immune system. TNFα is released from an activated T cell to start the process of an inflammatory response. By blocking this cytokine and preventing it 'locking into' key receptors, the inflammatory pathway cannot be activated effectively.

Five therapeutic options have been developed to block the mechanism of action of TNFα. These are:

- Adalimumab (Humira®), a subcutaneously administered therapy.
- Certolizumab pegol (Cimzia®), a subcutaneously administered therapy.
- Etanercept (Benepali®, Enbrel®), a subcutaneously administered therapy.
- Golimumab (Simponi®), a subcutaneously administered therapy.
- Infliximab (Flixabi®, Infectra®, Remicade®, Remsima®), delivered as an infusion every 8 weeks (once stabilized on treatment).

➲ Also see 'Infliximab (IV infusion)', p. 567; ➲ 'Adalimumab licensed indications (subcutaneous administration)', pp. 488–489 and 549; ➲ 'Etanercept licensed indications (subcutaneous administration)', p. 490 and pp. 549–550.

What is anti-TNFα?

All five current anti-TNFα therapies are developed from biotechnology using monoclonal antibodies.

Issues in treatment with anti-TNFα therapy

A national register in the UK collects evidence to examine the safety and efficacy of biologic therapies (BSR Biologics Register).[1] Screening and treatment eligibility criteria for anti-TNFα therapies have been developed for AS, JIA, PsA, and RA.[2]

➲ Also see 'Assessing the patient', Chapter 8, pp. 290–291; ➲ 'Clinical examination and history taking', Chapter 8, pp. 294–297.

Treatment is contraindicated if there is evidence of:

- Active infections. Screening for infections (bacterial, viral, or fungal) including prior contact with/or immunization against TB must be reviewed and discussed with prescribing physician. Note: remember to check for any current or recent sepsis of prosthetic joints.
- Moderate to severe heart failure. New York Heart Association (NYHA) class III/IV.
- Pregnant or breastfeeding.

Caution for patients who have:

- Caution for mild heart failure (NYHA class I/II).
- Demyelinating disorders—caution in those with pre-existing or recent-onset CNS demyelinating disorders.

- Caution for those prone to infections, e.g. chronic leg ulcers, persistent chest infections, and indwelling catheters.
- Patient who are positive for hepatitis B virus—guidelines advise a risk/benefit assessment should be undertaken. Biologic therapy may be appropriate if antiviral treatment is given. Liaise closely with hepatologist. Refer to BSR guidelines.[3]
- Hepatitis C—appears to show no deterioration in hepatitis or viral load following treatment.
- HIV infections—cannot be advised at present; minimal evidence available.
- Caution in patients with COPD or ↑ risk of malignancies due to heavy smoking.

Cautions in patients who have a prior history of malignancy (<10 years). International observational data will inform the debate about malignancy. Discuss with prescribing physician.

Screening patients

- Fulfils eligibility criteria, patient consents to treatment, and data collection for the BSR Biologics Register.[1]
- No contraindications as outlined earlier. Any areas of cautions, review and discuss with prescribing physician and patient.
- Screen for TB and risks related to prior TB contact or travel to areas of high risk, TB history, and prior immunization.[4]
  - Undertake screening as indicated and according to identified risks. Patients may require treatment if at high risk or suboptimal treatment in the past.
  - Chest X-ray if not undertaken in last 6 months or repeat if index of suspicion for infections or lung disease.
- Blood pressure, weight, and normal blood monitoring profile prior to commencement of therapy.
- Co-prescribed MTX:
  - Evidence suggests optimal response when co-prescribed.
  - Reduces risks of neutralizing antibodies against the monoclonal antibody therapy.
- Note history of atophy or previous allergic reactions—discuss with prescribing physician if patient has a history or severe allergic reactions.
- Preliminary observational data suggest anti-TNFα drugs are reassuring. Certolizumab pegol licence advocates using in pregnancy and breastfeeding if there is a clinical need. However, the patient should discuss their plans and evidence before making an informed decision about their treatment plans.
- Immunization status—if appropriate, update immunizations before starting treatment.
- Full patient assessment regarding consent and follow-up management including awareness of responsibilities to monitor and report any infections.

RA eligibility criteria for anti-TNFα therapy

- Fulfils diagnostic criteria for diagnosis of RA (ACR 1987 criteria).
- Active RA with a DAS28 joint count score >5.1.[2]
  - Disease has not responded to intensive therapy with a combination of conventional DMARDs.

For full details of treatment criteria and specific drug therapies refer to NICE guidance.[2,5]

➲ See Chapter 4, 'Rheumatoid arthritis', pp. 62–78.
➲ Also see Chapter 17, 'Blood tests and investigations', p. 505.

References

1. British Society for Rheumatology Biologics Register: https://www.bsrbr.org
2. NICE (2016). Adalimumab, etanercept, infliximab, certolizumab pegol, golimumab, tocilizumab and abatacept for rheumatoid arthritis not previously treated with DMARDs or after conventional DMARDs only have failed (TA195). https://www.nice.org.uk/guidance/ta195
3. Holroyd CR, Seth R, Bukhari M, et al. (2019). The British Society for Rheumatology biologic DMARD safety guidelines in inflammatory arthritis. *Rheumatology (Oxford)* 58:220–6.
4. British Thoracic Society Guidelines (2005): https://www.brit-thoracic.org.uk
5. NICE (2016). Tuberculosis (NG33). https://www.nice.org.uk/guidance/ng33

B-cell (CD-20) depletion therapies

B lymphocytes are a vital component of our immune system. T and B lymphocytes act in different ways to enable an appropriate immune response. B cells have a synergistic effect with T cells and are identified as playing a role in:

- T-cell activation and expansion.
- Production of antibodies such as RF and anti-CCP.
- Production of proinflammatory cytokines (TNFα), IL-6, and lymphotoxin.

B cells develop in sequential steps, from stem cells through to plasma cells that produce antibodies (immunoglobulins). B cells proliferate and when fully developed have the capacity to react to antigens and produce plasma membrane-bound antibodies. B cells that produce antibodies are in effect the memory of the immune system, recognizing and creating a specific antibody response to antigen attacks. This results in a faster and more targeted response when further exposed to the antigen.

Cell surface markers are expressed on precursor B cells. One of these markers, CD-20, is the focus of B-cell depletion therapy. Rituximab depletes B cells with the CD-20 marker, disabling those cells and reducing the B cells that produce antibodies. This approach does not compromise the patient's immune system as stem cells and plasma cells are unaffected. Rituximab has shown sustained benefits for RA patients with a reduction in radiological evidence, signs, and symptoms, and a good safety profile. Rituximab is the only licensed B-cell depletion therapy available. MabThera® is the originator drug. There are currently two biosimilars e.g. (Rixathon® and Truxima®) which although are generated in a different way work similarly to MabThera®.

➲ See 'Biosimilars', Chapter 18, pp. 538–540 and 533.

What is rituximab?

Rituximab is an anti-CD-20 B-cell depletion therapy developed as a monoclonal antibody. It is biologically engineered from part chimeric and part human antibody.

Rituximab in the treatment of MSCs

Rituximab has a long history in the treatment of non-Hodgkin's lymphoma (NHL). Early evidence has demonstrated that the level of infusion-related reactions is significantly lower in patients with IJD compared to NHL:

- RA: 30–35% first infusion reactions—severe infusion reactions are uncommon and rarely lead to withdrawal.
- NHL infusion-related reactions: >75% first infusion reactions:
  - Hypotension and bronchospasm seen in >10% of patients.
  - Cytokine release syndrome is rare (<10%) and occurs in association with load of anti-rituximab antibodies. This can be a delayed reaction 2–3 weeks after first dose and is managed with steroids.

Treatment

It is recommended in RA as a combination therapy with a once-weekly dose of MTX and administered as an IV infusion. It can also be used in combination with glucocorticoids for treating ANCA-associated vasculitis (➲ see 'Rituximab', Chapter 18, p. 574).

Although in routine clinical it is used for refractory SLE, NICE approval is limited to RA and ANCA-associated vasculitis.

Eligibility criteria

Patients with RA who have been treated with an anti-TNFα will have undertaken a rigorous screening process. If patients are being considered for rituximab without prior screening such as in ANCA-associated vasculitis or prior TNFα, a review of eligibility and screening criteria using the SPC and local guidelines should be adhered to.

- Severe active RA—adults only who have had an inadequate response or intolerance of other DMARDs including one TNF inhibitor.
- Adults with ANCA-associated vasculitis in combination with glucocorticoids, to induce remission, when cyclophosphamide is contraindicated, not tolerated, or the maximum cumulative dose has been reached. It can also be used in active or progressive disease despite a cyclophosphamide course lasting 3–6 months or if the patient has uroepithelial malignancy.

➲ Also see 'Anti-tumour necrosis factor alpha: overview', pp. 493–495; ➲ 'Treatment with biologic therapies: key points', pp. 488–492.

Treatment continuation criteria

In RA, treatment should be continued only if there is an adequate response following initiation of therapy and if an adequate response is maintained following retreatment with a dosing interval of at least 6 months. An adequate response is defined as an improvement in disease activity score (DAS28) of 1.2 points or more. Retreatment in ANCA-associated vasculitis is not defined in the SPC or NICE guidance.

Rituximab treatment issues that need to be considered

- Optimal treatment benefits are seen in patients who have seropositive RA.
- Currently there are no DAS28 criteria for commencing treatment but NICE criteria state use in severe active RA and that retreatment requires a DAS improvement of 1.2 or more.
- Anti-TNFα failure patients do not require additional TB screening prior to starting rituximab.
- Clinical history and screening to exclude chronic or recurrent infections/allergies. History of atophy should be noted prior to infusion.
- Review co-morbidity risk factors, e.g. cardiovascular and pulmonary disease.
- Viral hepatitis screening is recommended to monitor immunoglobulin levels and CD-19 levels, baseline and with each treatment cycle.

- Immunization (inactivated)—administer 1 month prior to treatment or 7 months after infusion provided B cells are detectable. Live vaccines should not be administered.
- Check concordance and prescription for MTX.

Questions and evolving issues

- Timing of DAS to evaluate response to rituximab not specified by NICE.
- Benefit of rituximab in other autoimmune diseases is available from uncontrolled studies, e.g. Sjögren's syndrome.
- During the first year, the serious infection risk is the same for rituximab and a second TNF inhibitor. The period of risk for rituximab should be 6 months or longer after last exposure. See 'Further reading'.

Further reading

British Society for Rheumatology Biologics Register: https://www.bsrbr.org

NICE (2014). Rituximab in combination with glucocorticoids for treating anti-neutrophil cytoplasmic antibody-associated vasculitis (TA308). https://www.nice.org.uk/Guidance/TA308

NICE (2016). Adalimumab, etanercept, infliximab, certolizumab pegol, golimumab, tocilizumab and abatacept for rheumatoid arthritis not previously treated with DMARDs or after conventional DMARDs only have failed (TA195). https://www.nice.org.uk/guidance/ta195

Silva-Fernandez L, De Cock D, Lunt M, et al. (2017). Serious infection risk after 1 year between patients with rheumatoid arthritis treated with rituximab or with a second TNF inhibitor after initial TNFi failure: resulted from the BSR Biologics Register for RA. *Rheumatology (Oxford)* 57:1533–40.

New biologic disease-modifying therapies

There is an intense interest in new therapies for MSCs following experiences with biologic treatments. These therapies have transformed the lives of patients and, importantly, have provided researchers with a greater insight into the disease themselves and how they can advance treatments based upon the knowledge gained.

The pace of research into further therapeutic options continues while national and international biologics registries regularly review observational data on safety and efficacy of licensed biologic therapies. These registries together with expert guidance documents produced by professional working groups and data surveillance by the pharmaceutical industry enhance our knowledge of the licensed therapies and inform us of ongoing pretreatment and monitoring issues.

The future challenge will be to develop therapies that can reduce the not insignificant costs related to producing biologics. bDMARDs are administered by the subcutaneous or IV route adding to the costs of treatment. More recently, targeted synthetic biologics have received marketing authorization to treat rheumatological conditions. Equally, the introduction of more biosimilars over time will provide less costly options for the clinician to consider.

More recently, oral tsDMARDs including apremilast, baricitinib, and tofacitinib are being used in clinical practice.

Follow-up care for those on biologic disease-modifying antirheumatic drugs

Generally speaking, patients who start bDMARDs gain a therapeutic benefit significantly greater than traditional therapies. These benefits appear to lift the sense of fatigue and reduce the pain—enabling patients to participate in normal ADLs. Biologics also reduce radiological progression (again, generally greater than those seen with cDMARDs). Observational registries (designed as research projects, to explore safety and efficacy of biologic therapies) have developed internationally. The UK BSR Biologics Register currently has a registry for RA and AS with a proposed registry for PsA soon to be implemented. It regularly publishes preliminary data.[1]

Examples of preliminary evidence published to date demonstrate:

- Patients with RA have an ↑ risk of myocardial infarction compared to those without RA. In the medium term, RA patients treated with TNFα have a significantly ↓ risk of MI compared with RA patients treated with cDMARDs.
- Pregnancy—early evidence appears to show that these therapies are not linked to infant mortality, deformity, or premature birth.[2] Please refer to the SPC for each individual biologic. ➲ See 'Pregnancy and long-term conditions', Chapter 14, pp. 419–421.
- In the RA patient group—the annual recurrent serious infections rate while treated with a biologic (cDMARD, TNFα, rituximab/tocilizumab) was estimated as 4.6% with respiratory tract infections being the most common. Those that experienced serious infection were generally older, seropositive, and steroid users and had a higher disability at baseline (assessed by the Health Assessment Questionnaire).
- Infections—↑ risk of skin and soft tissue infections. Some of the infections are food borne (e.g. *Listeria, Salmonella*).
- Infections—re-emergence of latent TB seen. Higher proportion of extra pulmonary presentations of TB. Lower rates seen with etanercept and rituximab compared to adalimumab and infliximab. However, recent evidence in the UK suggests rigorous screening approaches have reduced these rates in recent years.[2,3]
- Malignancy—incidence of malignancy remains difficult to interpret because patients with aggressive RA treated with cDMARDs have an ↑ malignancy rate; early data states that the addition of TNFα to cDMARDs does not alter the risk of cancer in RA patients selected for TNFα in the UK.
- Mortality data—it is known that patients with RA have a reduced life expectancy. Early follow-up of RA patients treated with anti-TNFα therapies still show this reduced life expectancy (compared to the general population). ♂ standard mortality rates of 1.99 and ♀ of 1.72. However, this reflects the reduced life expectancy seen in the pre-biologics era.
- Interstitial lung disease (ILD)—patients who have baseline ILD appear to show strong predictive trends that show ↑ all-cause mortality regardless

of treatment with anti-TNFα. However, those with ILD treated with anti-TNFα have higher mortality rates.

There are important issues to be considered from the patient's and HCP's point of view in follow-up care. However, patients can feel so well that occasionally they can forget the important safety issues while on treatment.

Patient responsibilities include:

- Having ready access to a telephone advice line or details of a first point of contact person in the event of a problem with treatment.
- Ensuring that they get prompt treatment of any infections.
- Attending for review appointments and blood monitoring requirements.
- Carrying a biologic 'alert card' to advise HCPs (including dentists, chiropodists, etc.) that they are receiving a treatment that significantly impairs their immunological response.
- Remembering to avoid live vaccines and plan their immunization strategies carefully with healthcare teams.
- Discuss family planning and contraception with the rheumatology team. See the SPC for each biologic therapy and for any concomitant medication such as MTX.[2]
- Avoidance of consumption of pâtés, unpasteurized milk, mould-ripened cheese, feta/goat's cheese, or raw foods (such as eggs) as an ↑ risk of opportunistic infections.
- Consideration of sunscreens and sun protection (↑ risk of skin melanomas particularly for PsA patients who have already been exposed to PUVA (psoralen plus ultraviolet A light) therapy).
- If co-prescribed with MTX, they should stay on treatment or discuss with their doctor or nurse before stopping their co-prescription.
- They may need to stop treatment a few weeks before surgery.
- That they remain on treatment providing they continue to fulfil the treatment criteria (benefit of treatment has to be demonstrated usually using the DAS 28).

The HCP's responsibilities include:

- Enabling patients to understand their treatment options throughout the course of their disease.
- Provision of an alert card and a first point of contact number for those on biologics.
- Provision of expert support and advice for other non-specialist practitioners in relation to patients receiving bDMARDs.
- Ensuring that the patient fulfils the eligibility criteria (or clinical need/ exception are documented in the notes).
- Documentation of assessments, eligibility, and treatment continuation criteria.
- Undertaking of regular reviews and reassessment of treatment benefit as outlined by NICE and national guidelines.[2]
- Reviewing blood monitoring and assess patients' general health prior to receiving treatment. If care is delivered by supporting organizations/1° care teams, build effective communication strategies to support review of patients' general health status and safety issues.

- Reiteration of safety messages and review patient knowledge on additional information needs in relation to:
  - A patient's general knowledge about their disease.
  - Specific information needs about biologics.
- If treatment fails, ensure patients are provided with up-to-date evidence-based information and advice on further treatment options or the next steps in their care.

References

1. British Society for Rheumatology Biologics Register: https://www.bsrbr.org
2. Flint J, Panchal S, Hurrell A, et al. (2016). BSR and BHPR guideline on prescribing drugs in pregnancy and breastfeeding—part I: standard and biologic disease modifying anti-rheumatic drugs and corticosteroids. *Rheumatology (Oxford)* 55:1693–7.
3. Royal College of Nursing (2017). *Assessing, Managing and Monitoring Biologic Therapies for Inflammatory Arthritis*, 4th edn. London: RCN.

Further reading

BNF: https://bnf.nice.org.uk/
BSR: https://www.rheumatology.org.uk
Summaries of Product Characteristics: https://www.medicines.org.uk

See also Chapter 14, p. 415.

Frequently asked questions

It seems like there are many more risks related to bDMARDs than a cDMARD is that right?

cDMARDs generally have stood the test of time and we know their strengths and weaknesses. They are not without risks but generally are less efficacious in the sense of reducing radiological progression and improving symptoms related to the disease compared to the newer biologics. Those who receive prompt treatment, particularly before joint damage has occurred, gain significant benefit.

Biologics are fairly new to clinical practice, they are currently categorized as black triangle therapies—that is, intensively monitored in order to confirm the risk/benefit profile of the products and require detailed reporting of any adverse events. However, it is important to know that the cell-to-cell interactions in blocking the inflammatory response are much more specifically targeted and ∴ the risks related to immunosuppression are probably greater. A high index of suspicion with patients presenting with infections/problems should be maintained. Seek medical advice if in doubt.

Will there be more of these more targeted biologics in the future?

Yes. There is ↑ recognition in many autoimmune LTCs that these biologic and more specifically targeted therapies are here to stay. Research in the development of these therapies and what we have learnt in using the treatments have helped us understand much more about the different disease mechanisms and the complex immune responses. We now understand that cytokines work like hormones and communicate with many other chemical 'messengers' that communicate with each other, sustaining inflammation.

Why is MTX co-prescribed with so many of the biologics?

Evidence in clinical trials and confirmed in clinical practice demonstrate that MTX enhances the effect of the biologics. This is because the biologics are monoclonal antibodies and the body can develop autoimmune responses to the monoclonal antibody itself. These responses to the biologic monoclonal antibody can be significantly reduced when co-prescribed with MTX. If antichimeric antibodies develop, they reduce the therapeutic benefit of the treatment.

Chapter 17

Blood tests and investigations

Investigation of the blood

Baseline investigations usually consist of a FBC, biochemical investigations, measurement of inflammatory markers, and an immunological screen.

Blood tests may be requested when a MSC is suspected; blood analysis can help to support the diagnosis. In many cases, positive results may aid (but not confirm) diagnosis. In the same light, negative results may not rule out a diagnosis. For example, the presence or absence of RF in the blood does not confirm or exclude the diagnosis of RA; it simply can act as one of many important prognostic indicators for disease severity. ~15% of the population are RF positive yet do not have an IJD and only 70–80% of the RA population are RF positive. In early disease, RF occurs less frequently. More recently, the anti-CCP test is recognized as the gold standard rather than RF. Anti-CCP antibodies are strongly predictive in the diagnosis of RA.

➲ See 'Autoimmune profiles', p. 513, for further discussion.

➲ See also 'Rheumatoid arthritis', Chapter 4, pp. 64–78.

Why do blood tests?

It is important to assess a FBC, renal function, and liver function before commencing medication to consider issues of pharmacokinetics (how the body deals with drugs) and pharmacodynamics (the likely effects a drug has on the body) as these will influence the drug choice or the dose prescribed.

When a diagnosis has been established and treatment has begun, blood tests are often required to monitor disease activity, assess efficacy of treatment, and to screen for unwanted, potentially life-threatening adverse drug reactions (➲ see Chapter 16, 'Pharmacological management: disease-modifying drugs', p. 452).

This section describes the most commonly requested investigations for MSCs, but it is not a comprehensive account of all the tests used in clinical practice.

- To establish a comprehensive clinical picture or fulfil diagnostic criteria. For example, if someone is seropositive for HLA B27—present in 95% of Caucasian patients with a diagnosis of AS. The result only has value if the history and clinical picture fits with the diagnosis. It should not be considered diagnostic but adds to the clinical picture.
- To aid in proactive management of early disease, e.g. to identify patients with non-specific joint problems, and before obvious clinical signs of an inflammatory disease can be confirmed, e.g. the use of anti-CCP has enabled early detection of those who have joint problems that might evolve into RA. This supports the 'treat to target' approach to management.[1]
- To identify prognostic indicators, e.g. high positive RF titres supported by evidence of joint erosions on X-ray or US are linked to poorer long-term outcomes for patients with RA. Anti-CCP can predict early erosive disease in RA.
- Adherence to treatment criteria, e.g. hypercholesterolaemia and treatment with statins.

- To address pharmacokinetics/pharmacodynamics issues that may affect drug dose or choice of drug, e.g. mild impairment of the renal function may alter the choice of drug if excreted via the kidneys or warrant a change of therapeutic approach or more rigorous monitoring regimens (e.g. NSAIDs). An estimated glomerular filtration rate is used to measure renal impairment.
- To evaluate current baseline status of other co-morbidities prior to starting treatment.
- As an early indicator of toxicity or side effects related to blood or organ functions.
- Enables an ongoing review of disease control and efficacy of treatment.

➔ See Chapter 16, 'Pharmacological management: disease-modifying drugs', p. 452.

Reference

1. NICE (2018). Rheumatoid arthritis in adults: diagnosis and management. Evidence review C: treat to target. https://www.nice.org.uk/guidance/ng100/evidence/c-treattotarget-pdf-4903172320

Further reading

Ledingham J, Gullick N, Irving K, et al. (2017). BSR and BHPR guidelines for the prescription and monitoring of non-biologic disease-modifying anti-rheumatic drugs. *Rheumatology (Oxford)* 56:865–8.

Watts R, Clunie G, Hall F, Marshall T (eds) (2011). Investigation of rheumatic diseases. In: *Oxford Desk Reference: Rheumatology*, pp. 23–46. Oxford: Oxford University Press.

Haematological investigations

Full blood count

The most common laboratory test is the FBC (Table 17.1) to examine different components of the blood, including red cells (erythrocytes), white cells (leucocytes), and platelets (thrombocytes). Blood test results are best interpreted based upon the reference levels of the laboratory that performed the tests

Haemoglobin

Measurement of Hb estimates the oxygen-bearing capacity of the RBCs. Anaemia (a low Hb level) is an important measure to consider in reviewing blood results. Smoking can ↑ Hb levels.

Anaemia

- Common feature in inflammatory conditions such as RA.
- Sometimes attributed to disease activity—anaemia of chronic disease.
- Anaemia may be as a result of an unwanted effect of medication or a combination of the disease and treatments, e.g. anaemia may be caused by GI bleeding from NSAIDs taken for pain relief. In young ♀, the most common cause is heavy menstrual loss.

Mean corpuscular volume (MCV)

This is a measure of the average size of RBCs. In patients with anaemia, the MCV classifies either microcytic anaemia, where MCV falls below the normal range, or macrocytic anaemia, where the MCV is above the normal range. The MCV may aid the clinician diagnostically, e.g.:

- A raised MCV may be related to vitamin B_{12} deficiency.
- A low MCV can be associated with thalassemia or iron deficiency.

Table 17.1 Normal FBC values

	♂	♀	Unit
Hb	13.5–18.0	11.5–16.4	g/dL
RBC count	4.5–6.5	3.9–5.6	$\times 10^{12}$/L
Haematocrit	0.40–0.54	0.36–0.47	Ratio
Mean corpuscular volume	78–96	78–96	fL
Platelet count	150–400	150–400	$\times 10^{9}$/L
WBC count	4.0–11.0	4.0–11.0	$\times 10^{9}$/L
Differential			
Neutrophils	2.0–7.5	2.0–7.5	$\times 10^{9}$/L
Lymphocytes	1.5–4.0	1.5–3.0	$\times 10^{9}$/L
Monocytes	0.2–0.8	0.2–0.8	$\times 10^{9}$/L
Eosinophils	0.04–0.4	0.04–0.4	$\times 10^{9}$/L
Basophils	<0.1–0.3	0–0.3	$\times 10^{9}$/L

White blood cell count

Leucocytes or WBCs develop in the bone marrow and lymph nodes. They are part of the body's defence mechanism against infectious disease and foreign materials. The number of white cells in the blood is often an indicator of the status of the immune responses. WBCs may also be affected by diseases or infections. Corticosteroids also raise the WBC count. The WBC count measures the total number of WBCs and estimates the numbers of each type of white cell, known as the differential count; these are:

- Neutrophils—defend against bacterial or fungal infection and inflammatory processes.
- Eosinophils—combat parasitic infections and control mechanisms associated with allergy.
- Basophils—are responsible for allergic response by releasing histamine.
- Monocytes—have a similar function to neutrophils but they have a longer life cycle. They also present pathogens to T cells, allowing the antibody response to begin.
- Lymphocytes—include:
  - B cells, which produce antibodies and react with pathogens to enable their destruction.
  - T cells, which help to coordinate the immune response.
  - Natural killer (NK) cells, which refer to a specific function rather than a specific cell type. NK cells can respond to and kill cells displaying signals of being infected by a virus or which have become cancerous.
- Raised WBC counts (leucocytosis) can be present during infection and are sometimes seen in active inflammatory conditions such as RA and gout.
- A low WBC count (leucopenia) can occur in certain conditions such as SLE or Felty's syndrome, or as a result of drug therapy.

➲ Also see 'Connective tissue diseases', p. 127.

Platelet count

Platelets are nuclear disc-shaped bodies circulating in the blood and are involved in the blood clotting process.

- Thrombocytosis (an ↑ platelet level). Although common in active RA, it is not associated with ↑ incidence of thrombotic events.
- Thrombocytopenia (a ↓ platelet count) is a feature of conditions such as Felty's syndrome and SLE. Thrombocytopenia can also occur as the result of drug therapy.

➲ Also see Chapter 16, 'Pharmacological management: disease-modifying antirheumatic drugs', p. 452.

Biochemical investigations

Liver function tests

LFTs are designed to indicate the state of hepatic function. Some laboratories may perform different groups of liver enzymes to others and ranges of values may vary. Refer to local laboratories to confirm normal ranges. Elevations of LFTs may be expressed as multiples of the upper limit of normal (e.g. three times upper limit of normal).

Baseline LFTs are essential to identify any prior hepatic disease which could potentially reduce drug metabolism and ↑ the risk of drug toxicity.

Alanine transaminase (ALT)

- Also called serum glutamic pyruvic transaminase (SGPT)
- Enzyme present in liver cells.
- Most sensitive indicator of liver injury (rather than biliary obstruction). When a liver cell is damaged it leaks this enzyme into the blood (Box 17.1).

Aspartate transaminase (AST)

- Also called serum glutamic oxaloacetic transaminase (SGOT)
- Enzyme that can be ↑ with liver damage. AST ↑ with MI.
- Usually very high in hepatocellular diseases such as viral hepatitis.

Alkaline phosphatase (ALP)

- Enzyme found in the biliary ducts.
- Can be ↑ with biliary obstructions but also ↑ with a number of inflammatory conditions.
- ALP is also present in bone and high levels are present in Paget's disease, fractures, and other diseases affecting the bones such as metastases (Box 17.1).

Box 17.1 Causes of high/low levels of some liver enzymes

Causes of high ALT

- Cirrhosis.
- Alcohol abuse.
- Congestive cardiac failure (hepatic congestion).
- Liver damage (drug induced) or hepatitis B or C.
- Medication.

Causes of low ALT

- Low ALT levels are rarely seen and usually insignificant.
- ❶ Note: strenuous exercise may cause elevation.

Causes of high ALP

- Bone disease—tumours, fractures, osteomyelitis, Paget's disease.
- Liver disease—liver tumours, biliary obstruction, cirrhosis.

Causes of low ALP

- Low ALP levels are rarely seen and usually insignificant.
- Note ALP specificity.

Total bilirubin (TBIL)

- ↑ levels of bilirubin can be present in various anaemias and reflect deficiencies in bilirubin metabolism such as cirrhosis or obstruction of the bile ducts

Gamma glutamyltranspeptidase (GGT)

- May be elevated even in minor levels of hepatic dysfunction or as a result of a number of non-specific causes.
- Mild levels of raised GGT can also be seen in inflammatory conditions such as SLE or RA.
- High levels of GGT can be associated with alcohol toxicity or liver disease.
- ❶ Grossly haemolysed bloods will produce spurious liver function results. ALP levels ↑ slowly with storage; preferably analyse on day of collection.

Renal function

Plasma concentrations of creatinine, urea, and the electrolytes (potassium, sodium, chloride, and bicarbonate) are useful indicators of kidney function. Creatinine is a sensitive estimator of function; raised creatinine can indicate renal damage although a calculated glomerular filtration rate expressed as mL/min gives a more precise indication of the state of the kidneys and is advocated for routine monitoring.

Renal disease potentially reduces the excretion of drugs. Kidney function deteriorates with age and caution should be applied when prescribing drug therapies or monitoring treatments for the older person where ↓ renal excretion can ↑ the potential for toxicities. Some therapies have an ↑ risk of nephrotoxicity and require extra vigilance in management and when monitoring.

Further reading

McGhee M (2014). *A Guide to Laboratory Investigations*, 6th edn. London: Radcliffe Publishing.

Inflammatory markers

The measurement of inflammatory markers in the blood, ESR, CRP, and PV can be very useful in assessing the activity of inflammatory diseases. ESR/CRP is an essential component of a DAS used in RA. All of these acute phase proteins ↑ in concentration in serum a few hours after initiation of an inflammatory process/injury. They are a class of proteins that derive from the liver as a response to injury/inflammation. The plasma concentrations respond to tissue injury, e.g. infection, trauma, malignancy, or inflammation.

➲ Also see 'Inflammatory joint disease: assessing the disease', Chapter 4, p. 62.

C-reactive protein

CRP is an acute phase plasma protein produced by the liver. CRP levels can rise to very high levels (>120 mg/L) after injury or during an inflammatory process. This is due to a rise in the plasma concentrations of IL-6, which is produced in macrophages, endothelial cells, and T cells. CRP is used as a marker of inflammation, and is useful in monitoring disease activity, but it must be remembered that CRP can be elevated in many conditions—including viral and bacterial infections. Fluctuations in CRP levels occur more quickly than in other markers of inflammation.

- Normal value: 0–10 mg/L.

Erythrocyte sedimentation rate

ESR is a non-specific measure of inflammation; levels are slightly higher in:

- Elderly people.
- People with anaemia.
- Black people.

The test uses anticoagulated blood placed in an upright test tube. The rate at which the RBCs fall is measured in mm/hour. If an inflammatory process is present, the ↑ fibrinogen levels cause the RBCs to clump together (rouleaux formation) and settle faster.

ESR can be elevated in inflammatory arthropathies such as RA, temporal arteritis, and PMR. ESR can also be elevated in bacterial infection and malignancies.

A general rule of thumb for the upper limit of normal value of ESR is

- ♂ = age in years divided by 2.
- ♀ = age in years plus 10 divided by 2.

Plasma viscosity

PV is another sensitive but non-specific marker of inflammation, which provides similar information to ESR. There is no specific difference in values between ♂ and ♀. PV results are not affected by anaemia (unlike ESR). PV:

- ↑ in parallel to ESR but is not affected by anaemia or by delay in analysis.
- Not affected by sex **but** is affected by age, exercise, and pregnancy.
- Some rheumatologists prefer to use PV as its sensitivity and specificity is better than ESR and CRP in discriminating between active and quiescent disease.
- Normal value: 1.50–1.72 mPa.

Further reading

McGhee M (2014). *A Guide to Laboratory Investigations*, 6th edn. London: Radcliffe Publishing.

Autoimmune profiles

Antibodies are proteins produced by WBCs to defend the body against toxins such as viruses and bacteria. Autoantibodies, instead of attacking the toxins, attack the body's own cells. Autoimmune diseases, such as RA, SS, systemic sclerosis, and SLE, are associated with circulating autoantibodies. However, these autoantibodies can also be found in healthy individuals. Autoantibodies are sometimes detected many years before the onset of signs and symptoms of disease.

Autoimmune screening includes:

Rheumatoid factor

RF is typically an IgM/IgG immunoglobulin complex found in about 70% of patients with RA at disease onset, and a further 10–15% becomes RF positive within the first 2 years. Such patients are said to be seropositive. However, the absence of RF in the serum does not exclude a diagnosis of RA, and those patients without RF are referred to as seronegative.

RF is present in about 5–15% of the general healthy population, and can be found in other conditions including SLE, SS, chronic liver disease, and acute viral infection, for example.

RA patients who are seropositive are likely to have more aggressive disease, with an ↑ risk of developing extra-articular manifestations.

Anti-CCP antibodies

The autoantibody anti-CCP should be tested in patients suspected of having RA. Anti-CCP may be detected in 50–60% of those presenting with early signs of RA. It appears that anti-CCP may pre-date arthritis symptoms by several years. The predictive value in early disease is of particular importance: ~85% of those positive for anti-CCP and RF will develop RA. In early RA, anti-CCP positive antibodies are strongly predictive of erosive disease. Optimal outcomes are achieved if these patients receive prompt DMARD therapy before irreversible joint damage occurs. This is an important test to be used in early arthritis clinics.

Anti-nuclear antibodies

ANAs (also known as antinuclear factor (ANF)) are antibodies that can attack the nucleus of cells. These antibodies are present in higher numbers than normal in autoimmune diseases, particularly in SLE.

The ANA test is requested when SLE or other autoimmune diseases such as SS are suspected. A positive ANA test is expressed as the titre of ANA that exceeds the level found in 95% of the normal population.

- 95% of patients with lupus have a positive ANA test.
- 20–40% of RA patients have positive ANA test.

❶ A positive ANA test in isolation does not confirm a diagnosis—see the next section on extractable nuclear antibodies (ENAs).

Extractable nuclear antibodies

An ENA test is usually requested following a positive ANA test or where clinical features strongly suggest a condition (such as SS). The blood sample will then be tested for reactivity using a combined ENA test. If the results are positive, further testing will identify specific antibodies to individuals

ENAs—which are outlined here together with the conditions, they are associated with.

- Ro—SS, SLE, neonatal lupus, and RA.
- La—SS, SLE, RA.
- RNP—mixed connective tissue disease, SLE.
- Scl-70—scleroderma.
- Jo-1—myositis.

ENA tests (positive or negative) do not indicate disease activity although different antibody profiles are associated with specific conditions. Repeated testing of ENA is not indicated unless there is a change in symptoms. The absence of an antibody does not exclude a clinical diagnosis, as ENAs are present only in a variable proportion of patients with the previously listed disorders.

► Individuals with SLE or SS should be screened for ENAs before considering pregnancy.

Immunoglobulins

Immunoglobulins form a major defence system of the body against foreign organisms and in mammals are divided into five subclasses (IgG, IgA, IgM, IgD, and IgE). Each immunoglobulin category has distinct groups of proteins and also has specific features. The value of such tests are chiefly to aid identification of an autoimmune disease.

Complement

The complement system is involved in the mediation of inflammation. Measurement of the complement components C3 and C4 aids in the diagnosis of immunological disorders, such as SLE, e.g. active SLE is usually associated with low complement levels. High complement levels occur as part of the acute phase response to inflammation.

► Rare hereditary deficiencies can be a cause for low complement levels.

Further reading

McGhee M (2014). *A Guide to Laboratory Investigations*, 6th edn. London: Radcliffe Publishing.

Blood test monitoring

When a patient attends a monitoring consultation, the blood test results are examined for improvements, or trends that may indicate adverse reactions to drugs. This helps to decide whether a medication should be stopped, or the dose adjusted. Many rheumatology patients have results that fall outside of the normal range. It is necessary to determine whether this is due to the patient's rheumatological condition, other co-morbidities, or due to the medications the patient is taking.

Haematological side effects

Anaemia

There are a variety of causes:

- Anaemia of chronic disease—where the cells are normal in size and colour (normocytic, normochromic) and the degree of anaemia seems to correspond to the activity of the arthritis.
- Anaemia due to DMARDs—e.g. due to bone marrow suppression with MTX, AZA, and sodium aurothiomalate (IM gold) or folate deficiency with MTX and AZA.
- Iron deficiency anaemia—microcytic, hypochromic, may be a consequence of poor diet or from GI bleeding due to NSAIDs. Rarely drug-induced haemolytic anaemia can occur which can be life-threatening if unrecognized. Usually occurs within 2 weeks of starting a new medication. A ↓ in Hb and an ↑ in bilirubin levels are seen. Can be confirmed by a positive Coomb's test/direct antiglobulin test (DAT).

Leucocytosis

↑ WBC count can be related to:

- Active inflammation such as RA or gout.
- Infection.

Leucopenia

↓ WBC count has many causes including:

- Conditions such as SLE and Felty's syndrome.
- Side effects of DMARDs (can be life-threatening).

Agranulocytosis

An acute condition due to bone marrow suppression leading to severe leucopenia, often attributed to medication.

Thrombocytopenia

- ↓ platelets.
- Thrombocytopenia is sometimes a feature of Felty's syndrome and can less commonly be seen in RA.
- Related to many of the DMARDs.

Idiopathic thrombocytopenic purpura

- Thrombocytopenia of unknown cause.

Biochemical side effects

- Abnormal LFTs can include:

  - Mild transient ↑ in liver enzymes are relatively common with DMARD use.
  - DMARDs should be withheld in marked ↑ in liver enzymes.
- Raised ALP and GGT—may also be raised in inflammation.
- Abnormalities in the U&Es associated with leflunomide and ciclosporin, penicillamine, and NSAIDs.

Key point: trends in results

It is important to observe for gradual changes in results over time. For example, there may be a slow ↓ in the number of white cells, although the white cell count remains within the normal range—the trend in results highlights the possibility of an adverse drug reaction. Vigilance and close monitoring are required as it may be necessary to withhold the drug.

- ➲ See Chapter 13, Rapid access and emergency issues', pp. 399–413.
- ➲ See Chapter 16, 'Pharmacological management: disease-modifying drugs', p. 452.
- ➲ See Chapter 18, 'Intra-articular, subcutaneous and intravenous therapies', p. 537.

Further reading

Ledingham J, Gullick N, Irving K, et al. (2017). BSR and BHPR guidelines for the prescription and monitoring of non-biologic disease-modifying anti-rheumatic drugs. *Rheumatology (Oxford)* 56:865–8.

Respiratory system

The baseline investigations in rheumatology usually include a chest X-ray. This is because in RA underlying pulmonary involvement is relatively common and includes interstitial fibrosis and pulmonary nodules. Pleurisy and pleural effusions can develop due to inflammation of the pleura. The lungs can also be adversely affected by some drugs used in rheumatology ∴ baseline evaluations are useful. Abnormalities found on chest X-ray should be investigated prior to treatment and will influence the choice of DMARD.

Drugs affecting the respiratory system

- *MTX*—pneumonitis is uncommon and pulmonary fibrosis is a rare complication of MTX. Pulmonary toxicity is rare and more likely to occur during the first year, but serious side effect can occur at any stage during treatment. Presents as dyspnoea and unproductive cough. Full PFTs may be required. Pneumonitis should be excluded by HRCT scan.
- *Sodium aurothiomalate* (IM gold)—hypersensitivity pneumonitis, dyspnoea, cough, pleuritic chest pain.
- *SAS*—eosinophilic pneumonitis, dyspnoea, fever.
- *D-penicillamine*—rare; bronchiolitis obliterans, dyspnoea late in therapy.
- *NSAIDs*—exacerbation of asthma, pneumonitis reported with naproxen.
- The emergence of latent TB has been associated with *anti-TNFα* therapies. It is ∴ essential to ensure adequate screening before initiating treatment—this includes a chest X-ray, TB prior contacts, risks and immunological status for TB. Screening for latent TB is advocated before all bDMARDs including tsDMARDs.
- Interstitial lung disease—may develop due an identifiable cause (e.g. underlying autoimmune conditions such as SLE or related to drug toxicity or chemical exposure), others may be idiopathic. Patients will need to be reviewed by a clinician and may require referral to a respiratory consultant before being considered for treatment.

Patients treated with DMARDs—in particular MTX or gold—complaining of dry cough, possibly accompanied by dyspnoea, should be urgently investigated to exclude drug-induced pneumonitis. Medication should be withheld until pneumonitis has been ruled out.

A productive cough in a patient, accompanied by a raised WBC count, is indicative of a chest infection, which will require investigating and treatment as necessary. Nurses should be vigilant about all forms of infection (including respiratory) for those treated with immunosuppressive agents as prompt treatment is essential.

Further reading

Ledingham J, Gullick N, Irving K, et al. (2017). BSR and BHPR guidelines for the prescription and monitoring of non-biologic disease-modifying anti-rheumatic drugs. *Rheumatology (Oxford)* 56:865–8.

Other tests

Serum urate—if a suspicion of gout

Serum urate (also referred to as uric acid) levels are age and sex dependent. Concentrations of uric acid ↑ with the onset of puberty in ♂ and menopause in ♀.

Uric acid is the end-product of protein metabolism and the breakdown of purines. An overproduction of uric acid is known as hyperuricaemia and this may result in gout. Hyperuricaemia is defined as a SUA concentration >7.0 mg/dL in ♂ and >6.0 mg/dL in ♀.

However:

- Not all people with hyperuricaemia have gout. Only 0.9 people per 1000/years of those with a serum urate (between 7 and 7.9 mg/dL) will present with gout.
- Not all people with gout have hyperuricaemia.
- During a flare of gout the tests may reveal high, normal, or low urate levels and SUA tend to ↓ during an attack of gout.

► This test may not be routinely available in all units.

➲ Also see 'Gout', pp. 118–119.

Thiopurine S-methyltransferase (TPMT)

TPMT is an important enzyme required to metabolize immunosuppressive drugs such as AZA from the body. About 1 in 300 people lack TPMT and would be at high risk of bone marrow suppression if treated with AZA. TPMT is therefore measured prior to commencing treatment with AZA and avoided in TPMT-deficient patients.

There are two types of TPMT deficiency that need to be considered for patients *who must be screened* prior to treatment with AZA.

- Homozygous state—AZA should be avoided and can be fatal (within 6 weeks).
- Heterozygous state—may be subject to delayed bone marrow toxicity (symptoms may not be evident until 6 months after starting treatment).

► Patients who are TPMT deficient are at greater risk of a catastrophic low white cell count early in treatment.

► Patients with normal TPMT levels can still develop leucopenia at any stage of treatment.

➲ See 'Pharmacological management: disease-modifying drugs', p. 452.

Human leucocyte antigen (HLA B27)

HLAs are proteins that assist the body's immune system differentiate between its own cells and harmful substances. HLA B27 is one of the HLA antigens. Estimates vary but it is thought that about 5–8% of the normal Caucasian population is HLA B27 positive. A positive HLA B27 test is not a good screening test but is linked to a greater risk of developing a seronegative spondyloarthropathy (e.g. AS). ➲ See 'Spondyloarthropathies', p. 93.

Key points and top tips in reviewing blood results

Blood tests are a valuable diagnostic tool but:

- Blood tests constitute only a part of a holistic assessment.
- A single result cannot confirm or exclude a diagnosis.
- A trend of ↓ or ↑ values is more valuable than a single result.
- Blood tests are affected by factors other than rheumatological disease.
- Consider co-morbidities and drug interactions.
- Treatment is not given on the basis of results alone.

Where possible, make use of a computerized database:

- Abnormal results may be usual for a particular patient.
- Trends in results are more easily visualized.
- Can identify key factors, e.g. relevance of starting on or ↑ DMARD dose, when drug toxicity is more likely.
- If no computer database available, a monitoring register/index cards/as well as a patient monitoring booklet are useful.
- Results outside of the normal range must be taken in context and may be of little clinical significance.

Remember:

- Vigilance is essential.
- Appropriate monitoring and action on abnormalities ↓ the risk of drug toxicity.
- Trends in results may signify drug toxicity before the blood test actually becomes abnormal.
- Drug toxicity can be fatal and happen at any stage during treatment.
- If in doubt, withhold DMARD until checked with prescribing clinician.

Remember: a trend of ↓ or ↑ values is more valuable than a single result and can identify the early signs of toxicity.

Further reading

Ledingham J, Gullick N, Irving K, et al. (2017). BSR and BHPR guidelines for the prescription and monitoring of non-biologic disease-modifying anti-rheumatic drugs. *Rheumatology (Oxford)* 56:865–8.

The disease in context with preparing the patient, treatment monitoring, and side effects

Patients will frequently be heard to say 'I don't like taking tablets; I worry about side effects'. While it is true that many drugs for MSCs are potentially toxic, this must be considered against the risk to the patient if the condition is left untreated. It is necessary to explain that the aim of treatment is to relieve symptoms, but, most importantly, to control and slow progression of the disease, which if left untreated, will have 'side effects' of its own, such as irreversible joint damage, functional decline, and other related conditions such as cardiovascular disease or osteoporosis.

The role of the rheumatology nurse

- Check all pre-screening assessments have been undertaken and results are available before starting treatment (e.g. ensuring that ♀ patients are not pregnant before starting treatment). Immunizations prior to commencing treatment if appropriate.
- Educate and empower patients about their condition and the various treatment options. Prompt and early treatment has been shown to be beneficial to patient outcomes, yet patients may need time to accept their diagnosis as well as to consider their wish to start a treatment. A shared decision-making approach can take time but needs to ensure the patient has had sufficient time to ask questions and consider the risks and benefits of treatment. The nurse's role is to present a balanced picture, empowering patients to make a shared informed choice.
- Reassure the patient that although there are risks associated with all drugs, the aim of regular monitoring is to detect any potential problems early.
- Some patients need a lot of support and counselling to maintain treatment, and many will try several different preparations before finding one that suits them and is effective. Ongoing education and support is vital.
- Providing clear information about the patient's responsibility while on treatment.
  - Attend for regular blood tests /keep a monitoring booklet.
  - Use effective precautions to prevent the risk of pregnancy while on DMARDs.
  - Contact the nurse advice line if they are concerned about side effects or stop taking treatment/need guidance on issues of contacts with infectious disease/travel immunizations, etc.

Why is monitoring so important?

The principal purposes of monitoring are patient safety and efficacy of treatment.

Rheumatology conditions are, by nature, unpredictable. It is very difficult to foresee how a patient will respond to treatment, or whether they are likely to develop side effects from medication.

By monitoring patients closely, it is possible to:

- Assess disease activity.
- Screen for toxicity.
- Detect trends in blood tests—e.g. a gradual ↓ in WBC count.
- Support the choice of medication.
- Adjust drug dosage according to disease activity.
- Ensure the patient is not overmedicated.

Many rheumatology patients are subject to polypharmacy and drug regimens may be complicated. For example, a fairly typical drug regimen for a patient with RA might include:

- MTX taken once a week.
- Folic acid taken once a week—3 days after the MTX.
- HCQ daily (note: the total dose of HCQ is calculated by body weight and might not be taken every day; be aware of possible variable doses).
- Prednisolone 5 mg and 7.5 mg on alternate days.
- A bisphosphonate taken once-weekly on an empty stomach in the middle of a fast.
- Analgesics taken when necessary.
- PPI to protect the stomach.

In terms of DMARD monitoring, most adverse reactions occur early, usually within the first few months of initiation of treatment, and ∴ monitoring is usually more frequent in the initial stages.

► Side effects may develop at any time and may be precipitated by the addition of a treatment affecting the pharmacokinetics of the original prescribed DMARD. In general, once treatment is established and monitoring is stabilized, the frequency of monitoring can be reduced, but must be continued as long as the patient is taking the DMARD or according to national guidelines.

Shared-care monitoring

It is important to ascertain who takes responsibility for DMARD monitoring. Ideally, 'shared-care' guidelines should be established, between 1° and 2° care. This sets out who is accountable for monitoring:

- The type and frequency of tests required.
- What to do when abnormalities are found.

Patients who take DMARDs are usually given shared-care patient-held monitoring booklets and educated on the medication, frequency of testing, and why the blood tests are needed. In some cases, patients are also educated on what to be aware of on each of the blood parameters measured.

➲ Also see 'Pharmacological management: disease-modifying drugs', p. 452; ➲ 'Nursing issues in patient-centred care', pp. 332–335; ➲ 'Infections', Chapter 13, pp. 400–401.

Radiological investigations

Radiological investigations play an important role in the diagnosis and ongoing management and review of many MSCs. Many nurses have undertaken additional training to request radiological investigations; usually these are confined to plain X-rays. There are three principles of radiation protection:

- Justification of the procedure—will it benefit the patient or lead to a change in treatment?
- Optimization—using the lowest dose necessary.
- Limitation—the dose should not exceed the agreed limits

Before requesting an X-ray, nurses must:

- Undertake relevant training and continually update their knowledge.
- Consider issues related to the use of ionizing radiations.
- Adhere to local and national guidance that outline best practice in protecting staff and patients from unnecessary exposure/harm.

Key aspects of radiological management include responsibilities for the:

Employer

- Written protocols for every standard investigation.
- Referral criteria should include clarity of referral pathways, radiation dose including limits, and quality issues.
- Ensure adequate training for all staff including continuing professional development.

Referrer

- Those entitled to refer for medical exposure.
- Responsible for providing sufficient clinical information to justify each exposure.

Practitioner

- Take responsibility for medical exposure. Must comply with trust procedures and ensure justification for exposure.

Operator

- Responsible for all practical aspects of performing procedure.
- Authorization of procedure.

Plain radiographic X-rays

- Specific positions may be required to identify pathology—e.g. standing X-rays to explore joint space narrowing on weight-bearing.
- Plain X-rays are helpful in identifying:
  - Erosions or fractures.
  - Baseline measurement, e.g. pretreatment chest X-ray. Exclude underlying pathology prior to treatment, e.g. TB. Calcification of ligaments, e.g. spinal. Joint-space narrowing or avascular necrosis or bone tumours.

- Limitations include superimposed structures obscuring the view to area of interest and are reliant on the different radiographic densities and quality of X-ray films and exposure.

Research trials use radiological evidence to evaluate changes in MSCs. In some cases, specific measurement tools have been developed to identify radiological changes using a composite score based on measurements at different points on a radiological film—e.g. the total Sharp's score measures key points in X-rays of the hand or feet.

Computerized tomography (CT) scanning & High Resolution CT (HRCT)

CT uses a moderate to high dose of radiation to provide an imaging technique that shows three-dimensional (3D) pictures of internal tissues. This is achieved by taking frequent 2D images while rotating around a single axis. Contrast enhancement enables greater clarity between tissues, demonstrating differences in their physical density. CT scans are valuable in assessment of areas such as the spine enabling an estimate of the quality and integrity of intervertebral discs.

HRCT (sometimes called thin-section CT) takes thin sections of internal tissues with high spatial frequency so very small interlobar fissures can be identified. It is used to clarify specific problems in more detail. The pattern of scanning may vary depending upon the clinical picture. HRCT is the investigation frequently used when there is a suspicion of interstitial lung disease.

Magnetic resonance imaging

MRI uses magnetic spinning and polarization of the magnetic fields to measure interactions between absorption and emission of energy to examine the tissues of the body. MRI utilizes the different densities of tissues (proportions of water or lipid/fats), using 3D visual 'cuts' or sliced selections to produce a visual result. It is a popular method for many musculoskeletal investigations including imaging joints, soft tissue, and early bone erosions.

Ultrasound

US plays an important role in current practice. It is a non-invasive technique that can be used in a clinical setting by trained clinicians to aid and inform treatment decisions. US uses a Doppler tool to beam sound waves through tissues. The early identification of erosions, synovitis, ganglion cysts, or osteopenia has particular value in treating early disease, allowing prompt treatment before long-term established damage takes place. US techniques, training, and research into optimizing its use in clinical and research settings is ongoing.

Health professionals are increasingly being trained to undertake US in Europe.

Isotope scanning

Isotope scanning uses a small dose of radioisotope that passes systemically through the body (via an oral or IV route) to scan target organs or tissues by emitting gamma rays which identify hot spots (high level of gamma rays) or cold spots (low levels of gamma rays). Time for the radioisotope to reach the target organ may vary and patients may have to wait before being scanned with a gamma camera that detects the rays emitted from the body. Isotope scanning is valuable for detecting infection, inflammation, and malignancies. Rarely, anaphylactoid reactions can occur from the injection.

DEXA scan

- Used to detect osteoporosis.
- Signs of osteoporosis may be detected on plain X-ray but do not provide an objective measure of the BMD.
- DXA uses low-energy X-rays to measure the density of bone. The results are given as T- or Z-scores in relation to calculated averages BMD scores (➔ see 'Osteoporosis', pp. 40–59).

Further reading

Department of Health (2017). *The Ionising Radiation (Medical Exposure) Regulations 2017*. London: DH. http://www.legislation.gov.uk/uksi/2017/1322/contents/made
Dougherty L, Lister S (eds) (2015). *The Royal Marsden Hospital Manual of Clinical Nursing Procedures*, 9th edn (Professional Edition). Oxford: Blackwell Publishing. http://www.rmmonline.co.uk
Also see local trust policies.

Respiratory investigations

This section outlines some of the standard tests for respiratory disease. For guidance on the different aspects of respiratory complications with MSCs, refer to ➲ 'Respiratory system', Chapter 17, p. 517.

Peak flow

Rarely useful as it is a measure of airways obstruction and has a wide normal range.

Spirometry

A simple test which can be performed in the clinic or ward. Will detect airways obstruction and also a restrictive problem due to interstitial lung disease. Spirometry is often normal in early interstitial lung disease.

Nursing point: the test should not be performed immediately after a full meal. If the patient is on an inhaled bronchodilator, they may be asked to withhold this before the test.

Full PFTs

Generally, a combination of a more complex description of lung volumes ('spirometry plus'), 'transfer factor', or 'diffusion coefficient'. A ↓ in transfer factor is usually the earliest indication of developing interstitial lung disease.

Nursing point: tests are undertaken in a pulmonary function laboratory. Similar preparatory issues to spirometry

Mouth pressure

A measure of the maximum negative pressure (inspiration) or positive pressure (expiration).

Blood gases and oxygen saturation

Always record inspired oxygen. This could be the room air or percentage of oxygen or flow rate plus device used.

Pulse oximetry

Measures oxygen saturation of arterial blood in the fingertip or ear lobe—the SaO_2. Simple to perform, non-invasive, and can be repeated as required. SaO_2 is variable and may fluctuate, e.g. at times of anxiety. Serial readings are ∴ helpful. Reduced in more severe interstitial lung disease but often normal in mild to moderate disease.

Nursing point: poor circulation in the fingers (e.g. systemic sclerosis, Raynaud's) may prevent satisfactory recording from fingers—consider measuring from ear lobe. Nail varnish may also affect results.

Pulse oximetry on exercise

A fall in SaO_2 on exercise is a more sensitive test of mild interstitial lung disease.

Nursing point: as for pulse oximetry. Usually a PT or nurse will undertake this investigation. Appropriate exercises need to be considered in the context of the patient. Record SaO_2 at rest, on cessation of exercise, and the lowest recorded level during observation, together with the exercise undertaken (e.g. distance travelled).

Arterial blood gases

Arterial blood samples are analysed for oxygen. Carbon dioxide acid–base status (pH, bicarbonate) rarely required in the outpatient context, unless coexistent COPD or severe respiratory muscle weakness. These might cause ventilatory failure, and therefore ↑ blood carbon dioxide ($PaCO_2$). Important in the assessment of the acutely ill patient as arterial blood gases can detect metabolic acidosis.

Nursing point: arterial blood gases are obtained via a needle from an artery, usually the radial artery at the wrist. Collected in a pre-heparinized syringe. Samples should be processed immediately or sent to the laboratory on ice. Once the sample is obtained, inform the pathology department immediately to avoid any delay in processing.

Radiology

Plain chest X-ray

An essential investigation for respiratory symptoms. May demonstrate evidence of pleural disease (effusion, thickening) or parenchymal (lung tissue) abnormalities of cardiac disease. However, it is usually normal in pulmonary hypertension (seen in systemic sclerosis or muscle disease) and often normal in milder interstitial lung disease.

CT

CT pulmonary angiogram (CTPA). Now the usual method to detect or exclude pulmonary hypertension.

MRI scan

Rarely helpful in lung disease.

Isotope lung scan

Used less frequently than CTPA in the diagnosis of PE. It gives less information than CTPA but a normal isotope lung scan does exclude PE. In the presence of other lung disease, it is less accurate in the diagnosis of PE.

Exclude cardiac involvement

The most usual set of initial investigations to rule out cardiac causes for breathlessness are:

- Chest X-ray.
- Electrocardiogram.
- Echocardiogram.

Tuberculosis and biologic disease-modifying antirheumatic drugs

Human TB is an infection caused by the bacterium *Mycobacterium tuberculosis*. Worldwide, there were ~10 million new cases in 2016, and 1.3 million deaths due to TB. The annual incidence of TB varies dramatically between countries. Examples for 2016 are Western Europe <10 cases/100,000 per annum; India, 211, and the Philippines, 554. TB rates vary between different communities, chiefly because of their links to high-prevalence areas around the world. In the UK, the rate for those born in the UK is 3.2/100,000, but 49.4 for those born abroad.

Active and latent TB infection

The numbers infected with the TB bacterium annually greatly exceeds the 10 million figure just mentioned. Fortunately, the majority of infected individuals will not become ill, will be unaware that they have been infected, and are therefore not part of the 10 million statistic. Three outcomes of the initial infection are possible:

- Some will successfully eradicate the TB bacterium.
- In others, the infection is contained by the host defence mechanisms within granulomatous lesions in the body, but these lesions continue to have viable bacteria within them. This state is known as latent TB. These individuals are at risk that their TB will reactivate in the future.
- In a minority of exposed individuals, the initial infection spreads within the lung as pulmonary TB, or via the bloodstream causing disseminated disease such as miliary TB or TB meningitis, or localized disease such as bone TB. These patients have clinical disease and are part of the 10 million statistic.

TB and bDMARDs

The risk of reactivation is ↑ by illnesses and therapies that suppress the immune system such as bDMARDs. The introduction of anti-TNFα therapies (e.g. etanercept, infliximab, and adalimumab) for RA revealed an ↑ incidence of TB. The risk is significantly lower with etanercept. It seems likely that the newer anti-TNFα agents certolizumab and golimumab also ↑ the risk of TB.

The risk of TB is highest in the first 6 months of treatment. This is due to reactivation of latent TB. This risk can be ↓ but not completely abolished by anti-TB drugs given prior to starting the anti-TNFα. The risk of TB does not go back to baseline over time, because patients on anti-TNFα remain more vulnerable to infection with TB on new exposure. When TB disease does develop in an immunocompromised patient, the presentation may be atypical, and the disease is more likely to be disseminated in nature and rapid in progression.

Screening for patients at risk of tuberculosis

Careful history plus examination of the chest to include:

Past or future exposure

- Living or born in a country or community with a high prevalence of TB.
- Frequent or prolonged travel overseas to area of high prevalence of TB.
- Family history of TB.
- Occupational risk, e.g. laboratory or health workers, prison staff.

Personal history of TB

- Previous TB and adequacy of any treatment.
- Prior bacillus Calmette–Guérin (BCG) vaccination and check for scar.
- Any symptoms suggestive of TB or active lung disease.
- Document current medical therapy noting any drugs which impair immunity.

Testing for TB

Chest X-ray (within the previous 3 months) is part of standard screening in most but not all protocols. The ACR only recommends chest X-ray if indicated by history or a positive test of immune reactivity to TB.

A chest X-ray may reveal features of possible active or past TB but may also show evidence of other pulmonary complications of the rheumatological disease. A normal chest X-ray does not exclude latent TB or extrapulmonary active TB.

If the patient's symptoms or chest X-ray suggest active TB, appropriate samples should be sent for TB culture.

In the absence of a past history of TB or evidence of active disease, latent TB is diagnosed by a positive immune reactivity to TB. Traditionally this has been achieved by a tuberculin skin test, usually a Mantoux.

> ❶ False positives and negatives can occur in those with a normal immune system.
>
> ❶ False negatives may also be seen with who are already taking drugs such as corticosteroids or MTX which impair immunity and ∴ reduce the size of the skin induration seen at 48–72 hours. In order to maintain sensitivity of the test, an induration of 5 mm or more is usually taken as positive in this context.

An alternative to a tuberculin skin test is a blood test—the interferon gamma release assay (IGRA). Examples include the QuantiFERON-TB Gold® and the T-spot TB® tests. Positive tests indicate active, latent, or treated infection, but again false negatives can occur, particularly in those who are significantly immunosuppressed. An IGRA is preferred to Mantoux testing in those who have had a BCG vaccination.

The choice between Mantoux testing or an IGRA is by local agreement, and some authorities suggest both should be done, accepting a positive by either test as evidence of past or present TB infection.

Referral to a TB specialist and treatment regimens

Referral is necessary if there is:

- Evidence of active infection or latent TB.
- Abnormality on chest X-ray.
- Doubt about the adequacy of past treatment of TB.

Treatment of active TB

- Treatment of active TB should follow local or national guidelines using at least three anti-TB drugs initially.
- Treatment of latent TB is usually with a single agent: isoniazid or rifampicin between 4 and 6 months, or a combination of rifampicin and isoniazid for 3–4 months. For more details of these and other regimens, see WHO guidelines.[1]
- Both isoniazid and rifampicin cause side effects with moderate frequency, particularly skin rash. Hepatotoxicity is seen with isoniazid. Rifampicin has a number of drug interactions. See: https://bnf.nice.org.uk/drug/rifampicin.html
- If a patient is currently prescribed corticosteroids, the dose of corticosteroids should be doubled for the duration of rifampicin therapy, or the single agent isoniazid used in preference.
- In active TB, the start of anti-TNFα treatment should be delayed until at least 2 months of fully compliant TB treatment has been achieved, and for latent TB treatment at least 1 month is needed. These decisions are made jointly by the rheumatologist and TB specialist.

➲ Also see 'Anti-tumour necrosis factor alpha: overview', Chapter 16, p. 493.

References

1. WHO (2018). *Latent Tuberculosis Infection: Updated and Consolidated Guidelines for Programmatic Management*. Geneva: WHO.
2. BNF/NICE. Rifampicin. https://bnf.nice.org.uk/drug/rifampicin.html

Further reading

British Thoracic Society Standards of Care Committee (2005). BTS recommendations for assessing risk and for managing Mycobacterium tuberculosis infection and disease in patients due to start anti-TNFα treatment. *Thorax* 60:800–5.

Royal College of Nursing (2017). *Assessing, Managing and Monitoring Biologic Therapies for Inflammatory Arthritis*, 4th edn. London: RCN.

Singh JA, Saag KG, Bridges SL Jr, et al. (2016). 2015 American College of Rheumatology guideline for the treatment of rheumatoid arthritis. *Arthritis Care Res (Hoboken)* 68:1–25.

Cardiovascular side effects

In recent years there has been ↑ evidence demonstrating that those with IJD have an ↑ risk of cardiovascular disease. The majority of the focus of this research has focused on RA but early evidence supports the additional risk in other IJDs. The ↑ risks appear to be attributed to early and more advanced blood vessel damage, due to high levels of inflammation. Swollen joint counts and ↑ CRP are associated with carotid plaque progression in RA.[1]

RA is associated with ↑ mortality, almost half of which is due to diseases of the heart and blood vessels, mainly heart attack and stroke. In many rheumatology departments, annual cardiovascular risk assessments are performed. However, many of the cardiovascular risk calculators inadequately consider the additional risk related to IJD. However, there is ↑ interest in developing risk calculators that adequately account for disease activity. Further education is required to ensure that patients with IJD receive the same level of care and assessment in cardiac risk management as other conditions, such as diabetes.

Patients should be encouraged to adopt healthy lifestyle measures such as stopping smoking, losing weight, eating a healthy diet, and taking measures to lower their blood pressure or cholesterol levels. Management of cardiovascular risk increasingly includes prescribing of antihypertensive and statin therapy.

Prompt disease control is an effective approach to reducing cardiovascular risk, supporting the principle, at least according to current research in RA, of the treat to target approach.

Some medication commonly used in rheumatology practice can have an adverse effect on the cardiovascular system. A recent focus has been on the potential risks related to cardiovascular risks with bDMARDs and in particular IL-6 therapies which ↑ lipid levels and anti-TNFα therapies; however, registry evidence suggests that those treated with biologics almost halved their risk of myocardial infarcts.

See Fig. 17.1.

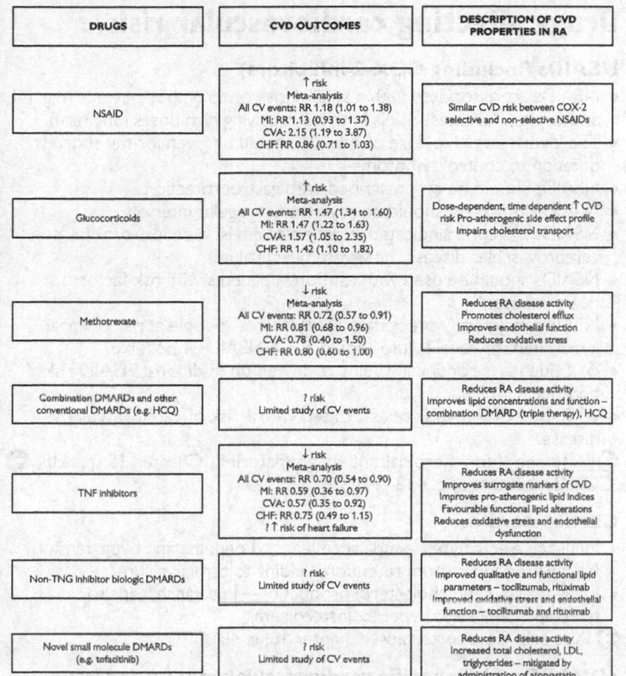

DRUGS
CVD OUTCOMES
DESCRIPTION OF CVD PROPERTIES IN RA
NSAID
↑ risk
Meta-analysis
All CV events: RR 1.18 (1.01 to 1.38)
MI: RR 1.13 (0.93 to 1.37)
CVA: 2.15 (1.19 to 3.87)
CHF: RR 0.86 (0.71 to 1.03)
Similar CVD risk between COX-2 selective and non-selective NSAIDs
Glucocorticoids
↑ risk
Meta-analysis
All CV events: RR 1.47 (1.34 to 1.60)
MI: RR 1.47 (1.22 to 1.63)
CVA: 1.57 (1.05 to 2.35)
CHF: RR 1.42 (1.10 to 1.82)
Dose-dependent, time dependent ↑ CVD risk Pro-atherogenic side effect profile
Impairs cholesterol transport
Methotrexate
↓ risk
Meta-analysis
All CV events: RR 0.72 (0.57 to 0.91)
MI: RR 0.81 (0.68 to 0.96)
CVA: 0.78 (0.40 to 1.50)
CHF: RR 0.80 (0.60 to 1.00)
Reduces RA disease activity
Promotes cholesterol efflux
Improves endothelial function
Reduces oxidative stress
Combination DMARDs and other conventional DMARDs (e.g. HCQ)
? risk
Limited study of CV events
Reduces RA disease activity
Improves lipid concentrations and function – combination DMARD (triple therapy), HCQ
TNF inhibitors
↓ risk
Meta-analysis
All CV events: RR 0.70 (0.54 to 0.90)
MI: RR 0.59 (0.36 to 0.97)
CVA: 0.57 (0.35 to 0.92)
CHF: RR 0.75 (0.49 to 1.15)
? ↑ risk of heart failure
Reduces RA disease activity
Improves surrogate markers of CVD
Improves pro-atherogenic lipid indices
Favourable functional lipid alterations
Reduces oxidative stress and endothelial dysfunction
Non-TNG inhibitor biologic DMARDs
? risk
Limited study of CV events
Reduces RA disease activity
Improved qualitative and functional lipid parameters – tocilizumab, rituximab
Improved oxidative stress and endothelial function – tocilizumab and rituximab
Novel small molecule DMARDs (e.g. tofacitinib)
? risk
Limited study of CV events
Reduces RA disease activity
Increased total cholesterol, LDL, triglycerides – mitigated by administration of atorvastatin

Fig. 17.1 Drugs used for treatment of rheumatoid arthritis and their cardiovascular risk. CHF, congestive heart failure; CV, cardiovascular; CVA, cerebrovascular accident; CVD, cardiovascular disease; RR, relative risk.
Reprinted from BR England et al. (2018) 'Increased cardiovascular risk in rheumatoid arthritis; mechanisms and implications' *BMJ* 36: doi;10.1136/bmj.K1036 with permission from the BMJ Publishing Group.

Reference

1. Low AS, Symmons DP, Lunt M, et al. (2017). Relationship between exposure to TNFi therapy and incidence and severity of myocardial infarction in patients with rheumatoid arthritis. *Ann Rheum Dis* 76:654–60.

Drugs affecting cardiovascular risk

NSAIDs (including COX-2 inhibitors)

- NSAIDs are associated with a small ↑ risk of thrombotic events (e.g. MI and stroke). Greatest risk is in those receiving high doses long term.
- The lowest effective dose of NSAID should be given for the shortest duration to control symptoms.
- NSAIDs should be co-prescribed with gastroprotection.
- NSAIDs long term should be reviewed at regular intervals.
- NSAIDs are contraindicated in patients with ischaemic heart disease, cerebrovascular disease, or severe heart failure.
- NSAIDs should be used with caution in patients with risk factors for heart disease.
- NSAIDs may rarely precipitate renal failure—people at risk of renal impairment or renal failure should avoid NSAIDs if possible.
- Evidence is continually being reviewed on traditional NSAID risks/ benefits.
- Raised CRP levels are associated with ↑ risk of cardiovascular disease.

Also see 'Non-steroidal anti-inflammatories', Chapter 15, p. 438, 'COX-2 inhibitors', pp. 438–441.

Corticosteroids

- Influence electrolytes—imbalance leads to oedema and hypertension from water and sodium retention, leading to cardiac failure.
- Influence lipid and cholesterol production—imbalance leads to hyperlipidaemia and hypercholesterolaemia.

Also see 'Corticosteroids', Chapter 16, p. 481.

cDMARDs with specific cardiovascular monitoring issues

Ciclosporin

- Hypertension—blood pressure should be measured prior to treatment and continue regularly during treatment.
- Discontinue if hypertension develops during treatment that cannot be controlled by antihypertensive therapy.

Also see 'Ciclosporin', Chapter 16, p. 456.

Leflunomide

- Hypertension is a recognized side effect of leflunomide.
- Blood pressure should be monitored twice before starting treatment (2 weeks apart) and blood pressure >140/90 mmHg should be treated before commencing treatment.
- Monthly monitoring of BP thereafter or at least at every visit—every 2 weeks for the first 6 months then once every 8 weeks.

Also see 'Leflunomide', Chapter 16, p. 464.

bDMARDs, biosimilars, and tsDMARDs

Anti-TNFα: adalimumab, etanercept, infliximab, golimumab, certolizumab pegol

- Patient's cardiac status should be screened prior to treatment with anti-TNFα (contraindicated in NYHA class III/IV).
- Anti-TNFα should be used with caution in heart failure (NYHA class I/II) and should be discontinued if symptoms develop or worsen.
- IL-6 therapies—tocilizumab, sarilumab
- IL-6 agents have been shown to raise cholesterol and triglycerides. Monitor lipid profiles and treat if required according to national guidelines.

Inhibitor of Janus-associated tyrosine kinase (JAK1, JAK2, JAK3): baricitinib and tofacitinib

- Monitor lipid profiles and treat if required according to local/national guidelines

➜ See 'New biologic disease-modifying therapies', p. 485.

Rituximab (MabThera®) and biosimilars

- Hypertension and hypotension have been reported.
- Patients who normally take antihypertensives should withhold them for 12 hours prior to infusion.
- Rituximab should be used with caution in patients with known heart disease.

➜ Also see 'Intravenous therapies', Chapter 18, p. 554.

Further reading

BNF: https://bnf.nice.org.uk/

BSR: https://www.rheumatology.org.uk

England BR, Thiele GM, Anderson DR, Mikuls TR (2018). Increased cardiovascular risk in rheumatoid arthritis: mechanisms and implications. *BMJ* 36:k1036.

Simon LS, Hochberg MC (2016). Non-steroidal anti-inflammatory drugs. In: Doherty M, Hunter DJ, Bijlsma H, et al. (eds) *Oxford Textbook of Osteoarthritis and Crystal Arthropathy*, 3rd edn, pp. 297–304. Oxford: Oxford University Press.

Other side effects

The major adverse reactions to rheumatology drugs have been detailed elsewhere (➔ see 'Pharmacological management: disease-modifying drugs' chapter 16, p. 542). There is, however, a wide range of other recognized side effects; briefly this includes:

GI tract

- Analgesics—constipation.
- NSAIDs—indigestion and peptic ulceration. All NSAIDs are associated with GI toxicity, especially in the elderly. Selective COX-2 inhibitors have a lower risk of upper GI side effects than non-selective NSAIDs. All NSAIDs and COX-2 inhibitors are contraindicated in patients with active peptic ulceration.

► Note: risks and benefits of NSAIDs including cardiovascular risks are discussed in ➔ 'Pain relief: non-steroidal anti-inflammatory drugs', Chapter 15, p. 438.

Skin (drug reactions)

- DMARDs—rashes and pruritus.
- NSAIDs—hypersensitivity, rashes can be severe.
- Corticosteroids—atrophy, bruising, acne, striae.

Headaches

- Most DMARDs—stop drug if severe.

Eyes

- HCQ—rare retinopathy.
- Corticosteroids—cataracts, glaucoma.

Hypersensitivity

- Most DMARDs.
- Anti-TNFα/rituximab.

Malignancy

- DMARDs, e.g. AZA, ciclosporin.
- Cyclophosphamide—↑ risk of haemorrhagic cystitis and bladder cancer. The higher the cumulative dose the greater the risk.
- Anti-TNFα—theoretical ↑ risk

💣 Lymphoma risk appears to be related to contributing factors such as uncontrolled inflammation, duration, and aggressiveness of disease rather than drug therapy.

Fertility

- Limited evidence for most DMARDs with regard to fertility and pregnancy outcomes. Review SPC and discuss in detail with prescribing clinician.
- SAS—oligospermia.
- MTX—avoid pregnancy, contraceptive measures for ♂ and ♀—potential fetal abnormality, may induce spontaneous abortion.

- Leflunomide—effective contraception is vital during treatment and for 2 years following treatment for ♀ and 3 months for ♂. Drug washouts may be necessary
- NSAIDs—long-term use is associated with reversible but reduced ♀ fertility. Can affect closure of fetal ductus arteriosus *in utero* and the possibility of pulmonary hypertension of the newborn. May cause delayed onset of and ↑ the duration of labour.

➲ See 'Pharmacological management', Chapter 16, pp. 429–444; ➲ 'Pregnancy and fertility', Chapter 14, pp. 415–425 for detailed information.

Metabolic disturbance

- Corticosteroids—hyperglycaemia may occur due to the effect of corticosteroids on the metabolism of glycogen. Known diabetics may require an adjustment of their diabetic therapy.
- Cushingoid features—e.g. 'moon face'.

Musculoskeletal

- Corticosteroids—osteoporosis, muscle wasting.

This is not a comprehensive list of all the known adverse reactions to rheumatology drugs. More in-depth information can be found in individual drug data sheets and the *BNF*.

Further reading

Flint J, Panchal S, Hurrell A, et al. (2016). BSR and BHPR guideline on prescribing drugs in pregnancy and breastfeeding—part I: standard and biologic disease modifying anti-rheumatic drugs and corticosteroids. *Rheumatology (Oxford)* 55:1693–7.

Flint J, Panchal S, Hurrell A, et al. (2016). BSR and BHPR guideline on prescribing drugs in pregnancy and breastfeeding—part II: analgesics and other drugs used in 90 rheumatology practice. *Rheumatology (Oxford)* 55:1698–702.

Chapter 18

Intra-articular, subcutaneous, and intravenous therapies

Overview of treatment options

This introduction aims to provide a brief overview of the change in treatment options available for a number of rheumatological conditions and importantly, some of the issues that had to be considered in the development of services. This is of particular relevance as many of the newer therapies introduced over the last 20 years have been administered by IV or subcutaneous injection.

The development of services in the provision of new therapies

In the last 20 years, treatment approaches for patients with rheumatological conditions have improved significantly, particularly for those with inflammatory forms of joint disease such as AS, RA, and PsA.

The changes are chiefly as a result of a wealth of extensive research over the last 30–40 years. The insights have enabled us to have a greater understanding of the cell-to-cell interactions that are implicated in an inflammatory process but ultimately, mechanisms that contribute to the immune responses we see in many rheumatological conditions. At the end of the 1990s, the first biologic therapy was introduced and set the path for a new approach to treatment. The small molecules (cytokines) involved in the inflammatory response were rapidly identified and researched. The first of these therapeutic options used small molecules (cytokines), biologically engineered to act as an inhibitor of the proinflammatory cytokines such as TNFα. From that moment onwards, rheumatology care changed rapidly. Patients, their families, and healthcare teams went on a journey—experiencing impressive benefits to patients' quality of life and disease control. However, in routine clinical practice there were many issues to consider:

- Patients with long-standing disease have a range of co-morbidities and extensive disease—these issues raised some complexities in their management with anti-TNFα therapies.
- The need for additional team support to ensure patients received adequate counselling, disease assessment, screening, and monitoring, and administering initially IV infusions but subsequently subcutaneous therapies, required services to examine how they could improve care and reduce any potential risks.
- In addition, biologically engineered therapies are expensive to prescribe and place an ↑ financial pressure on the NHS and other healthcare provisions internationally. NICE sets cost-effective, evidence-based guidelines for the use of treatments within the NHS; such guidelines are now integral to any new expensive therapy introduced.
- Research evidence combined with clinical experience and evidence from an observational study collected by the BSR Biologics Registry[1] identified early issues and as a result robust approaches for screening and monitoring were implemented nationally.
- As part of robust screening and evaluation criteria:
  - Patients can be disappointed if they are not eligible for the new therapies.

- Patients must be reassessed for eligibility criteria regularly—and potentially come off a treatment if it is not showing sufficient benefit.
- Detailed counselling was required to ensure patients understood their responsibilities while on therapy including continuing their current medication (e.g. MTX) and reporting infections promptly.

The role of the nurse specialist became pivotal to the provision of many of the above-listed service needs. They have had to enhance their abilities to train patients to self-administer subcutaneous therapies, coordinating IV administration, and importantly monitoring for safety and efficacy of treatments alongside their consultant colleagues. Additional follow-up clinics were developed to specifically review patients on biologic therapies and telephone support was vital as the 1° care teams had little experience of biologic therapies and did not feel confident in advising patients. The RCN Rheumatology Forum played an early pivotal role in supporting nurses by developing a comprehensive biologics guidance document. This document is now in its fourth edition[2] and remains a key resource for nurses.

Moving forward

Treatment options for rheumatological conditions have been transformed with a range of biologic therapies available (refer to the range available in this chapter). In recent years, research has also confirmed the 'treat to target' approach in RA and further disease areas are being scrutinized as to the feasibility of undertaking a 'treat to target' approach. This involves early aggressive treatment of the disease and a regular review to assess achievement of agreed targets for disease control.[3] ➔ Also see treat to target in Chapter 4, 'Rheumatoid arthritis', Chapter 4, p. 62.

Today, patients are trained to self-administer subcutaneous therapies; patient organizations are readily available and support patient knowledge and empowerment for managing their own condition more effectively.

We now also have the emergence of new targeted synthetic therapies that are administered orally and still expensive, but early evidence has demonstrated their efficacy in disease control with similar safety issues to consider in monitoring and screening. Equally, there are now a wide range of new therapies that are copies of the early licensed drug therapies (e.g. anti-TNFα therapies). These drugs are referred to as biosimilars.

What is a biosimilar?

Biosimilars are therapies that have been developed to produce a replica of the originator biologic therapy with a focus on determining a comparability of the molecule's characteristics; in essence, this means that it must demonstrate pharmacokinetic equivalence and be demonstrated to be consistently comparable in terms of efficacy, safety, tolerability, and of course immunogenicity.[4]

The use of biosimilars for infliximab, etanercept, and rituximab is outlined in this chapter. However, there are important issues to be aware of in daily clinical practice:

- Biosimilars are not interchangeable with the originator drug—patients can be switched to the biosimilar (following a shared decision-making consultation with the specialist team).
- The prescribing and issuing of a drug must specifically name the drug to be prescribed and a biosimilar cannot be interchangeable with a prescription for the originator drug (e.g. a prescription for infliximab cannot be replaced by Remsima®).
- Currently there is a significant cost saving when patients are treated with a biosimilar and starting new patients on biosimilars may enable significant cost savings to healthcare services.

References

1. BSR Biologics Register: https://www.bsrbr.org/
2. Royal College of Nursing (2017). *Assessing, Managing and Monitoring Biologic Therapies for Inflammatory Arthritis*, 4th edn. London: RCN.
3. NICE (2018). RA in adults: diagnosis and management. Evidence C: treat to target (NG100). https://www.nice.org.uk/guidance/ng100/evidence/evidence-review-c-treattotarget-pdf-4903172320
4. Schulze-Koops H, Skapenko A (2017). Biosimilars in rheumatology: a review of the evidence and their place in the treatment algorithm. *Rheumatology (Oxford)* 56:iv30–48.

Intra-articular injections: overview

In countries with fairly well-developed healthcare systems, experienced rheumatology specialist nurses may be trained in the administration of IA joint injection. This allows for a more holistic approach to the patient with the complete episode of care delivered by one person at one clinical appointment.

In order to undertake the additional training and responsibility of administering joint injections, as with other advanced roles, nurses must to be aware of their professional code of conduct. They should also ensure that their organization has recognized their advanced role and agreed to provide vicarious liability.

The following section provides an outline of IA injections and is aimed at providing the nurse on a ward or a clinic area an insight into the care of patients who receive an IA joint injection. A nurse who observes or supports the patient receiving a joint injection can play an important role in advising and caring for the patient. Some of the principles and practicalities of joint injections and care of the patient are outlined.

Joint aspiration is the removal of fluid from the joint space. Aspiration and injection is an essential procedure for the diagnosis and treatment of joint disease. *US or X-ray guidance* may be used in some cases to aid precision of the injection or where locating the exact site to inject is difficult (e.g. X-ray guidance is often used for hip injections)

Indications for joint aspiration and injection

- Diagnostic to identify the cause of the problem, e.g.:
  - Sepsis.
  - Crystals—monosodium urate, calcium pyrophosphate.
  - Haemarthrosis.
- Treatment:
  - To reduce IA pressure by removing fluid thus relieving pain and ↑ mobility.
  - To inject steroid.
  - Recurrent aspiration for sepsis.
  - The use of IA steroid may avoid the need for systemic use.

Key issues in preparing the patient for joint or soft tissue injection

Before undertaking the procedure, the person performing the aspiration and/or injection should provide a full explanation to the patient to outline the procedure and gain the patient's consent. This should include:

- Checking that contraindications to an IA injection have been checked (➔ see 'Contraindications to intra-articular steroid injections and post-treatment advice', Chapter 18, p. 547).
- A full explanation of the procedure, to include the effects and possible side effects of IA injection.
- A clear outline of the level of discomfort to be expected during the procedure:
  - This is usually minor and short-lived; in experienced hands, a joint injection should be no more painful than venepuncture.

  - It is helpful if the patient can be more relaxed as perceptions of pain may be reduced.
- The effects of the injection should be seen fairly quickly; if local anaesthetic is used there is an immediate effect. However, this wears off in 2–4 hours and patients should be advised to take additional analgesia before the steroid effects are felt.
- The steroids usually take effect within 24 hours and may persist for 2 months or more. In a small minority of patients, it can take up to a week to see the full effect of the steroid injection.
- Rest is advocated for between 24–48 hours, particularly in weight-bearing joints, so that the patient gets the maximum benefit from the steroid.
- Some patients can experience a post-injection flare. This may be as a result of a reaction to the microcrystalline suspension of the corticosteroid used. The patient should be given information to deal with this, such as rest following the injection, using analgesia as the local anaesthetic wears off. Ice or hot packs to help relieve post-injection flare pain may be helpful.
- The potential benefits of IA injection can last up to 2 months or longer.
- It is generally recommended that a joint is not injected more frequently than once every 3–4 months.
- A full explanation of potential side effects of IA injections should be given in written form for the patient to take home.

Side effects of IA steroid injections

- Post-injection flare varies but is seen in 1–2% of IA injections; it may be slightly higher for soft tissue injections. Very rarely an allergic reaction can occur and an anaphylaxis kit should always be at hand.
- Facial flushing occurs in 5–12%.
- Joint infection is rare if aseptic technique is used (risk of 0.01–0.03%).
- Rarely, subcutaneous fat atrophy can occur (more frequent with periarticular injections) and is seen as a whitening or depigmentation of the skin. This does resolve with time.
- Tendon rupture can occur if the drug is injected into a tendon.
- Some ♀ may experience disruption of their menstrual cycle, with either spotting, prolonged menstrual bleeding, or may miss a period as a result of steroid being injected.
- Patients with diabetes can experience a temporary rise in blood glucose levels and should be warned that this can happen and to adjust their diet and medication if necessary.

Further reading

Elmadbouh H (2016). Musculoskeletal injections. In: Hutson M, Ward M (eds) *Oxford Textbook of Musculoskeletal Medicine*, 2nd edn, pp. 236–59. Oxford: Oxford University Press.

Sabanthan A, Dunkley L (2015). Survey of joint injection procedure in the Yorkshire and Humber Area. *Rheumatology (Oxford)* 54 Suppl 1:i146–7.

Drugs used in administrating intra-articular injections

Steroids are the most commonly used preparation for IA injections, frequently administered with a local anaesthetic such as lidocaine.

IA steroids

- Have an anti-inflammatory effect.
- Superior to NSAIDs.
- Rapid onset, reliable, and effective for treating synovitis.
- ↓ pain and deformity, ↑ mobility and function.
- Useful in patients where systemic steroids would normally be contraindicated, e.g. diabetes and osteoporosis.

Commonly used injectable steroids

There are a number of IA steroids on the market; they are relatively insoluble and as a consequence are longer-acting and not absorbed systemically to a great degree.

The commonly used preparations are listed here in order of ↑ potency and length of action:

- Hydrocortisone acetate 25 mg/mL (Hydrocortistab®).
- Prednisolone acetate 25 mg/mL (Deltastab®).
- Methylprednisolone acetate 40 mg/mL (Depo-Medrone®).
- Triamcinolone acetonide 40 mg/mL (Kenalog®).
- Local anaesthetic.

Prevents pain by causing reversible block of nerve conduction along nerve fibres.

Lidocaine

Lidocaine is often mixed with the injectable steroid preparation (as described in the previous subsection) prior to injecting. This is probably the most effective and commonly used local anaesthetic for the following reasons:

- Rapid onset of action.
- Lasting effect of between 2 and 4 hours.
- Incidence of side effects is low in local injection.
- Available in a range of strengths from 0.1% to 2%.

Most common side effects are headache, light headedness, and drowsiness. Rarely, anaphylaxis, numbness of the tongue, anxiety, restlessness, or blurred vision can occur.

Other drugs used in IA injections

Yttrium-90

Yttrium-90 is a radioisotope used for the treatment of severe, chronic synovitis when IA steroids have failed to help. It is rarely used nowadays and the value of such an approach remains controversial.

- Yttrium is used as an alternative to surgical synovectomy.
- The joint is aspirated, injected with steroid, followed by yttrium-90.

- Strict immobilization of the joint is required to prevent extra-articular leakage of the radioisotope.
- The joint is splinted following the procedure and the patient is kept on bed rest for 48 hours following the procedure.

Hyaluronic acid (HA)

A high-molecular-weight polysaccharide that is a major component of synovial fluid and cartilage.

- In OA the molecular weight and concentration of HA is reduced.
- 'Viscosupplementation' with an IA injection of HA, it is claimed, helps to normalize the viscoelasticity of the synovial fluid.
- HA is licensed for symptom relief in OA of the knee when other conservative treatments have failed.
- In about 2% of patients there is an ↑ in pain and swelling following injection.
- Research evidence for knee and hip injections remains mixed as to the benefits of HA versus other injectable steroids for pain relief.

Further reading

Elmadbouh H (2016). Musculoskeletal injections. In: Hutson M, Ward M (eds) *Oxford Textbook of Musculoskeletal Medicine*, 2nd edn, pp. 236–59. Oxford: Oxford University Press.

Paskins Z, Dziedzic K, Leeb B (2015). Osteoarthritis: treatment. In: Bijlsma JWJ, Hachulla E (eds) *Eular Textbook on Rheumatic Diseases*, Chapter 31. London: BMJ.

Preparation and management of those receiving intra-articular joint injections

Nurses and allied HCPs involved in assisting with IA joint aspirations and injections have important roles to play in the procedure in the following ways:

- Preparation of the equipment.
- Preparation of the patient.
- Care of the patient during and after the procedure.
- Dealing with samples and disposal of fluid.

Preparation of equipment

An aseptic, no-touch technique is mandatory for any joint aspiration and injection.

Assemble equipment needed:

- Alcohol swabs for cleaning the skin.
- Syringes—an assortment of various sizes depending on the joints to be injected.
- If the joint needs aspiration, a 10–30 mL syringe may be required.
- For the injection either a 2 or 5 mL syringe is used.
- Needles—21-gauge green needles for large joints, 23- or 25-gauge (blue or orange) for smaller joints.
- Specimen bottles for the aspirate.
- Local anaesthetic—lidocaine 1% or 2% depending on the preference of the operator.
- Steroid for injection—a selection is best so that the person performing the injection can choose the most appropriate steroid for the joint to be injected (two registered practitioners should check the prescription).
- Gloves may be worn to protect the operator, especially in high-risk situations.
- Swabs and adhesive dressings.
- Alcohol hand gel.
- Anaphylaxis kit.

Preparation of the patient

- The nurse should put the patient at ease by explaining the procedure and checking that the patient fully understands what will be happening to them and confirm the patient's identification and the prescription.
- Consent would normally be taken by the person performing the procedure and can be taken in the form of written or verbal consent but must be clearly documented.
- If necessary the patient should be helped to undress and to expose the area to be injected, while maintaining their dignity.
- The patient should be comfortably positioned on a couch with the area to be injected exposed and, if necessary, supported sufficiently so that the muscles are relaxed.
- Tense muscles can make the injection impossible; for this reason, it is extremely important to try and get the patient to relax. If guided imagery is used this can give the patient a pleasant image to focus on, aiding relaxation.

Care of the patient during the procedure

- The nurse should remain with the patient throughout the procedure for moral support and reassurance as required.
- The nurse can assist the injector as necessary with opening of packets, and passing equipment as necessary.
- Most procedures are uneventful but occasionally the patient may feel a little faint following the procedure; if this happens, lie the patient down and where possible elevate the feet.
- Following the procedure offer the patient assistance to dress if necessary.
- Written information should be provided on aftercare following the injection.
- The nurse should reinforce information regarding rest following the injection and provide a contact number for the patient to ring should there be any concern or complications.

Dealing with samples of synovial fluid

- If the joint is aspirated, it is usual for the fluid to be examined for colour, clarity, and viscosity.
- If there is inflammation, such as RA, within the joint, the fluid is much more yellow and volume is high.
- In OA, the volume of fluid is often lower, the fluid clearer, and much more viscous (like egg white).
- The amount of fluid aspirated should be recorded as this can give an indication of the amount of inflammation that was present in the joint.
- Low volumes do not necessarily indicate that there is no IA process; in some cases, when there is a large amount of inflammation the synovial membrane is thrown up into villous-type folds and the fluid becomes loculated or trapped in these folds. Fibrin and rice bodies and other debris may hinder aspiration.
- Specimens can be sent in a universal container for Gram stain, microscopy, culture, and sensitivity (MC&S), as routine; these investigations are mandatory if infection is suspected. (Request a Gram stain and MC&S on the microbiology form.)
- The universal container should be labelled with the patient's name, date of birth, hospital number, and a description of the site of fluid aspiration and other essential information requested by the laboratory.
- Polarized light microscopy is the routine examination in an acute red joint as this identifies crystals. (Requested as crystals on the microbiology form.)
- Gout crystals (monosodium urate) show up under polarized light as long needle-shaped crystals that have a strong (negative) birefringence.
- Calcium pyrophosphate crystals are seen as short, thick, rhomboid-shaped rods and show a weak (positive) birefringence.

Contraindications to intra-articular steroid injections and post-treatment advice

It is important to assess patients prior to undertaking or supporting the administration of a joint injection. Patients should not receive a joint injection if there is:

- Evidence of any active infection, e.g. fever, coloured sputum, urinary tract infection, or skin infection, as the infection can spread to the joint.
- Joint sepsis—aspiration of the joint is mandatory, with specimens being sent for Gram stain, culture, and sensitivity.
- Previous infection in the joint to be injected in the past 6 months. There is a risk of a continued presence of a small pocket of subclinical infection which may flare as a result of the steroid injection.
- Patient currently taking antibiotics.
- Broken, damaged, or ulcerated skin near or at the injection site, as there is a route in for infection and ∴ the patient is at ↑ risk of infection.
- Prosthetic joints are never injected in routine clinical practice.
- Unstable coagulopathy; patients on warfarin need a stable international normalized ratio.
- Planned surgery in the next 2 weeks.
- Unstable diabetes (warn diabetic patients of the potential effect on the blood glucose level).
- Fracture in or near the joint as steroids can impair the local healing process.
- Active TB.
- Ocular herpes.
- Acute psychosis or strong history of previous steroid psychosis.
- Severe local osteoporosis near the joint.
- When joint destruction is severe and there is marked instability.
- Hypersensitivity to any of the components of the injection.

► Pregnancy: a review on the use of corticosteroids state there is no convincing evidence that systemic corticosteroids ↑ the risk of congenital abnormalities, ∴ the use of short-term treatments such as IA injections should **not** be considered a contraindication. Treatment as with all patients should be taken by the prescribing clinician based upon a risk benefit analysis (refer to the *BNF*).

Post-treatment advice

- Usually the very early analgesic effects of lidocaine will wear off in about 2–4 hours and **some** patient may feel an initial 'post-injection flare' over the next 2–3 days but this will dissipate as the steroid starts to work. Some patients feel no flare and prompt benefit from the injections. Advise that the use of paracetamol or cold packs might relieve the initial post-injection flare discomfort.
- Rarely (~4%) there will be skins changes or skin depigmentation (seen more frequently in dark-skinned patients).

- Advice on resting after a joint injection varies but usually the patient is advised to rest the joint for the next 24–48 hours—normal movements but not strenuous activity.
- There is no consensus on driving immediately after an injection and in the UK there appears to be no specific barrier to driving post injections from an insurance perspective. Country to country this may vary and ∴ written guidance should be offered to patients based upon national guidelines/insurer's policy.
- The patient should take note of how long they receive benefit from the injection.
- All patients who receive an IA injection should have a patient information leaflet outlining when to seek medical advice and including other important information. For example:
    - Diabetics should monitor their blood sugars more often for a week after the injection and may need to seek guidance if the blood sugar levels are high.
    - If the injected joint becomes more painful, red, and swells further and is hot (or have a high temperature), seek urgent medical advice. This is incredibly rare (➔ see 'Joint injections: overview', Chapter 18, p. 541).
    - About 5% of people experience facial flushing in the first 2 days.
    - Menstrual disturbance can occur after the injection, especially if more than one joint is injected. It should last no longer than one cycle. Seek medical advice otherwise.
    - The information sheet should have a specialist nurse or department contact telephone number.

Further reading

Elmadbouh H (2016). Musculoskeletal injections. In: Hutson M, Ward M (eds) *Oxford Textbook of Musculoskeletal Medicine*, 2nd edn, pp. 236–59. Oxford: Oxford University Press.

Paskins Z, Dziedzic K, Leeb B (2015). Osteoarthritis: treatment. In: Bijlsma JWJ, Hachulla E (eds) *Eular Textbook on Rheumatic Diseases*, Chapter 31. London: BMJ.

Price Z, Murphy D, Mackay K (2011). Intra-articular injection and driving advice: a survey of UK Rheumatologists' current practice. *Musculoskeletal Care* 9:188–93.

Subcutaneous therapies: overview

Medications can be delivered via a number of different routes depending upon the pharmacodynamics of the drug and the prescriber must consider:

- How the drug is absorbed and distributed.
- The processes involved in metabolizing and excreting the drug.

The subcutaneous route is used to enable a slow but sustained absorption of a drug therapy. However, the rate of absorption will depend upon the site of the injection. Diffusion through the tissues and removal/transportation of the drug by local blood supply are essential for the drug to have the planned treatment effect. Absorption from the abdomen is considered the fastest route. However, it is essential that injection sites are rotated to prevent fat atrophy, induration, or scarring. Sites that can be used for safe subcutaneous administration include:

- Abdomen.
- Outer aspect of the thigh and buttocks.
- The upper outer aspect of the top of the arm.

Drugs are delivered subcutaneously because they would be significantly altered by the oral route or need a greater 'steady state' in the sense of slow and sustained release. Examples of therapies administered via the subcutaneous route include:

- Insulin.
- Vaccines.
- Sustained pain relief (e.g. using a syringe driver pump).
- MTX.

Therapies that are administered via the subcutaneous route for MSCs include:

- Biological therapies:
  - Anti-TNFα therapies (e.g. adalimumab, certolizumab pegol, etanercept, and golimumab).
  - Anti-IL-1 receptor agonist (anakinra).
  - Anti-IL-6, e.g. tocilizumab and sarilumab.
  - Anti-IL-12/23, e.g. ustekinumab.
  - Anti-IL-17, e.g. secukinumab.
  - Anti-IL-17A, e.g. ixekizumab.
- Denosumab—a monoclonal antibody for the treatment of osteoporosis.
- Parathyroid (PTH)—an anabolic treatment for osteoporosis; a synthetic version of human PTH is teriparatide (Forsteo®).
- MTX—a cytotoxic immunosuppressant therapy that can be co-prescribed with biologic therapies. Prefilled injection pens of MTX are available in a variety of dosing regimens, e.g. Methofill®, Metoject®, Nordimet®, and Zlatal®
- ► Subcutaneous MTX is an important therapeutic option for patients:
  - Who have intolerance due to GI symptoms.
  - Who require greater bioavailability.
  - If nurses are administering subcutaneous therapies (rather than patient self-administered), this may be used to resolve some issues in relation to concerns about compliance of oral therapies.

Note: where possible, it is usual to encourage and support patients (or a carer) to be trained to self-administer subcutaneous injections to optimize efficiency of service/resources and cost-effectiveness of nurse time.

➲ See 'Further reading', Chapter 16, p. 455; for monitoring regimens and Table 16.1.

Community support for patients receiving subcutaneous therapies

There are a number of organizations that can provide community support for patients requiring subcutaneous therapies. These organizations can provide:

- A package of care as part of the purchase of the treatment. For some therapies this service is integral to the prescribing and offers a service that can train the patient to self-administer or check their technique and deliver subcutaneous therapies to the patient's home on a regular basis.
- Regular prearranged deliveries that ensure the treatment is managed and stored at the correct temperature while in transit for those therapies that require specific temperature control.
- Continuity of service.

Further reading

BNF: https://bnf.nice.org.uk/

Electronic Medicines Compendium. Summaries of product characteristics. http://www.medicines.org.uk

Holroyd CR, Seth R, Bukhari M, et al. (2019). The BSR DMARD safety guidelines in inflammatory arthritis—executive summary. *Rheumatology (Oxford)* 58:220–6.

NICE—topics on arthritis: https://www.nice.org.uk/guidance/conditions-and-diseases/musculoskeletal-conditions/arthritis

Royal College of Nursing (2017). *Assessing, Managing and Monitoring Biologic Therapies for Inflammatory Arthritis*, 4th edn. London: RCN.

Versus Arthritis. Biological therapy alert card. https://www.versusarthritis.org/order-our-information

Patient self-administration of subcutaneous therapies

Patients can self-administer subcutaneous injections providing they:

- Consent to being trained and take responsibility for the treatment and equipment in their own home. In some cases, a patient unable to inject themselves may nominate a close relative or partner to be trained to inject.
- Have the ability to recall and sustain the steps involved in self-administration including:
  - Applying appropriate hygiene techniques in preparing to inject.
  - Maintaining trained techniques in administering treatment, ensuring aseptic technique.
  - Having the functional ability to administer the treatment (or have a nominated carer who can be trained).
  - Being able to maintain concordance with monitoring and treatment regimens.
  - Recognizing the risks related to home administration and storage of drugs and equipment (including responsible disposal of equipment and spillage).

Detailed guidance on patient self-administration for biologic therapies and MTX has been developed.[1,2]

Benefits of patient self-administration

- Independence for the patient—flexibility for work and social activities.
- Can encourage the patient to perceive themselves as having an enhanced ability to self-management and reduce perceptions of reliance on healthcare support.
- ↓ nursing activity costs/resources.

Risks related to patient self-administration

- ↓ patient contact and times to carry out opportunistic review/ education/support.
- ↓ vigilance by team with regard to disease activity/infections or side effects.
- Risks related to poor concordance to monitoring/failure to adhere to standards of self-administration/drug storages and management.

Training patients to self-administer subcutaneous therapies

Training patients to self-administer subcutaneous injections has been undertaken for a number of years and much of the expertise in this field has been developed from the field of diabetes and patient-administered subcutaneous injections of insulin.

A step-wise approach to training patients to self-administer subcutaneous therapies has been specifically developed for patients with MSCs. Documentation and frameworks for nursing practice, patient training tools, and checklists are available. They include:

- MTX—a cytotoxic drug administered at doses <25 mg.[1]
- Biologic therapies—monoclonal antibodies (anti-TNFα).[2]

Key issues in patient-administered subcutaneous therapies

- Patients must express an interest in participating in the training and consent to treatment.
- Select patients who fulfil the criteria for treatment.
- Provide a comprehensive training programme for patients (and partner/carer). Review patient's confidence and technique before home administration.
- Must be able to adhere to aseptic techniques and recommended storage of treatments in home environment.
- Encourage rotation of injection sites.
- Ensure monitoring and co-prescriptions of drug therapies are considered, e.g.:
  - Patient may be self-administering two different subcutaneous therapies, such as adalimumab (biologic) and MTX (cytotoxic therapy). Disposal for MTX requires a cytotoxic storage and disposal policy.
- Provide written and verbal information on key point of contact (e.g. telephone advice line).
- If receiving a biologic therapy, ensure patient 'alert card' is issued—advising patient of when to receive prompt medical advice.[3]
- Review patients on at least an annual basis to check subcutaneous injection technique.
- Training must be provided by competent nurses who can:
  - Provide evidence-based drug information, including risks and benefits of treatment.
  - Demonstrate the procedure with clarity and tailor education according to the individual patient's learning needs.
  - Ensure adequate documentation of processes.
  - Recognize limitations of their practice.

References

1. Royal College of Nursing (2016). *Administering Subcutaneous Methotrexate for Inflammatory Arthritis*, 3rd edn. London: RCN.
2. Royal College of Nursing (2017). *Assessing, Managing and Monitoring Biologic Therapies for Inflammatory Arthritis*, 4th edn. London: RCN.
3. Versus Arthritis. Biological therapy alert card. https://www.versusarthritis.org/order-our-information

Further reading

Electronic Medicines Compendium. Summaries of product characteristics. http://www.medicines.org.uk

Frequently asked questions: subcutaneous therapies

Should subcutaneous injections be injected at 45° or 90°?

Evidence supports a 90° angle. You should use a 26-gauge needle, with an 8 mm length and then pinch the skin so you can then insert the needle at a 90° angle. The decision to pinch or not to pinch relies upon the needle length (shorter needle will not require a pinch technique) and angle of injection (45° will require a pinch technique).

Are there any specific issues I need to consider for patients who are obese or thin when administering subcutaneous injections?

Studies demonstrate that patients who are obese or thin still receive the drug into the subcutaneous tissues if injected as recommended.

Do patients self-administering MTX need to wear masks, goggles, and aprons?

It is important that routine cytotoxic management and disposal of used equipment are adhered to according to local trust or organizational policy. Patients do not need to wear masks or goggles. Aprons may be appropriate to protect clothing or accidental spillage depending upon the site they are injecting (e.g. an apron will not be appropriate when injecting into the abdomen).

Why are patients giving subcutaneous MTX when it can be taken orally?

MTX is an inexpensive therapy and research has not been commissioned by the pharmaceutical companies to demonstrate the benefits of the subcutaneous route of administration for IJDs. However, the pharmacokinetics show that MTX is more readily absorbed and reduces some of the unacceptable side effects some patients experience taking MTX orally. A licensed prefilled subcutaneous MTX is available at different dosing regimens although is costlier than the oral route.

Is it common for patients to get reactions following subcutaneous administration of biologic therapies?

Biologic therapies are foreign proteins and have the potential to cause a reaction to treatment in the same way that a blood transfusion can. However, the most commonly reported problem for subcutaneous therapies is that of injection site reactions (>10%), although it is relatively uncommon for patients to discontinue treatment due to injection site reactions.

Why are patients treated with bDMARDs advised to carry an 'alert card'?

The 'alert card' is to remind patients to tell all HCPs that they are receiving a bDMARD and highlights the need to treat all infections seriously and to seek specialist guidance on bDMARDs.

Intravenous therapies: overview

Issues related to infusions and good practice

Nurses are responsible for the correct administration of prescribed medicines to patients in their care at all times, being guided by the Nursing and Midwifery Council standards. The nurse should have knowledge of the use, action, dosing regimens, side effects, and interactions of any medicines being administered and be competent to prepare and administer the infusion.

Local policies and procedures should be in place to assist the nurse in safe preparation and administration of IV medicines and should be adhered to at all times. Pharmacists should provide appropriate information and advice to all staff and in some cases will have responsibility for preparing medicines to be administered by the parenteral route.

Checklist for preparation and administration of IV medicines

- Preplan before drawing up doses.
- Be sure of local protocols.
- Check medicine against prescription—check that the dose, time, and route are correct.
- Check patient identification.
- Check IV site.
- Check that any equipment required is working.
- Know how to administer each medicine, e.g.:
  - Calculation of concentration and rate.
  - Reconstitution.
  - Addition of medicines to recommended diluents.
  - Check package insert, SPC, and local medicines information pharmacist.
- Use aseptic technique during reconstitution steps, addition of medicine to diluents, and care of the line.
- Maintain a sterile, particle-free solution.
- Thoroughly mix any additions, checking for precipitation or particles.
- Complete infusion additive label and attach to infusion.
- Understand how the medicine works and explain this to the patient if appropriate.
- Continue to monitor for precipitation, patient response, or adverse effects, where appropriate.

Further reading

Dougherty L, Lister S (eds) (2015). *The Royal Marsden Hospital Manual of Clinical Nursing Procedures*, 9th edn. Chichester: Wiley-Blackwell Publishing.

Electronic Medicines Compendium. Summaries of product characteristics. ☞ http://www.medicines.org.uk

Royal College of Nursing (2016). *Standards for Infusion Therapy*, 4th edn. RCN, London.

Holroyd CR, Seth R, Bukhari M, et al. (2019). The BSR DMARD safety guidelines in inflammatory arthritis—executive summary. *Rheumatology (Oxford)* 58:220–6.

Abatacept

Abatacept selectively modulates the activation of T cells involved in the immune system's inflammatory response which can lead to joint pain, swelling, and ultimately damage in IJDs. It is licensed for the treatment of RA in combination with MTX, with or without MTX in PsA, and with MTX in polyarticular JIA. Current NICE guidance are available for RA and JIA. It is currently being reviewed by NICE for PsA.

Pretreatment screening

- Detailed history and physical examination.
- Chest X-ray.
- TB screening.
- Viral hepatitis screening.
- Check previous history of varicella zoster (VZ)—if no previous history, a VZ antibody test should be undertaken—for those >50 years of age with a negative test and no contraindications, a single VZ vaccination should be offered at least 14 days prior to biologic commencement.
- Routine blood tests.
- Baseline disease assessment: (e.g. DAS28 or Psoriatic Arthritis Response Criteria (PsARC)).

Contraindications

- Hypersensitivity to abatacept or to any of the excipients.
- Active acute or chronic infection.
- Concomitant use of other biologic agents.
- Demyelinating disease.
- Pregnancy.
- Use in children (safety not yet established).
- Live vaccines at time of treatment or within 3 months of use.

Cautions

- COPD.
- Any underlying condition that predisposes to infection.
- History of recurrent or persistent infection.

Treatment regimen

- Infusion given at weeks 0, 2, 4, and then every 4 weeks thereafter (Table 18.1) (➲ see 'Administration/nursing care', pp. 556 and 557).
- MTX weekly.
- For drugs which may be needed at time of infusion, see Table 18.2.

Practical considerations

- *Equipment*: full resuscitation facilities and infusion pump are required. A sterile, non-pyrogenic, low-protein-binding filter (pore size 0.2 μm to <1.2 μm) is essential. A silicone-free disposable syringe is provided and this must be used to reconstitute each vial.
- *Time and nursing resources*: infusions take 30 min. Close monitoring is required.
- *Handling*: abatacept does not require any special handling precautions.

Table 18.1 Abatacept infusion

Body weight	Dose (mg)	Number of 250 mg vials
<60 kg	500	2
≥60 kg to ≤100 kg	750	3
>100 kg	1000	4

Table 18.2 Drugs that may be needed at the time of infusion

Chlorpheniramine	10 mg IV three times daily
Hydrocortisone	100 mg IV three times daily
Metoclopramide	10 mg IV three times daily
Paracetamol	1 g orally four times daily (max. 4 g in 24 hours)

Administration/nursing care

Prior to treatment

- Check there are no contraindications to treatment (➔ see 'Contraindications', p. 555).
- Check any recent blood tests are within satisfactory parameters.
- Record baseline observations of temperature, pulse, and blood pressure.
- Urinalysis if symptoms of infection are reported.

Preparation

Prepare the infusion according to the manufacturer's guidelines. Abatacept is supplied in 250 mg vials as a dry powder. Each vial is reconstituted with 10 mL of sterile water for injections using the silicone-free disposable syringe provided with each vial and an 18–21-gauge needle.

The reconstituted solution must be immediately diluted to 100 mL with sodium chloride 0.9% solution, i.e. withdraw the equivalent volume of fluid from a 100 mL bag (20 mL for two vials; 30 mL for three vials; 40 mL for four vials) and replace with the abatacept solution.

Administering the infusion

- Abatacept is infused through a filter into a peripheral cannula using an IV pump with a primed line.
- Abatacept should be administered over 30 min.

Clinical observations during infusions

No routine observations during the infusion are required; however, in the event that the patient reports feeling unwell, observations should be monitored and recorded. Observe for any signs of respiratory deterioration in those with COPD.

Repeat baseline observations 1 hour after the infusion starts (➔ see 'Post-infusion care', p. 557).

Observe for side effects throughout—take appropriate action as listed next and record any adverse events in the patient's notes:

- ❗ Anaphylactic reactions have been reported. In this event:
  - Stop infusion.
  - Call physician.
  - Administer IV hydrocortisone, IV chlorpheniramine, and/or any emergency treatment as indicated.
- Acute infusion-related events (i.e. those that occur within 1 hour of the infusion) are most commonly dizziness, headaches, and hypertension.
- Headache and nausea are the most common side effects occurring in ≥1/10 patients following the infusion.
- For a full list of adverse effects, see the SPC.

Post-infusion care and advice to patients

- Discharge patient post infusion providing observations taken 1 hour after the infusion start time are satisfactory.
- Advise patient to:
  - Seek medical advice if any symptoms develop that are suggestive of an infection, e.g. fever in the hours or days after the infusion (provide contact numbers for the rheumatology department or first contact point, e.g. GP and/or attend ED).
  - If monotherapy, FBC, U&Es, and LFTs—every 3–6 months.
  - Maintain regular MTX monitoring according to BSR and local guidelines.
  - If diabetic, patients need to be aware that abatacept interferes with blood glucose monitoring strips (GDH-PHQ) resulting in falsely elevated blood glucose readings on the day of the infusion.
- Ensure follow-up for assessment or next infusion has been arranged.
- Ensure patient has a biologics alert card.

Patient information

Patient information leaflets are available from:

- National Rheumatoid Arthritis Society: http://www.rheumatoid.org.uk
- Versus Arthritis: https://www.versusarthritis.org/

Further reading

BNF: https://bnf.nice.org.uk/

BSR: https://www.rheumatology.org.uk

Electronic Medicines Compendium. Summaries of product characteristics. http://www.medicines.org.uk

Holroyd CR, Seth R, Bukhari M, et al. (2019). The BSR DMARD safety guidelines in inflammatory arthritis—executive summary. *Rheumatology (Oxford)* 58:220–6.

NICE (2010). Adalimumab, etanercept, infliximab, rituximab and abatacept for the treatment of rheumatoid arthritis after the failure of a TNF inhibitor (TA195). https://www.nice.org.uk/guidance/ta195

NICE (2015). Abatacept, adalimumab, etanercept and tocilizumab for treating juvenile idiopathic arthritis (TA373). https://www.nice.org.uk/guidance/ta373

NICE (2016). Adalimumab, etanercept, infliximab, certolizumab pegol, golimumab, tocilizumab and abatacept for rheumatoid arthritis not previously treated with DMARDs or after conventional DMARDs only have failed (TA375). https://www.nice.org.uk/guidance/ta375

Royal College of Nursing (2017). *Assessing, Managing and Monitoring Biologic Therapies for Inflammatory Arthritis*, 4th edn. London: RCN.

Belimumab

Belimumab is a fully humanized monoclonal antibody directed against soluble B lymphocyte stimulator (BLyS). It is licensed as an add-on treatment for active autoantibody-positive SLE in adults who are receiving standard therapy. Current NICE guidance is available for SLE.

Pretreatment screening

- Detailed history and physical examination.
- Chest X-ray.
- TB screening.
- Viral hepatitis screening.
- Check previous history of VZ—if no previous history, a VZ antibody test should be undertaken—for those >50 years of age with a negative test and no contraindications, a single VZ vaccination should be offered at least 30 days prior to belimumab infusion.
- HIV screening.
- Routine blood tests.
- Check for hypogammaglobulinaemia.

Contraindications

- Hypersensitivity to belimumab or to any of the excipients.
- Severed active central nervous system lupus.
- Severe active lupus nephritis.
- HIV.
- Past or current hepatitis B or C.
- History of renal or major organ transplant, or haematopoietic stem cell/marrow transplant.
- Active acute, chronic, or recurrent infection.
- Concomitant use of cyclophosphamide or B-cell targeted therapy.
- Pregnancy.
- Use in children.
- Live vaccines for 30 days prior to treatment or within 3 months of use.

Cautions

- History of malignancy.
- Any underlying condition that predisposes to infection.
- Breastfeeding (case-by-case consideration of risk:benefit ratio for both the patient and baby).

Drugs which may be needed prior to infusion

- Chlorpheniramine: 10 mg IV three times daily.
- Paracetamol: 1 g orally four times daily (maximum 4 g in 24 hours).

Treatment regimen

- Infusion given at weeks 0, 2, 4, and then every 4 weeks thereafter (➲ see 'Administration/nursing care', p. 560).
- 10 mg/kg.

Practical considerations

- *Equipment*: full resuscitation facilities and infusion pump are required. A sterile, non-pyrogenic, low-protein-binding filter (pore size 0.2 μm to <1.2 μm) is essential. A silicone-free disposable syringe is provided, and this must be used to reconstitute each vial.
- *Time and nursing resources*: infusions take 60 min. Close monitoring is required.
- *Handling*: belimumab does not require any special handling precautions.

Administration/nursing care

Prior to treatment

- Check there are no contraindications to treatment (➔ see 'Contraindications', p. 559).
- Check any recent blood tests are within satisfactory parameters.
- Record baseline observations of temperature, pulse, and blood pressure.
- Urinalysis if symptoms of infection are reported.

Preparation

Prepare the infusion according to the manufacturer's guidelines. Belimumab is supplied in 5 mL vials (120 mg) or 20 mL vials (400 mg). Allow 10–15 min for the vial to warm to room temperature (15–25°C).

The 120 mg vial is reconstituted with 1.5 mL of sterile water for injections and the 400 mg vial is reconstituted with 4.8 mL of sterile water for injections to make a final concentration of 80 mg/mL using the silicone-free disposable syringe provided with each vial and an 21–25-gauge needle. The reconstituted solution must be diluted to 250 mL with sodium chloride 0.9% solution or sodium chloride 4.5 mg/mL (0.45%), or lactated Ringer's solution for injection, i.e. withdraw the equivalent volume of fluid, e.g. 1.5 mL for 120 mg dose and 5 mL for 400 mg dose.

Administering the infusion

- Belimumab is infused through a filter into a peripheral cannula using an IV pump with a primed line.
- Belimumab should be administered over 60 min.

Clinical observations during infusions

Repeat baseline observations every 30 min during the infusion (➔ see 'Post-infusion care', p. 561).

Observe for side effects throughout—take appropriate action as listed next and record any adverse events in the patient's notes:

- ❗ Anaphylactic reactions have been reported. In this event:
  - Stop infusion.
  - Call physician.
  - Administer IV hydrocortisone, IV chlorpheniramine, and/or any emergency treatment as indicated.
- ❗ Hypersensitivity and infusion reactions have been reported in 0.9% of patients, up to several hours after the infusion. The risk is greatest after the first two infusions and ∴ patients should remain under clinical supervision for several hours after at least the first two infusions.

- Acute infusion-related events (i.e. those that occur within 1 hour of the infusion) are most commonly dizziness, headaches, and hypertension.
- For full list of adverse effects, see the SPC.

Post-infusion care and advice to patients

- Discharge patient post infusion providing observations taken 1 hour after the infusion start time are satisfactory.
- Advise patient to:
  - See medical advice if signs of delayed hypersensitivity reactions which may occur in the hours or days after the infusion.
  - Seek medical advice if any symptoms develop suggestive of an infection, e.g. fever in the hours or days after the infusion (provide contact numbers for the rheumatology department or first contact point, e.g. GP and/or attend ED).
- Ensure follow-up for assessment or next infusion has been arranged.
- Advise the patient that a disease assessment and review of effectiveness of treatment will be undertaken at 24 weeks after treatment.
- Women of childbearing age must ensure effective means of contraception for at least 4 months post infusion.
- Ensure patient has a biologics alert card.

Patient information

Patient information leaflets are available from:

- Versus Arthritis: ☞ https://www.versusarthritis.org/

Further reading

BNF: ☞ https://bnf.nice.org.uk/

Electronic Medicines Compendium. Summaries of product characteristics. ☞ http://www.medicines.org.uk

NICE (2016). Belimumab for treating active autoantibody-positive systemic lupus erythematosus (TA397). ☞ https://www.nice.org.uk/Guidance/TA397

Royal College of Nursing (2017). *Assessing, Managing and Monitoring Biologic Therapies for Inflammatory Arthritis*, 4th edn. London: RCN.

Ibandronate

Ibandronate is a bisphosphonate licensed in 2005 to treat osteoporosis in postmenopausal ♀. It selectively inhibits osteoclast activity without affecting bone formation, leading to an ↑ in bone mass. NICE has published guidelines on the use of ibandronate.

➔ See also Chapter 3, 'Osteoporosis', pp. 39–59.

Contraindications (*BNF*)

- Hypersensitivity to ibandronate or to any of the excipients.
- Hypocalcaemia (see following list of cautions).

Cautions

- Renal impairment.
- Uncorrected hypocalcaemia—this should be treated before starting ibandronate therapy.
- Rarely, osteonecrosis of the jaw has been reported in patients receiving IV bisphosphonates for the treatment of cancer and also in some patients taking oral bisphosphonates with concomitant corticosteroids. Most cases are linked with invasive dental procedures. Patients with risk factors (e.g. corticosteroids, cancer, chemotherapy, poor oral hygiene, etc.) should have a dental examination prior to treatment and avoid invasive procedures during treatment.

See the *BNF* or SPC for a full list of cautions.

Treatment regimen

- Ibandronate IV injection 3 mg every 3 months.
- Calcium and vitamin D supplementation.

Practical considerations

- *Equipment*: access to resuscitation facilities.
- *Time and nursing resources*: given over 15–30 sec as bolus IV injection.
- *Handling*: no special precautions required.

Administration/nursing care

- *Preparation of ibandronate*: ibandronate is supplied as prefilled syringes.
- *Administering the infusion*: given over 15–30 sec as bolus IV injection.
- *Observations*: not required unless the patient reports feeling unwell.

Post-infusion care and advice

- Advise patient to take any calcium and vitamin D supplements at least 60 min after the infusion.
- The patient should remain in the department for 20 min after the first injection in case of allergic response. They may then be discharged if there are no reported side effects. Subsequently they may be discharged as soon as the infusion is completed in the absence of side effects.
- Advise the patient that they may have transient flu-like symptoms particularly after the first injection. Paracetamol can be taken to relieve these symptoms. Occasionally there is temporary pain in bones and muscles and, rarely, nausea and/or abdominal pain.

Patient information

Patient information leaflets are available from:

- Royal Osteoprosis Society: https://www.nos.org.uk
- Paget's Society: https://www.paget.org.uk
- Versus Arthritis: https://www.versusarthritis.org/

Further reading

BNF: https://bnf.nice.org.uk/

BSR: https://www.rheumatology.org.uk

Electronic Medicines Compendium. Summaries of product characteristics. http://www.medicines.org.uk

NICE (2017). Bisphosphonates for treating osteoporosis (TA464) [updated 2019]. https://www.nice.org.uk/guidance/ta464

Iloprost

Iloprost is licensed for the treatment of some types of pulmonary hypertension and recently a nebulized version has been introduced for the treatment of pulmonary hypertension (Ventavis®). However, it may only be used under specialist supervision. The use of iloprost infusions for the treatment of Raynaud's syndrome and scleroderma remain unlicensed indications.

Contraindications (*BNF*)

- Unstable angina.
- Within 6 months of MI or 3 months of cardiovascular events.
- Pulmonary occlusive disease.
- Cardiac failure.
- Severe arrhythmias.
- Heart valve defects.
- Conditions which ↑ risk of bleeding.
- Pregnancy or breastfeeding.

Interactions/cautions

↑ risk of bleeding if given with NSAIDS, aspirin, phenindione, clopidogrel, eptifibatide, tirofiban, and anticoagulants. Caution with antihypertensives. See the *BNF* or SPC for a full list.

Treatment regimen for Raynaud's syndrome and scleroderma

- IV iloprost 100 mcg in 500 mL sodium chloride or glucose 5% (0.2 mcg/mL).
- To be infused continuously for up to a maximum of 6 hours daily (as tolerated) on 3–5 consecutive days (Fig. 18.1).

Drugs which may be needed at time of infusion

Paracetamol (or other analgesic) and antiemetics as required.

Practical considerations

- *Equipment*: full resuscitation facilities and infusion pump required. Bed or fully reclining chair.
- *Time and nursing resources*: each infusion lasts for 6 hours and ∴ may be given on an outpatient basis. Close monitoring is required.
- *Handling*: iloprost must be correctly diluted before being administered. If the solution comes in contact with skin or eyes, wash off immediately with large amount of water and rinse thoroughly. Contact with skin may cause a long-lasting but painless erythema.

Administration/nursing care

Preparation of iloprost solution for use with infusion pump

Add 1 mL (100 mcg) iloprost to 500 mL infusion fluid (sodium chloride 0.9% or glucose 5%) and mix well. The resulting solution of iloprost is at a concentration of 0.2 mcg per millilitre. In units where the staff are using a syringe driver, make up according to the manufacturer's guidelines.

Start the infusion at 10 mL/hour Check heart rate and blood pressure after 30 min		
↓		
If previous dose has been tolerated, ↑ to 20 mL/hour Check heart rate and blood pressure after 30 min	→	If unacceptable adverse effects[a] reduce rate by 10 mL/hour
↓		
If previous dose has been tolerated, ↑ to 30 mL/hour Check heart rate and blood pressure after 30 min	→	If unacceptable adverse effects[a] reduce rate by 10 mL/hour
↓		
If previous dose has been tolerated, ↑ to 40 mL/hour Check heart rate and blood pressure after 30 min	→	If unacceptable adverse effects[a] reduce rate by 10 mL/hour
↓		
Continue as above, ↑ **the rate by 10 mL/hour** every 30 min (providing the previous dose has been tolerated) until the optimal rate is established[b] Continue observations every 30 min	→	If unacceptable adverse effects,[a] reduce rate by 10 mL/hour
↓		
Stop the infusion after 6 hours[c]		

Fig. 18.1 Iloprost infusion.

Figure 18.1 notes: iloprost infusion treatment issues

[a]Adverse effects

- Common adverse effects: facial flushing, headache, nausea and vomiting, abdominal cramps.
- If these are considered unacceptable by the patient, reduce the rate as above.
- Give analgesics and/or antiemetics as required.
- Serious adverse effects: persistent clinically significant drop in blood pressure, persistent clinically significant tachycardia, vagal reaction with bradycardia, nausea, and vomiting.
- If these occur, *stop the infusion*. The infusion may be restarted 1 hour after the symptoms have resolved at HALF the previous rate.

[b]Optimal rate/dose

- The infusion rate is ↑ by 10 mL/hour every 30 min as detailed above until unacceptable adverse effects occur. The infusion rate is then reduced by 10 mL/hour. This reduced rate is the optimal infusion rate.
- For the majority of patients the optimal infusion rate will not exceed 50 mL/hour. For patients weighing <75 kg the optimal infusion rate will rarely exceed 40 mL/hour. A small proportion of patients may tolerate higher rates.

[c]Length of infusion

- The total maximum length of the infusion, including the rate titration, is 6 hours.

Administering the infusion/observations

Take baseline observations of temperature, pulse, and blood pressure.

- Days 1–3 (dosage titration): see Fig. 18.1
- Day 4 to the end of treatment (infusion of optimal dose): start the infusion at the optimal rate (see Fig. 18.1 footnote b) and infuse at this rate for 6 hours.

Post-infusion care

The patient may be discharged at the end of the infusion providing they are not experiencing any adverse effects and observations at the end of the infusion are satisfactory.

Patient information

Patient information leaflets are available from:

- Scleroderma and Reynaud's UK: https://www.sruk.co.uk/
- Scleroderma Society: http://www.sclerodermasociety.co.uk
- Versus Arthritis: https://www.versusarthritis.org/

Further reading

BNF: https://bnf.nice.org.uk/

Denton CP, Hughes M, Gak N, et al. (2016). BSR and BHPR guideline for the treatment of systemic sclerosis *Rheumatology (Oxford)* 22:1906–10.

Electronic Medicines Compendium. Summaries of product characteristics. http://www.medicines.org.uk

Infliximab

Infliximab is a biologically engineered monoclonal antibody inhibiting activation of TNFα, an important cytokine implicated the inflammatory responses. It is licensed for use in RA (in combination with MTX), AS, and PsA (with or without MTX). In the UK, Remicade® is the original licensed infliximab treatment. There are currently three licensed biosimilars (Flixabi®, Inflectra®, and Remsima®) although further biosimilars may well become available and options may vary regarding access in different countries.

NICE guidance for infliximab is available for RA, PsA, and AS.

➲ See 'Biosimilars', Chapter 16, p. 499.

Pretreatment screening

- Detailed history and physical examination.
- Chest X ray and TB screening.
- Routine blood tests.
- Baseline outcome measures (e.g. DAS28, BASDAI, and PsARC).
- ANA and double-stranded DNA.
- Viral hepatitis screening.
- Check previous history of VZ—if no previous history, a VZ antibody test should be undertaken—for those >50 years of age with a negative test and no contraindications, a single VZ vaccination should be offered at least 14 days prior to biologic commencement.
- Consider HIV screening.

Contraindications

- Hypersensitivity to infliximab or other murine proteins.
- Active acute or chronic infection.
- Consider previous sepsis in prosthetic joints if remains *in situ*.
- Severe heart failure NYHA class III/IV (caution in NYHA class I/II).
- Demyelinating disease.
- Pregnancy.
- Use in children <18 years of age (safety not yet established).
- Live vaccines.

Treatment regimen

- RA—initial dose 3 mg per kg body weight.
  - Infusions at weeks 0, 2, 6, and then every 8 weeks.
- PsA—initial dose 5 mg per kg body weight.
  - Infusions at weeks 0, 2, 6, and then every 8 weeks.
- AS—initial dose 5 mg per kg body weight.
  - Infusions at weeks 0, 2, 6, and then every 6–8 weeks.
- All indications—dose ↑ may sometimes be considered for inadequate response (see the SPC).
- Table 18.2 shows drugs to be available during the infusion.

Practical considerations

- *Equipment*: full resuscitation facilities and infusion pump are required. A sterile, low-protein-binding filter (pore size <1.2 μm) is essential.

- *Time and nursing resources*: infusions take between 1 and 2 hours. Close monitoring is required. Patient must be observed for 2 hours following first four infusions, and then for 1 hour following subsequent infusions.
- *Handling*: infliximab does not require any special handling precautions.

Administration/nursing care

Prior to treatment

- Check that there are no contraindications to treatment.
- Check recent blood tests are within satisfactory parameters.
- Urinalysis.
- Record baseline observations of:
  - Temperature, pulse, and blood pressure.
- Prepare the infusion according to the manufacturer's guidelines. It is supplied in vials as a dry powder. One vial mixed with 10 mL sterile water equates to 100 mg infliximab. The prescribed dose is added to 250 mL 0.9% sodium chloride. Vials should not be shared between patients as this can ↑ the risk of contamination.

Administering the infusion

Infliximab is infused through a filter (➔ see 'Equipment', Chapter 18, p. 554) into a peripheral cannula using an IV pump with a primed line.

Clinical observations during infusions

- Every 30 min—temperature, pulse, and blood pressure.
- Observe for side effects throughout: take appropriate action as shown in the following subsections and record any adverse events in the patient's notes.

Infusion reactions and adverse events

See Table 18.3.

Table 18.3 Infliximab infusion reactions and adverse events

Infusion reaction	Action
Mild fever, chills, pruritus	• Slow down rate of infusion
Chest pain, hypertension, hypotension, and/or dyspnoea	• Stop infusion • Alert physician—consider use of IV hydrocortisone and/or IV chlorpheniramine • Review with physician—consider restarting infusion after 20 min at a slower rate
Anaphylactic reaction	• Stop infusion • Call physician—administer IV hydrocortisone, IV chlorpheniramine, and any emergency treatment as indicated

Post-infusion care and advice to patients

Monitor blood pressure, temperature, and pulse every 30 min for 2 hours following first four infusions, and then for 1 hour following subsequent infusions. Discharge patient post infusion providing all observations are satisfactory.

Advise patient to seek medical advice for symptoms of infection and to maintain their regular monitoring and clinical attendances.

- Maintain regular MTX monitoring according to BSR and local guidelines.
- If monotherapy, blood monitoring (FBC, U&E, and LFTs) every 3–6 months.

Ensure next infusion date booked and patient has a biologics alert card. Provide first contact point telephone numbers to the patient.

Patient information

Patient information leaflets are available from:

- National Ankylosing Spondylitis Society (NASS): ☞ http://www.nass.co.uk
- National Rheumatoid Arthritis Society: ☞ http://www.nras.org.uk
- Versus Arthritis: ☞ https://www.versusarthritis.org/

Further reading

BNF: ☞ https://bnf.nice.org.uk/

BSR: ☞ https://www.rheumatology.org.uk

Holroyd CR, Seth R, Bukhari M, et al. (2019). The BSR DMARD safety guidelines in inflammatory arthritis—executive summary. *Rheumatology (Oxford)* 58:220–6.

Electronic Medicines Compendium. Summaries of product characteristics. ☞ http://www.medicines.org.uk

NICE (2010). Adalimumab, etanercept, infliximab, rituximab and abatacept for the treatment of rheumatoid arthritis after the failure of a TNF inhibitor (TA195). ☞ https://www.nice.org.uk/guidance/ta195

NICE (2010). Etanercept, infliximab and adalimumab for the treatment of psoriatic arthritis (TA199). ☞ https://www.nice.org.uk/guidance/ta199

NICE (2016). Adalimumab, etanercept, infliximab, certolizumab pegol, golimumab, tocilizumab and abatacept for rheumatoid arthritis not previously treated with DMARDs or after conventional DMARDs only have failed (TA375). ☞ https://www.nice.org.uk/guidance/ta375

NICE (2016). TNF-alpha inhibitors for ankylosing spondylitis and non-radiographic axial spondyloarthritis (TA383). ☞ https://www.nice.org.uk/guidance/TA383

Royal College of Nursing (2017). *Assessing, Managing and Monitoring Biologic Therapies for Inflammatory Arthritis*, 4th edn. London: RCN.

Methylprednisolone

IV methylprednisolone is given to patients in a number of rheumatological conditions to suppress inflammation.

Contraindications

- Active infection.

Cautions

- Unstable diabetes mellitus.
- Unstable cardiac conditions.
- Avoid concomitant use of live vaccines.
- Recent contact with shingles/chickenpox.

Refer to the *BNF* for complete listings.

Treatment regimen

- Methylprednisolone 500 mg or 1 g in 250 mL 0.9% sodium chloride.
- Three infusions may be prescribed to be given over a 3-day period.

Practical considerations

- *Equipment*: full resuscitation facilities and infusion pump required.
- *Time and nursing resources*: infusions usually last for 60 min. Close monitoring is required.
- *Handling*: no special precautions required.

Administration/nursing care

- Prepare the infusion according to the manufacturer's guidelines.

Administering the infusion

As prescribed on the drug chart. Commonly, the infusion will be given over a period of 60 min.

Clinical observations during infusions

Prior to infusion: record pulse and blood pressure as a baseline. Further observations are not required unless the patient reports feeling unwell.

Infusion reactions and adverse events

- Rare cases of anaphylaxis have been reported.
- Rarely, cardiac arrhythmias and/or circulatory collapse and/or cardiac arrest can occur. Usually associated with rapid administration of large doses (>500 mg in <10 min).
- Refer to the *BNF*/SPC for a complete list.

Post-infusion care

The patient should remain in the day unit for 1 hour after the first infusion for observation. If further infusions are given, the patient may be discharged as soon as the infusion is completed, providing there are no reported side effects.

Patient information

Patient information leaflets are available from:

- Versus Arthritis: https://www.versusarthritis.org/

Further reading

BNF: https://bnf.nice.org.uk/

Electronic Medicines Compendium. Summaries of product characteristics. http://www.medicines.org.uk

Pamidronate

Pamidronate is a bisphosphonate used to treat the overproduction of bone and relieve pain associated with Paget's disease. It is given to treat osteoporosis when oral preparations are not deemed appropriate or cannot be tolerated. Other licensed uses include tumour-induced hypercalcaemia and metastatic bone pain.

Contraindications

- Clinically significant hypersensitivity to pamidronate disodium or other bisphosphonates.

Cautions

- Should not be given with other bisphosphonates.
- Rarely, osteonecrosis of the jaw has been reported in patients receiving IV bisphosphonates for the treatment of cancer and also in some patients taking oral bisphosphonates with concomitant corticosteroids. Most cases are linked with invasive dental procedures. Patients with risk factors (e.g. corticosteroids, cancer, chemotherapy, poor oral hygiene, etc.) should have a dental examination prior to treatment and avoid invasive procedures during treatment.
- In patients with Paget's who may be at risk of calcium or vitamin D deficiency, oral supplementation should be considered.

See the *BNF* or SPC for a full list.

Treatment regimen for Paget's

Pamidronate 60 mg in 250 mL sodium chloride 0.9% is often prescribed but other regimens may be used. See the *BNF* and SPC for complete listings.

Practical considerations

- *Equipment*: full resuscitation facilities and infusion pump required.
- *Time and nursing resources*: infusions may last for 1–3 hours.
- *Handling*: no special precautions required.

Administration/nursing care

Preparation of pamidronate

Pamidronate is supplied as a dry powder and should be prepared according to the instructions given by the manufacturer. It should never be given as a bolus injection.

Administering the infusion/observations

- In order to minimize local reaction, a large vein should be selected for cannula insertion.
- Infusion rate should not exceed 60 mg per hour and in renal impairment, the rate should not exceed 20 mg hour.
- Prior to infusion: record pulse and blood pressure as a baseline.
- These observations do not need to be repeated unless the patient reports feeling unwell.

Post-infusion care and advice

- The patient should remain in the department for 1 hour after the first infusion in case of an allergic response. They may then be discharged if there are no reported side effects. Subsequently they may be discharged as soon as the infusion is completed in the absence of side effects.
- Serum electrolytes, calcium, and phosphate should be monitored as levels may fall 24–48 hours post infusion; normalization is achieved between 3–7 days. It is ∴ suggested that blood levels are checked prior to the infusion and after 1 week.
- Advise the patient that they may have a rise in body temperature in the next 24–48 hours and/or flu-like symptoms. Paracetamol can be taken to relieve these symptoms. Occasionally there is temporary pain in bones and muscles and, rarely, nausea and/or abdominal pain.
- There are rare cases of somnolence and/or dizziness after the infusion ∴ the patient should be advised not to drive home.

Patient information

Patient information leaflets are available from:

- Royal Osteoprosis Society: https://www.nos.org.uk
- Paget's society: https://www.paget.org.uk
- Versus Arthritis: https://www.versusarthritis.org/

Further reading

BNF: https://bnf.nice.org.uk/

Electronic Medicines Compendium. Summaries of product characteristics. http://www.medicines.org.uk

Rituximab

Rituximab is a genetically engineered chimeric mouse/human antibody designed to deplete precursor B cells. It is indicated for use in severe active RA in combination with MTX in adult patients and in ANCA-associated vasculitis in combination with glucocorticoids. NICE has published guidance for the treatment of RA and ANCA-associated vasculitis. MabThera® is the original rituximab treatment. There are currently two biosimilars available (Rixathon® and Truxima®) although more may become available and others may be available in different countries.

Pretreatment screening

- Detailed history and physical examination.
- Chest X-ray.
- Routine blood tests.
- Viral hepatitis screen.
- Immunoglobulin levels. Repeat prior to each cycle.
- Baseline DAS28.
- CD19 may be considered.
- Any inactivated vaccinations should be given 1 month prior or at least 7 months after treatment (no live vaccines).
- Check previous history of VZ—if no previous history of VZ, an antibody test should be undertaken—for those >50 years of age with a negative test and no contraindications, a single VZ vaccination (live vaccine) should be offered at least 1 month before treatment is initiated. Discuss with the rheumatologist.
- Patients who are taking antihypertensive therapies may need to withhold their treatment for 12 hours prior to the infusion.

Contraindications

- Hypersensitivity to rituximab or other murine proteins.
- Active acute or chronic infection.
- Severe heart failure NYHA class IV.
- Pregnancy.
- Use in children (safety not yet established).

Treatment regimen

- IV 1000 mg rituximab on day 1 and day 15.
- MTX weekly.

Further courses of may be considered 6–12 months after initial course.

- Table 18.4 shows drugs given 60 min prior to infusion.
- Table 18.2 shows drugs to be available during the infusion.

  NB: in patients with an acute flare of GPA or microscopic polyangiitis:
- Methylprednisolone given intravenously for 1–3 days at a dose of 1000 mg per day is recommended prior to the first infusion of MabThera® (the last dose of methylprednisolone may be given on the same day as the first infusion of MabThera®).
- This should be followed by oral prednisone 1 mg/kg/day (not to exceed 80 mg/day and tapered as rapidly as possible based on clinical need) during and after MabThera® treatment.
- ➲ See Chapter 5, 'Connective tissue diseases', pp. 127–184.

Table 18.4 Drugs given 60 min prior to infusion

Methylprednisolone	100 mg IV (100 mg in 100 mL normal saline infused over 30 min)
Paracetamol	1 g orally
Chlorpheniramine	10 mg IV

Practical considerations

- *Equipment*: full resuscitation facilities and infusion pump required.
- *Time and nursing resources*: first infusion may take between 6 and 7 hours, the second can be completed more quickly if no adverse effects during first one. Close monitoring is required.
- *Handling*: as rituximab is not an irritant there are no special handling precautions in the case of extravasation.

Administration/nursing care

- Check no analgesics containing paracetamol have been taken within the last 4 hours and that any morning dose of an antihypertensive has been omitted.
- Take baseline observations of temperature, pulse, blood pressure, and oxygen saturation levels.
- Administer pre-infusion medications as per drug chart 60 min before rituximab.
- In units where the staff prepare the infusion, make up rituximab according to the manufacturer's guidelines.

Administering the infusion

- Rituximab is infused through a peripheral cannula using an IV pump with a primed line.
- The following regimen is based on a concentration of 2 mg/mL, i.e. 1000 mg in 500 mL.
- The rate of the infusion will depend on the concentration of the rituximab and whether it is the first or second infusion. In the event of a reaction to the first infusion, the second infusion should be administered as per instructions for the first infusion (Tables 18.5–18.7).

Clinical observations during infusions

- Blood pressure.
- Pulse.
- Temperature.
- Oxygen saturation levels.

First hour every 15 min then every 30 min (prior to ↑ the rate of infusion and until infusion completed).

NB: most reactions have been noted during the first few minutes of the infusion so observe the patient carefully during this time and following each ↑ in infusion rate.

Table 18.5 Rituximab infusion rate for day 1

Time	mg/hour	mL/hour
1st 30 min	50	25
2nd 30 min	100	50
Then the rate can be ↑ by 50 mg/hour (25 mL/hour) every 30 min to a maximum rate of 400 mg/hour (200 mL/hour) providing no adverse reactions occur		

Table 18.6 Rituximab infusion rate for day 15—if the patient had no reaction to the first infusion

Time	mg/hour	mL/hour
1st 30 min	100	50
2nd 30 min	200	100
Then the rate can be ↑ by 100 mg/hour (50 mL/hour) every 30 min to a maximum rate of 400 mg/hour (200 mL/hour) providing no adverse reactions occur		

Table 18.7 Rituximab can be diluted to a concentration of between 1 and 4 mg/mL normal saline

Concentration (mg/mL)	1	2	4
Volume of fluid (mL)	1000	500	250

Infusion reactions and adverse events

Acute infusion reactions may occur within 1–2 hours of the first rituximab infusion (Table 18.8). These may include:

- Fever.
- Headache.
- Rigors.
- Flushing.
- Nausea.
- Rash.
- Upper respiratory tract infection symptoms.

Transient hypotension and bronchospasm are usually related to the infusion rate. A small ↑ in serious infections has been noted (not opportunistic infections such as TB).

Table 18.8 Rituximab infusion reactions

Reaction	Action to take
Mild-to-moderate reactions (30–35% at 1st infusion; less with the 2nd)—e.g. low-grade fever; hypotension <30 mmHg from baseline	• Halve the infusion rate • Consider giving medication as needed
Moderate-to-severe reactions (uncommon: frequency is reduced by the concomitant use of IV steroids)—e.g. fever >38.5°C; chills; mucosal swelling; SOB; hypotension by >30 mmHg from baseline	• STOP the infusion and treat the symptoms • Contact the doctor • The infusion should be restarted at half the previous rate only when the symptoms have resolved

Post-infusion care advice for the patient

- Can leave the department once infusion is complete and observations are satisfactory.
- Seek medical advice if any symptoms suggestive of an infection, e.g. fever in the hours or days after the infusion (provide contact numbers for the rheumatology department or first contact point, e.g. GP and/or attend ED).
- Women of childbearing age should not become pregnant within 12 months of their last infusion. Advise effective use of contraception.
- Restart any antihypertensive drugs on next day.
- Maintain regular MTX monitoring according to BSR and local guidelines.
- If monotherapy monitoring of FBC, U&E, and LFTs—every 3–6 months.
- Ensure follow-up assessment at 16 weeks to assess response.

Patient information

Patient information leaflets are available from:

- National Rheumatoid Arthritis Society: http://www.nras.org.uk
- Versus Arthritis: https://www.versusarthritis.org/

Further reading

BNF: https://bnf.nice.org.uk/

BSR: https://www.rheumatology.org.uk

Holroyd CR, Seth R, Bukhari M, et al. (2019). The BSR DMARD safety guidelines in inflammatory arthritis—executive summary. *Rheumatology (Oxford)* 58:220–6.

Electronic Medicines Compendium. Summaries of product characteristics. http://www.medicines.org.uk

NICE (2010). Adalimumab, etanercept, infliximab, rituximab and abatacept for the treatment of rheumatoid arthritis after the failure of a TNF inhibitor (TA195). https://www.nice.org.uk/guidance/ta195

NICE (2014). Rituximab in combination with glucocorticoids for treating anti-neutrophil cytoplasmic antibody-associated vasculitis (TA308). https://www.nice.org.uk/guidance/ta308

Tocilizumab

Tocilizumab is a monoclonal antibody which targets IL-6. Tocilizumab IV is licensed for the treatment of RA either as monotherapy or in combination with MTX. It is also indicated in JIA (see the SPC for full details). The subcutaneous version is also licensed for GCA (➔ see Chapter 5, 'Connective tissue disease', Chapter 4, p. 115). ➔ Also see sections on JIA in Chapter 4, 'Inflammatory joint diseases', Chapter 4, pp. 81–91 and p 62.

NICE has published guidance for the treatment of RA and JIA.

Pretreatment screening

- Detailed history and physical examination.
- Chest X-ray.
- TB screening.
- Viral hepatitis screening.
- Check previous history of VZ—if no previous history, a VZ antibody test should be undertaken—for those >50 years of age with a negative test and no contraindications, a single VZ vaccination should be offered at least 14 days prior to biologic commencement.
- Consider HIV screening.
- Routine blood tests.
- Lipid blood tests.
- Baseline outcome measurement (e.g. DAS28).

Contraindications

- Hypersensitivity to the active substance or to any of the excipients.
- Active acute or chronic infection.
- Concomitant use of other biologic agents.
- Pregnancy and breastfeeding.
- Use in children <6 years old.
- Live vaccines at time of treatment (see current vaccination guidelines for interval between vaccination and starting tocilizumab).

Cautions

- History of recurrent or persistent infection.
- Any underlying condition that predisposes to infection (e.g. diverticulitis, diabetes, and interstitial lung disease).

Treatment regimen

- 8 mg/kg body weight (doses >800 mg are not recommended in individuals who weigh >100 kg).
- The dose should be adjusted in the case of liver enzyme abnormalities, low absolute neutrophil counts, and low platelets; please see the SPC and BSR/BHPR guideline for more information.
- Infusion given at 4-weekly intervals.
- MTX weekly if on combination therapy.
- Table 18.2 shows drugs which may be needed at the time of infusion.

Practical considerations

- *Equipment*: full resuscitation facilities and infusion pump are required. A sterile, non-pyrogenic, low-protein-binding filter (pore size 0.2 μm to <1.2 μm) is essential. A silicone-free disposable syringe is provided, and this must be used to reconstitute each vial.
- *Time and nursing resources*: infusions take 60 min. Close monitoring is required.
- *Handling*: tocilizumab does not require any special handling precautions.

Administration/nursing care

Prior to treatment

- Check there are no contraindications to treatment (➔ see 'Contraindications', p. 578).
- Check any recent blood tests are within satisfactory parameters.
- Record baseline observations of temperature, pulse, and blood pressure.
- Urinalysis if symptoms of infection are reported.

Preparation

Prepare the infusion according to the manufacturer's guidelines. Tocilizumab is supplied in vials containing 20 mg/mL of either 4 mL (80 mg), 10 mL (200 mg), or 20 mL (400 mg).

In adult patients, it should be diluted to a final volume of 100 mL with sterile non-pyrogenic sodium chloride 0.9% solution, i.e. withdraw the equivalent volume of fluid from a 100 mL bag. In children, it should be diluted to a final volume of 50 mL, please see the SPC for full details.

Administering the infusion

- Tocilizumab should be administered over 60 min.

Clinical observations during infusions

- Observations of temperature, pulse, and blood pressure every 30 min.
- Observe for side effects throughout—take appropriate action and record any adverse events in the patient's notes.

For a full list of adverse effects, see the SPC.

Post-infusion care and advice to patients

- Advise patient:
  - To seek medical advice if any symptoms develop suggestive of an infection, e.g. fever in the hours or days after the infusion (provide contact numbers for the rheumatology department or first contact point, e.g. GP and/or attend ED).
  - If taking MTX, maintain regular monitoring according to BSR and/or local guidelines.
  - If tocilizumab monotherapy blood tests should be repeated in the week prior to the next infusion.
- Ensure follow-up for assessment or next infusion has been arranged.
- Ensure patient has a biologics alert card.
- Ensure regular lipid parameters at 3 months then at physician's discretion.

Patient information

Patient information leaflets are available from:

- National Rheumatoid Arthritis Society: http://www.nras.org.uk
- Versus Arthritis: https://www.versusarthritis.org/

Further reading

BNF: https://bnf.nice.org.uk/

BSR: https://www.rheumatology.org.uk

Electronic Medicines Compendium. Summaries of product characteristics. http://www.medicines.org.uk

Holroyd CR, Seth R, Bukhari M, et al. (2019). The BSR DMARD safety guidelines in inflammatory arthritis—executive summary. *Rheumatology (Oxford)* 58:220–6.

NICE (2011). Tocilizumab for the treatment of systemic juvenile idiopathic arthritis (TA238). https://www.nice.org.uk/guidance/ta238

NICE (2014). Tocilizumab for the treatment of rheumatoid arthritis. https://www.nice.org.uk/guidance/ta247

NICE (2015). Abatacept, adalimumab, etanercept and tocilizumab for treating juvenile idiopathic arthritis (TA373). https://www.nice.org.uk/guidance/ta373

NICE (2016). Adalimumab, etanercept, infliximab, certolizumab pegol, golimumab, tocilizumab and abatacept for rheumatoid arthritis not previously treated with DMARDs or after conventional DMARDs only have failed (TA375). https://www.nice.org.uk/guidance/ta375

Royal College of Nursing (2017). *Assessing, Managing and Monitoring Biologic Therapies for Inflammatory Arthritis*, 4th edn. London: RCN.

Zoledronic acid

Zoledronic acid is a bisphosphonate licensed to treat osteoporosis in postmenopausal ♀ and adult ♂, and treatment of osteoporosis associated with long-term systemic glucocorticoid therapy in postmenopausal ♀ and adult ♂. It is also for the treatment of Paget's disease in adults. It selectively inhibits osteoclast activity without affecting bone formation, leading to an ↑ in bone mass. NICE guidelines on bisphosphonates for treating osteoporosis are available.

➲ See Chapter 4, 'Osteoporosis', pp. 39–59.

Contraindications (*BNF*)

- Hypersensitivity to zoledronic acid, any bisphosphonate, or to any of the excipients.
- Hypocalcaemia (see following list of cautions).
- Severe renal impairment (creatinine clearance <35 mL/min).
- Pregnancy and breastfeeding.

Cautions

- Renal impairment (see the SPC).
- Uncorrected hypocalcaemia—this should be treated before starting ibandronate therapy.
- Rarely, osteonecrosis of the jaw has been reported in patients receiving IV bisphosphonates for the treatment of cancer and also in some patients taking oral bisphosphonates with concomitant corticosteroids. Most cases are linked with invasive dental procedures. Patients with risk factors (e.g. corticosteroids, cancer, chemotherapy, poor oral hygiene, etc.) should have a dental examination prior to treatment and avoid invasive procedures during treatment.

See the *BNF* or SPC for a full list.

Treatment regimen

Osteoporosis

- Zoledronic acid IV injection 5 mg every 12 months.
- Calcium and vitamin D supplementation.

Paget's disease

- Initial dose of zoledronic acid by IV injection 5 mg, retreatment after 1 year or longer in patient who have relapsed.
- Adequate supplemental calcium corresponding to at least 500 mg elemental calcium twice daily is ensured for at least 10 days following zoledronic acid administration.

Practical considerations

- *Equipment*: access to resuscitation facilities.
- *Time and nursing resources*: given over not less than 15 min as an IV infusion (5 mg in 100 mL).
- *Handling*: no special precautions required.

Administration/nursing care

- *Preparation of zoledronic acid*: as infusion.
- *Administering the infusion*: given over not less than 15 min as IV infusion.
- *Observations*: not required unless the patient reports feeling unwell.

Post-infusion care and advice

- Advise patient to take any calcium or calcium and vitamin D supplements as prescribed.
- The patient should remain in the department for 20 min after the first infusion in case of an allergic response. They may then be discharged if there are no reported side effects. Subsequently they may be discharged as soon as the infusion is completed in the absence of side effects.
- Advise the patient that they may have transient flu-like symptoms particularly after the first injection. Paracetamol or ibuprofen can be taken to relieve these symptoms. Occasionally there is temporary pain in bones and muscles and, rarely, nausea and/or abdominal pain.

Patient information

Patient information leaflets are available from:

- Royal Osteoprosis Society: ℘ https://www.nos.org.uk
- Paget's society: ℘ https://www.paget.org.uk
- Versus Arthritis: ℘ https://www.versusarthritis.org/

Further reading

BNF: ℘ https://bnf.nice.org.uk/

BSR: ℘ https://www.rheumatology.org.uk

Electronic Medicines Compendium. Summaries of product characteristics. ℘ http://www.medicines.org.uk

NICE (2017). Bisphosphonates for treating osteoporosis (TA464) [updated 2019]. ℘ https://www.nice.org.uk/guidance/ta464

Chapter 19

Non-pharmacological therapies

Joint protection

What is joint protection? Why use it?

The pain, strain, and frustration of undertaking daily activities are common features in many types of arthritis, back pain, and soft tissue conditions (e.g. CTS, de Quervain's tenosynovitis, and repetitive strain injury). Joint protection is used to:

- Protect joints that are vulnerable as a result of pain, swelling, or weakness of the ligaments and muscles.
- Provide improved movement patterns and activities to conserve energy and protect the joints.
- Ensure correct posture and positioning when undertaking activities.
- Restructuring activities to improve function, reduce pain, swelling, risk of deformities, and maximize independence.

► For people with inflammatory arthritis or hand OA, refer to an OT for detailed advice and training to preserve joint function long term. If they have lower limb OA, refer to a PT.[1]

Joint protection, pacing, and exercise

People can be confused why they are recommended to protect joints and pace activities and yet to exercise. It can seem contradictory. Joint protection is not about stopping activity but doing it differently. Pacing reduces fatigue so they can exercise. Exercise builds muscle and endurance to protect joints and reduce fatigue. Present these strategies as working together (Table 19.1).

Making changes

Research supports the value of joint protection[2,3] and exercise[4,5]. Finding easier ways of carrying out tasks makes common sense and over time people will naturally find ways to ease pain and avoid activities that produce pain. There are benefits in convincing patients early on of the benefits of joint protection.

Adjusting to change

Many people find change difficult, experience frustrations, and find the 'need' to change like feeling as if they have 'given in'. Patients may need time and support to adapt to these changes. They should be encouraged to recognize that they are taking control, not giving in. Start by asking about:

- Everyday problems they experience and how their arthritis limits the activities they value (e.g. at work, hobbies, socially, sex life and in the home). Encourage them to review the way they use their affected joints and note which activities and movements cause them aches, pain, stiffness and/or fatigue.
- How they see being able to do these things in 5 years' time?
- The pros and cons of making changes to help them achieve what they want to do. Reiterate that adapting is not giving in.
- When they have accepted the principles of change and benefits, advise them of the value of joint protection, how it works, and key principles (Table 19.1). Provide practical ideas and help them set achievable goals to practise using the solutions outlined.

Table 19.1 Key joint protection principles

Principle	Example
1. Reduce force and effort	Use levers, labour-saving devices, slide, or wheels to move objects, or assistive technology (➜ see Chapter 11, 'Care in the community', p. 351)
2. Spread load over several joints	Use palms of 2 hands to carry, not fingertips (use a cloth for hot items)
3. Use larger, stronger joints	Hold bags over forearm/shoulder or use backpack not hands; use hip/shoulder to open/close doors/drawers
4. Use joints in stable positions; avoid positions of potential deformity (e.g. bent sideways or down)	Avoid twisting at knee: stand up with knees facing forward, not to side; push up with palms of hands, not knuckles. Avoid lifting heavy objects with wrists bent down. Avoid pushing fingers towards little finger
5. Avoid strong pinch and grip	Enlarge and pad handles, pens, and tools; use gadgets for easy grip, e.g. jar openers (➜ see Chapter 11, 'Care in the community', pp. 351–383). Don't press hard on thumb
6. Correct posture	Avoid poking head and leaning forward when active or sitting. Use supportive seating and beds

- Then progress to ask about activities they have difficulty with and/or find painful. Encourage them to problem-solve and propose alternative solutions by listing on paper the different stages in the activity; analyse how they do each stage—discuss movements and equipment used and which aspects cause difficulty, aches, or pain. Focus on changing the elements of a problem; use the principles in Table 19.1 to jointly brainstorm different ways of doing these stages. Note these on paper and give the person a copy to help them remember.
- At the next follow-up appointment, review their progress and encourage them to try problem-solving again for another problem—and repeat if you have time.

References

1. Versus Arthritis. Looking after your joints when you have arthritis. https://www.versusarthritis.org/order-our-information
2. Hammond A, Bryan J, Hardy A (2008). Effects of a modular behavioural arthritis education programme. *Rheumatology (Oxford)* 47:1712–8.
3. Oppong R, Jowett S, Nicholls E, et al. (2014). Joint protection and hand exercises: an economic evaluation. *Rheumatology (Oxford)* 54:876–83.
4. Lamb SE, Williamson EM, Heine PJ, et al. (2015). Strengthening and Stretching for Rheumatoid Arthritis of the Hand Trial (SARAH) Trial Team. *Lancet* 385:421–9.
5. Dziedzic K, Nicholls E, Hill S, et al. (2015). Self-management approaches for osteoarthritis in the hand. *Ann Rheum Dis* 74:108–18.

Why splint joints?

Hand/wrist splints are commonly provided for RA, thumb OA, and repetitive strain injuries such as CTS and other types of tenosynovitis. They are provided to:

- Reduce pain.
- Improve function.
- Reduce inflammation.
- Realign or correct deformity.

When to splint?

Indications for splint referral are given in Table 19.2. Referral to OT is recommended for splints as an individual assessment is often needed and is best combined with joint protection and hand exercise training. The provision of splints must meet Medical Devices Agency regulations. Splint adherence is significantly improved by effective patient education.

Wrist working splints

(See Fig. 19.1a.)

There are many commercial, working splint designs and they are made out of a range of products including elasticated fabric, neoprene, or elastane with aluminium or plastic support inserts. It is essential that the splint is the correct size and fit. If one design does not suit, try another. The insert should be moulded according to individual need:

- 20–30° extension for a functional splint.
- Or neutral–10° extension in CTS for symptom relief.

The splint straps should be firm enough to control wrist movement. The splint should not impede hand movement at the transverse palmar or thenar creases as this may cause stiffness. Patients should be informed that these splints initially will reduce grip strength as they take 1 or 2 weeks to get used to. After this, most benefits are gained in moderate to heavy activities (e.g. vacuuming, ironing, gardening, and lifting) as grip improves and pain reduces. They should not be worn for long periods or a stiff wrist may develop. Splints need replacing every 6 months or so as they wear out.[1]

Table 19.2 Indications for hand splints

Splint type	Indication
Wrist working	RA: wrist pain limiting hand function; weak grip CTS: wrist pain (day or night); pins and needles; weak grip
Hand resting	RA: night-time hand/wrist pain; acute inflammation wrist/MCP joints
Thumb	RA or OA: CMC joint or first MCP joint pain-reducing function
Figure of 8/silver ring	RA: correctable swan neck/boutonnière deformity
MCP ulnar deviation	RA: correctable MCP joint deformity (to realign fingers for improved function).

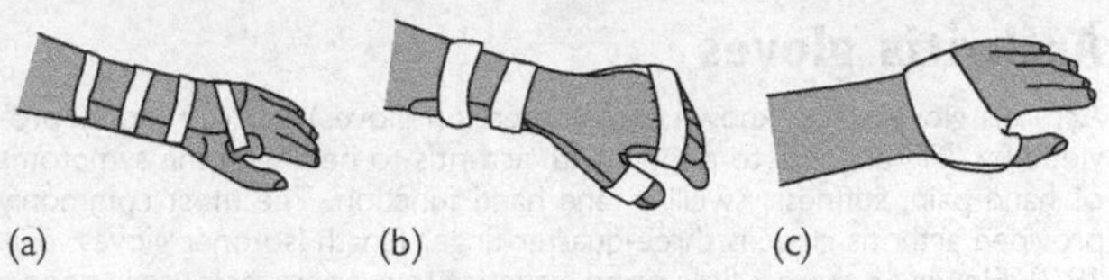

Fig. 19.1 Joint protection splints. (a) Elastic wrist working splint; (b) hand resting splint; (c) thumb splint.

Hand resting splints

(See Fig. 19.1b.)

These are usually custom-made in thermoplastic, placing the hand in a comfortable rest position. They are most beneficial in RA, other inflammatory diseases, and repetitive strain injuries if the person is being kept awake at night by pain. If two splints are necessary, it might be more appropriate to recommend alternate use or a modified design with finger/thumb ends free to enable hand function, e.g. pulling covers or flipping light switches.

Thumb splints

(See Fig. 19.1c.)

The thumb contributes 60% of hand function. Thumb pain and instability can significantly affect daily activities and work. OA of the CMC joint affects >30% of postmenopausal women ♀. Many do not realize that a splint and therapy would help. There are many designs:

- Hand-based C bar.
- Elasticated thumb wrap.
- Thumb/wrist splints.

The choice will be dependent on the extent of the problem—to effectively reduce pain. Early splint provision may avoid the need for later surgery.

MCP and finger deformity splints

Custom-made splints can correct early finger deformities and realign MCP joints for improved hand function in RA. These may avoid the need for later surgery.

Reference

1. Adams J, Hammond A, Burridge J, Cooper C (2005). Static orthoses in the prevention of hand dysfunction in rheumatoid arthritis: a review of the literature. *Musculoskeletal Care* 3:85–101.

Arthritis gloves

Arthritis gloves (also known as compression gloves) are commonly provided by OTs and PTs to people with arthritis to help with the symptoms of hand pain, stiffness, swelling, and hand function. The most commonly provided arthritis glove is three-quarter-finger length Isotoner gloves[1] (Fig. 19.2). However, there is little or no evidence to support their use in people with arthritis.[2,3] Isotoner gloves had comparable effects on hand symptoms and hand function to placebo gloves and are not cost-effective.[3]

If people with arthritis want to wear arthritis gloves to provide warmth and light support, they could be recommended to purchase mid-finger length gloves, typically containing 3–5% elastane themselves. Alternatively, they could try versions of arthritis gloves available at lower cost than Isotoner gloves. Overall, treatment strategies should focus on providing hand self-management education (joint protection and hand exercises) using cognitive behavioural approaches, as this is already proven to be effective in reducing hand pain and improving hand function.[3–5]

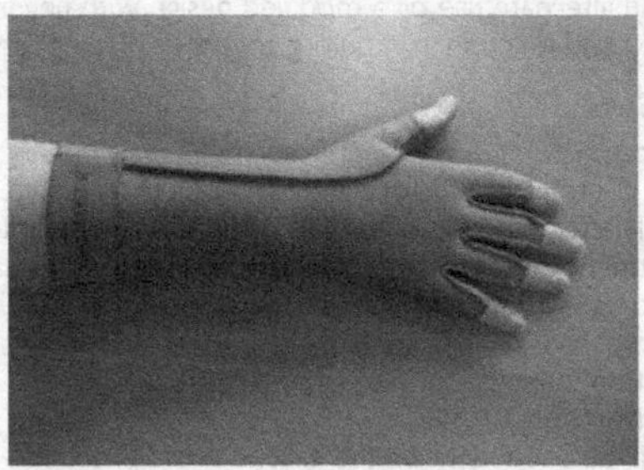

Fig. 19.2 Three-quarter-finger length Isotoner gloves: 80% nylon; 20% elastane (Lycra®); manufacturer states that they apply 23–32 mmHg pressure at MCP joints. Although there is no empirical evidence to support this.

References

1. Prior Y, Arafin N, Bartley C, Hammond A (2018) Inflammatory Or Rheumatoid Arthritis Patients' Perspectives On The Effect Of Arthritis Gloves On Their Hand Pain And Function (A-Gloves Trial): A Qualitative Study. *Annals of the Rheumatic Diseases* 77:1866-1867. Available at: http://dx.doi.org/10.1136/annrheumdis-2018-eular.5980
2. Hammond A, Jones V, Prior Y (2015). The effects of compression gloves on hand symptoms and hand function in RA and hand OA: a systematic review. *Clin Rehabil* 30:213–24.
3. Hammond A, Prior Y, Sutton C, et al. (2018). The effects of arthritis gloves on people with rheumatoid or inflammatory arthritis with hand pain: a randomised controlled trial (A-GLOVES TRIAL). *Ann Rheum Dis* 77 Suppl:A204.
4. Lamb SE, Williamson EM, Heine PJ, et al. (2015). Strengthening and Stretching for Rheumatoid Arthritis of the Hand Trial (SARAH) Trial Team. *Lancet* 385:421–9.
5. Oppong R, Jowett S, Nicholls E, et al. (2014). Joint protection and hand exercises: an economic evaluation. *Rheumatology (Oxford)* 54:876–83.

6. Hammond A, Prior Y (2016). A systematic review of the effectiveness of hand exercise interventions in Rheumatoid Arthritis. *British Medical Bulletin*, Advanced Access Published June 30, 2016:1–14. doi:10.1093/bmb/ldw024

Further reading

van Eijk-Hustings Y, van Tubergen A, Boström C, et al. (2012). EULAR recommendations for the role of the nurse in the management of chronic inflammatory arthritis. *Ann Rheum Dis* 71:13–9.

Vegt AE, Grond R, Grüschke JS, et al. (2017). The effect of two different orthoses on pain, hand function, patient satisfaction and preference in patients with thumb carpometacarpal OA: a multicentre, crossover, randomised controlled trial. *Bone Joint J* 99-B:237–44.

Fatigue and stress

Fatigue in arthritis

Fatigue is common in inflammatory forms of arthritis and OA and is increasingly recognized as an important factor affecting quality of life of those with long-term MSCs. Pacing uses the principle that regular short rests help 'recharge batteries' when fatigue, pain, and stress are factors in disease. However, there are many contributing factors and possible solutions to pacing. See Table 19.3 for ideas.

Activity pacing

Adjusting to limitations of a condition such as arthritis can frustrate people. As they attempt to maintain activities they used to be able to achieve easily, they may state that they do not wish to be 'beaten' by their condition and may overdo things on 'good days' and suffer for it later: the 'boom and bust' cycle. People may fail to accept the condition and restrictions (e.g. the over-doers) or become fearful of damaging joints or pain and become 'deconditioned' by a cycle of muscle weakness and loss of vitality (insufficient activity).

Research shows that pacing achieves effective outcomes for those who adapt to these frustrating limitations. Activity pacing works on the links between activity levels, fatigue, and pain and the use of simple principles such as pacing techniques (Table 19.3) and an activity diary.

Rest

Research shows 'over-doers' who pace are *more* active—and do not get exhausted so rapidly. Daily, 30–60 min of rest is effective but many find this difficult, with short breaks feeling more acceptable than longer periods.

Table 19.3 Pacing techniques

Use of pacing to take:	Activity: advise patients to use an alarm or timer to prompt them to take breaks. Encourage adhering to time allocation
Micro breaks	Stretch and relax: 30–60 sec breaks every 5–10 min
Short breaks	Every 1–2 hours take a 5–10 min break
Measure	How long an activity can be carried out before pain/fatigue starts (reduce 25% off the set quota) and review ability with 25% reduction in task
Measure	If under active; gradually ↑ activity quota by goal setting
Plan ahead	Break activities into smaller components to enable rest breaks; plan the same amount of activity and rest each day; balance heavier and lighter activities out through the day and week
Prioritize	Carry out essential activities. Ensure time and energy left for hobbies, and social and family activities. Are there activities that can be ↓ or omitted/delegated?
Problem solve	Identify ways to make activities easier by using joint protection and correct positioning

Table 19.4 Possible causes and solutions for fatigue

Possible cause	Possible solutions
The disease itself	Fatigue and pain are common in RA, Fibromyalgia, and OA. Ensure prescribed appropriate drug therapy
Overdoing activities	Activity pacing. Refer to OT for joint protection, activity pacing, and relaxation training and education/support groups (➲ see 'Expert patient programme', Chapter 10, pp. 350–351) Encourage positive approach to condition
Underactivity/ over resting	Activity pacing. Refer to OT and to PT Pacing training; arthritis education or EPP Encourage more activity; explain consequences of resting too much; dispel myth that activity will cause damage
Deconditioning/ lack of fitness	Support to enable ↑ activity/fitness programme. Refer to OT for pacing and/or PT for exercise training Arthritis education or EPP
Stress/depression	Assess the person's mood state. If clinically anxious/ depressed, refer to mental health practitioner. Provide support and self-help references, e.g. Versus Arthritis booklet 'Feelings matter: emotional wellbeing and arthritis'[a]
Poor sleep	Assess cause. If nocturnal pain—review analgesia prescribed prior to bedtime. For insomnia and sleep management advice: NHS Information: 'Sleep and tiredness'[b]; '10-tips to beat insomnia'[c] Sleepio—an online sleep improvement programme[d]

[a] https://www.versusarthritis.org/about-arthritis/managing-symptoms/emotional-well-being/; [b] https://www.nhs.uk/live-well/sleep-and-tiredness/; [c] https://www.nhs.uk/live-well/sleep-and-tiredness/10-tips-to-beat-insomnia/; [d] https://go.bighealth.com/sleepio_nhs

Ideally, they should progress to longer rests which are *relaxing*—in a comfortable chair, head and shoulders supported or lying; relaxing music or deep breathing to mentally and physically slow down (they should not keep busy watching TV/reading). They should also aim for at least 8 hours of sleep a day (Table 19.4).

Relaxation

Some people find relaxation CDs/apps helpful. This can be combined with the use of deep breathing (as a quick stress buster): advise patients to sit with arms and head relaxed, eyes closed, and listen to the sound of their breath. They should breathe in slowly through the nose (count of 4), breathe out slowly through slightly parted lips (count of 6), while thinking 'relax' (or other phrase that would help visualization of something pleasant, e.g. favourite place). Repeat breaths 6–10 times.

Further reading

McCabe C, Haigh R, Cohen H, et al. (2013). Pain and fatigue. In: Watts R, Conaghan P, Denton C, et al. (eds) *Oxford Textbook of Rheumatology*, 4th edn, pp. 93–9. Oxford: Oxford University Press.

Thermotherapy

Thermotherapy is the application of heat or cold to alter cutaneous temperature, IA temperature, and core temperature. It has been self-administered for millennia and is widely recommended for many MSCs because it is a safe, effective, popular, and easy way to apply treatment that does not require complex, expensive equipment. It also enhances the individual's perceptions of control and adds a simple approach to self-management strategies (Table 19.5).

There are a number of ways thermotherapy can be applied. Warmth can reduce pain considerably: examples include commercially available hot packs, a hot water bottle wrapped in a towel, hot baths, or wearing thermal clothing or bandages. Cooling can be achieved using cool packs, coolant sprays, or a homemade ice pack (a bag of frozen peas wrapped in a towel). Either heating or cooling can be chosen according to patient preference.

❗ Simple forms of thermotherapy (heat/ice packs) are safe for people with normal vasculature and neurological sensation. Care should be taken with patients who have diabetes, peripheral vascular disease, or peripheral neuropathies. It is appropriate for patients who can adhere to simple guidelines. The patient can be advised to:

- Heat or cold packs preferable to these for risk management.
- Lie or sit down and relax. Place the hot/cold pack on the painful joint for 10 min.
- Remove the pack and gently move the joint.
- Replace the hot/cold pack on the joint for another 5–10 min.

Whether heat or cold packs are used it should never become uncomfortably hot or cold.

Table 19.5 Effects of thermotherapy

	Heating	Cooling
'Shutting the pain gate'	Yes	Yes
Muscle relaxation	↑	↓
Tissue temperature	↑	↓
Blood flow	↑ (vasodilation)	↓ (vasoconstriction), followed by ↑ to prevent hypoxic damage
Metabolic rate	↑	↓
Neuronal excitability	↑	↓
Neuronal conduction rate	↑	↓
Tissue extensibility	↑	↓

Transcutaneous electrical nerve stimulation

TENS is a form of electrotherapy usually administered by PTs in the first instance. Studies suggest that TENS works by blocking pain pathways by inhibiting nociceptive at the presynaptic level, inhibiting the central transmission of pain sensations. It is often used to relieve pain, reduce inflammation, and improve muscle function. Indications for TENS include:

- Neurogenic or post-herpetic pain.
- Mild to moderate musculoskeletal pain (e.g. low back pain).

TENS is an easily applied, non-invasive modality; the only adverse effect is occasional, mild skin irritation. A small, inexpensive, battery-operated TENS machine delivers a low-frequency electrical impulse via surface skin electrodes. Patients can be easily instructed on placement of electrodes to self-administer treatment.

There are five TENS protocols—the choice is based upon the underlying condition and which pain relief mechanism is required (Table 19.6). The waveform, pulse duration, pulse frequency, intensity, and electrode position

Table 19.6 The treatment plans for TENS—rationale for pain relief

Indication	Definition	Treatment parameters
Conventional		
• Rationale: via pain gate • Indication: less severe pain	• High frequency 90–130 Hz • Pulse width <100 µsec	• Time: 30 min periods applied regularly as needed • Intensity: feel comfort-able buzz
Acupuncture		
• Rationale: via opioid • Indication: chronic conditions	• Low frequency 2–5 Hz • Pulse width >200 µsec	• Time: 30 min • Intensity: strong but comfortable buzz
Burst		
• Rationale: via all pain • Indication: long-term use	• Low frequency 10 Hz • Burst impulses, 2–3 per sec	• Intensity: strong but comfortable buzz
Brief intense		
• Rationale: via pain gate • Indication: short term for severe pain	• High frequency >80 Hz • Pulse width >150 µsec	• Time: 15–30 min • Intensity: close to maximum tolerance
Modulation		
• Rationale: all pain relief • Indication: long-term use	• All characteristics are varied throughout application	• Intensity: strong but comfortable buzz

can be adjusted to achieve optimal pain relief. High-frequency, 'strong-burst' TENS for >4 weeks has been shown to be most effective.

However, there were no additional benefits of TENS over and above group education and exercise programme in people with knee OA, failing to support its use as a treatment adjunct within this context.[1] Similarly, it was not cost-effective as an adjunct to 1° care management of tennis elbow.[2]

References

1. Palmer S, Domaille M, Cramp F, et al. (2014). Transcutaneous electrical nerve stimulation as an adjunct to education and exercise for knee osteoarthritis: an RCT. *Arthritis Care Res (Hoboken)* 66:387–94.
2. Lewis M, Chesterton LS, Sim J, et al. (2015). An economic evaluation of TENS in addition to usual primary care management for the treatment of tennis elbow: results from the TATE Randomized Controlled Trial. *PLoS One* 10:e0135460.

Further reading

Arthritis Foundation (2018). Fast and easy joint pain relief. https://www.versusarthritis.org/about-arthritis/managing-symptoms/emotional-well-being/

Beasley J (2012). Osteoarthritis and rheumatoid arthritis: conservative therapeutic management. *J Hand Ther* 25:163–71.

Brosseau L, Wells GA, Tugwell P (2004). Ottawa panel evidence based clinical practice guidelines for electrotherapy and thermotherapy interventions in the management of rheumatoid arthritis. *Phys Ther* 8:1016–43.

Chapter 20

Assessment tools and outcome measures

Assessment and outcome tools: overview

Most aspects of care start with some form of consultation with the patient to explore the patient's problem, clinical history taking, and assessments (health/disease assessment), followed by a treatment or management plan, and finally reviewing the outcome of the treatment or management plan. Measurement is fundamental to clinical practice and research. Assessment, diagnosis, and evaluation of care depend on measurements or a set of criteria. In a simple form consider:

Individual in a health or disease state: assessment → intervention → outcome.

Tools come in different forms. Some are physical measures, some are a set of criteria (when met, they imply/define a condition or health state), and some come in the form of a questionnaire. Any good measurement tool is expected to measure what it is meant to measure accurately and consistently. This is true for physical measures and validated questionnaires. A validated tool should work as a ruler or a scale, providing valid and reliable measurements. That is why validated questionnaires are referred to as 'scales' or 'measures'.

A validated questionnaire may measure a single concept or a concept comprising multiple subconcepts (referred to as a multidimensional tool). Multidimensional tools usually provide a global score (all the scores are combined to give a total score) and each subscale can provide a separate score if desired. In some cases, a mixture of both scoring systems will be used depending on the research question or the clinical goal. For example, the Hospital Anxiety and Depression Scale can be used to assess psychological distress (using the global score) or anxiety and depression (using the subscale scores) separately.

Validated tools are vital if the aim is to assess changes in health or disease status from baseline. Increasingly, tools are used for diagnostic or treatment criteria and are frequently incorporated into ICPs. Future evaluations may include measures to assess outcomes at specific points in the patient pathway of care.

Tools can be used as part of an assessment prior to treatment or intervention (assessment tool) to establish disease/health states at baseline and following treatment or intervention to assess the effects (outcome measure). They could also be used to assess benefits of services (e.g. benefits of a nurse-led clinic for tight control of disease activity in RA). The data collected may need to include a combination of clinical indicators and outcome measures (such as the Pain VAS, Quality of Life questionnaire for disease impact, and the Health Assessment Questionnaire-Disability Index for functional ability).

➲ Also see 'Selecting the right tool for the job', pp. 597–599.

Selecting the right tool for the job

See Fig. 20.1.

Tools can be used as:

- A validated method of evaluation using clearly defined parameters—assessment tools.
- A validated method of measuring changes as a result of a specific intervention/treatment/time frame—outcome measure.

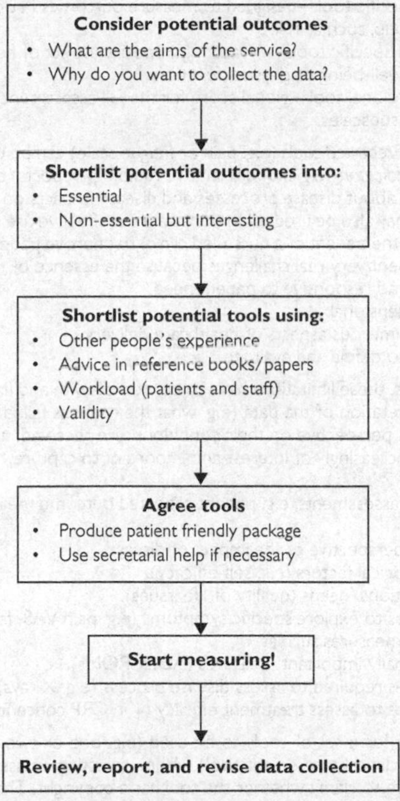

Fig. 20.1 The process of selecting the right tools.

Adapted with permission from Oliver S (ed.) (2004). *Chronic Disease Nursing: A Rheumatology Example*. Chapter 5, Nurse clinics: not just assessing patients' joints. John Wiley & Sons Ltd: Chichester.

The decision about what type of tool to use (assessment or outcome) will rely on:

- The aim of the study (why data are being collected).
- What is being measured (nature of the data).
- Whether a potential treatment or effect (change over time) is being expected.

Consideration should be given to whether there is a need to use a:

- Generic tool— designed to compare outcomes across different disease groups such as diabetes, cardiovascular diseases, and rheumatic and musculoskeletal diseases.
- Disease-specific tool—designed to measure outcomes in only one disease group, such as RA.
- Dimension-specific tools—measuring a specific aspect of health status, e.g. social well-being or physical function.
- Multidimensional tool—global score for the full assessment or broken down into subscales.

Individual *self-reported* tools (e.g. pain or fatigue scale) can be used together with *clinical indicators* (e.g. blood results or radiology reports) to inform clinical decisions about disease processes and disease impacts on the patient.

The data may also be used to demonstrate the effective use of specific resources (e.g. the benefit of a nurse-led clinic) to improve patient outcomes. This can present very real challenges because the essence of nursing:

- Is holistic and responsive to patient need.
- Is multidimensional.
- Crosses numerous aspects of healthcare delivery.
- Is difficult to define and evaluate.

In many cases, these limitations have to be worked with and flaws identified in the interpretation of the data (e.g. what the tool has failed to measure). The patient's perspective on their condition, care received, and outcomes of care are increasingly of interest and important to capture.

Consider:

- Subjective assessments, e.g. patient-reported outcome measures (PROMs):
  - Patient perspective of the impact of disease.
  - Psychological factors (e.g. self-efficacy).
  - Expectations/needs (quality of life issues).
  - Measures to explore specific symptoms (e.g. pain VAS, fatigue VAS).
- Objective measures such as:
  - Functionally important measures (ADLs, ROMs).
  - Measures required to assess disease process (e.g. X-rays).
  - Measures to assess treatment efficacy (↓ in CRP concentration).

It is common for a set of tools to be used (e.g. one or two PROMs with an objective clinical assessment tool). When selecting an assessment tool it is imperative to clarify whether the tool has a copyright. There are useful websites that can provide this information or your local audit department will be able to provide information.[1]

Reference

1. GL Assessment: https://www.gl-assessment.co.uk

Further reading

Bowling A (2001). *Measuring Disease*, 2nd edn. Buckingham: Open University Press.

Bowling A (2005). *Measuring Health: A Review of Quality of Life Measurement Scales*, 3rd edn. Buckingham: Open University Press.

Hewlett S (2004). Nurse clinics: using the right tools for the job. In: Oliver S (ed) *Chronic Disease Nursing: A Rheumatology Example*, pp. 41–59. London: Whurr Publishers.

OMERACT (Outcome Measures in Rheumatology)—an excellent resource with a wealth of information for all practitioners and patients: https://omeract.org/resources

Assessment tools: are they valid?

Is it a valid tool?

- Covers the relevant aspects of the concept.
- Is consistent and accurate.
- Is sensitive to change.

All outcome measures must be valid, reliable, and responsive.

In essence, they must be reliable and have credibility in the context of evidence-based care. This means that measures should demonstrate meaningful criteria to assess outcomes (from patient, clinician, and/or provider perspective).

For clinical use or research, it is strongly recommended that a well-validated tool is used unless the research is about developing the tools. Designing tools requires a sound knowledge of measurement. Key aspects that must be considered to ensure an effective and valuable tool are listed in Table 20.1.

Table 20.1 What you need to consider in selecting a tool

Choosing tools	Consider
Face validity	Is it credible from a clinician/patient perspective? Has the tool been validated in the disease area?
Construct validity	Does the tool measure the true biological aspects (psychological concept) of the condition?
Content validity	Does it cover all the relevant aspects needed to evaluate? Is it measuring the aspect of the disease you need to measure?
Responsiveness	Can it measure change in the concept that it purports to measure (i.e. is it sensitive to change)?
Reliability	Is it stable and consistent and accurate when repeated?
Language	Has it been validated in the same patient population (language, community, and culture)?
Ease of use	Is it easy to use? If a patient-completed tool, is the tool relevant and not too long? Is it easy to score and analyse?
Is it the best tool for job?	Are there better tools that will cover the topic more succinctly or reduce the overall number of tools to be used? Is it best to use a disease-specific or a generic tool?
Strengths and weaknesses	All tools have strengths and weaknesses—it helps to know what they are when using and analysing the results
Permission	Is the tool copyrighted? If yes, you may need to request permission for use
Cost	Some tools require access fees—check with your organization/institution if they already have a licence. Some tools are free for academic, research, and clinical (not-for-profit) use

Using a combination of assessments and tools can help provide a holistic view of the patient and help plan care. To select correct tools, the purpose of the measure must be clear. The purpose can be specified as:

- To demonstrate improvements in quality of life.
- To assess if a disease state (such as RA remission) has been achieved.
- To evaluate changes in psychological factors following an intervention (e.g. in self-efficacy following a patient education programme) (Fig. 20.1).

Data collection using non-validated tools can lead to inappropriate clinical decisions or misleading conclusions in research.

➲ Also see 'Selecting the right tool for the job', pp. 597–599.

Further reading

Bowling A (2001). *Measuring Disease*, 2nd edn. Buckingham: Open University Press.

Bowling A (2005). *Measuring Health: A Review of Quality of Life Measurement Scales*, 3rd edn. Buckingham: Open University Press.

De Vet HCW, Terwee CB, Mokkink LB, et al. (2011). *Measurement in Medicine*. Cambridge: Cambridge University Press.

Hewlett S (2004). Nurse clinics: using the right tools for the job. In: Oliver S (ed) *Chronic Disease Nursing: A Rheumatology Example*, pp. 41–59. London: Whurr Publishers.

Examples of assessment tools

The following selection of tools is not by any means exhaustive but aims to outline some examples of the types of tools that are available and may be useful to consider for MSCs.

Some diseases have mild, self-limiting symptoms and have a short duration, while others are incurable and will require continuing care and treatment. It might be useful to consider some key health issues that are common to all conditions (in varying degrees) and which might be considered 'core' data sets to measure because of their common presentation in many MSCs:

- Pain.
- Physical function.
- Quality of life (including social participation, independence, and well-being).
- Psychological factors that affect the individual in coming to terms with or managing their conditions (e.g. self-efficacy, self-esteem, and helplessness).

Health state measures

Health is considered an essential and valued concept that affects quality of life (social, emotional, and physical well-being not just the absence of disease). There is a plethora of tools to explore different components of quality of life in relation to changes in perceived or actual health or disease states. Many of these are generic and have a value in identifying differences in health status across a number of diseases.

Examples include:

- *Short form 36* (SF36®) (Ware and Sherbourne, 1992)[1]: there are nine health concepts (physical function, physical role, emotional role, social function, pain, mental health, vitality, general health, health transition). This is not a simple tool to score yourself but a good tool to use if you want to assess or compare quality of life scores across conditions. A computer package is available with the questionnaire to help scoring.[2]
- *Health Perceptions Questionnaire and General Health Rating Index © Algorithmic Medicine* (Ware, 1976)[3]: a tool that consists of 32 questions divided into eight subscales related to a patient's perception of health. A subset of 22 questions make up the General Health Rating Index, with subsets used for faster evaluations. The questionnaire is simple and fast to administer and has been widely studied.

Quality of life measures

Generic quality of life tools assess the physical, psychological, social, and environmental factors affecting the person while disease-specific quality of life tools assess how the condition has impacted each area of the patient's life.

- *European Quality of Life Questionnaire (EuroQoL EQ-5D)* (EuroQoL Group, 1990)[4,5]: a generic, patient self-completed tool that can be used for clinical, economic, and population health state assessments. The tool has two systems: descriptive and VAS (thermometer). The descriptive section contains five domains: anxiety and depression, mobility, pain

and discomfort, self-care, and usual activities. The thermometer is a vertical 20 cm VAS for the patient to self-rate their health (from worst imaginable state to best imaginable state). The weighting of the tool and each health state were determined by exploring a view of the general population (societal preference weights) and the weighting given may not be the same if explored with a patient who has a LTC. The tool is widely used to generate 'quality-adjusted life years' (QALYs) for use in economic evaluations. EuroQoL is also used to complement other disease specific quality of life tools.
- *Rheumatoid Arthritis Quality of Life Questionnaire (RAQoL)* (De Jong et al., 1997)[6]: the RAQoL is a disease-specific measure to assess the impact of RA on quality of life. It has 30 items categorized in the following subdimensions: sleep, mood and emotions, social life, hobbies, tasks of daily living, personal and social relationships, and physical contact. Respondents select (yes/no) whether or not each item applies to them. Scores can range from 0 to 30 with a high score representing a poor QoL. The tool has been validated in several languages, it is responsive, and takes only 5–6 min to complete.
- *Systemic Sclerosis Quality of Life Questionnaire (SScQoL)* (Reay et al., 2007)[7]: the SScQoL is a disease-specific measure to assess the impact of systemic sclerosis on health and well-being. It has 29 items addressing activity limitation, emotional factors, sleep, social (participation restrictions), and pain. Scores range from 0 to 29, a high score representing a poor quality of life. The SScQoL has been validated and translated into six languages.[8]
- *Osteoarthritis Quality of Life Questionnaire (OAQoL)* (Keenan, 2007)[9]: the OAQoL is a disease-specific measure assessing the impact of OA on a patient's life. It is a simple and easy to use 22-item unidimensional questionnaire. The items have true/not true responses and scores range from 0 to 22, with high scores indicating a poor quality of life.
- *Ankylosing Spondylitis Quality of Life Questionnaire (ASQoL)* (Doward et al., 2003)[10]: the ASQoL is an 18-item disease-specific measure to assess the impact of AS on a patient's life. Each item has a dichotomous 'yes/no' response scored '1' and '0,' respectively. The total scores range from 0 to 18, with a high score indicating a poor quality of life.
- *Psoriatic Arthritis Quality of Life Questionnaire (PsAQoL)* (McKenna et al., 2004)[11]: the PsAQoL is a 20-item disease- specific instrument to measure quality of life in people with PsA. Each item has a dichotomous (yes/no) response. Score range from 0 to 20 with a high score indicating poor quality of life. PsAQoL has been validated in several languages.

References

1. Ware JE, Sherbourne CD (1992). The MOS 36-Item Short-Form Health Survey (SF-36®): I. conceptual framework and item selection. *Med Care* 30:473–83.
2. RAND Health Care: ↗ https://www.rand.org/health-care/surveys_tools/mos/36-item-short-form.html
3. Ware JE (1976). Scales for measuring general health perceptions. *Health Serv Res* 11:396–415.
4. Herdman M, Gudex C, Lloyd A, et al. (2011). Development and preliminary testing of the new five-level version of EQ-5D (EQ-5D-5L). *Qual Life Res* 20:1727–36.
5. EuroQoL: ↗ https://euroqol.org/

6. De Jong Z, Van Der Heijde D, McKenna S (1997). The reliability and construct validity of the RAQoL: a rheumatoid arthritis-specific quality of life instrument. *Br J Rheumatol* 36:878–83.
7. Reay N (2008). *The Quality of Life in Patients with Diffuse and Limited Systemic Sclerosis.* Leeds: University of Leeds.
8. Ndosi M, Alcacer-Pitarch B, Allanore Y, et al. (2018). Common measure of quality of life for people with systemic sclerosis across seven European countries: a cross-sectional study. *Ann Rheum Dis* 77:1032–8.
9. Keenan AM, McKenna SP, Doward LC, et al. (2008). Development and validation of a needs-based quality of life instrument for osteoarthritis. *Arthritis Rheum* 59:841–8.
10. Doward LC, Spoorenberg A, Cook SA, et al. (2003). The development of the ASQOL: a quality of life instrument specific to ankylosing spondylitis. *Ann Rheum Dis* 62:20–6.
11. McKenna SP, Doward LC, Whalley D, et al. (2004). Development of the PsAQoL: a quality of life instrument specific to psoriatic arthritis *Ann Rheum Dis* 63:162–9.

Further reading

Doward LC, McKenna SP, Whalley D, et al. (2009). The development of the L-QoL: a quality-of-life instrument specific to systemic lupus erythematosus *Ann Rheum Dis* 68:196–200.

Assessment tools: clinical indicators and disease-specific tools

The decision to review patient outcomes must consider the appropriate tools to use. Assessment tools are often combined with clinical indicators.

The clinical indicators may include:

- An individual's health status over time (with or without an underlying disease state) (e.g. monitoring blood pressure, body weight).
- Monitoring disease activity (or disease state) as a result of treatment. The monitoring may be to assess changes to the individual (from baseline) as part of disease management to help clinical decisions such as stepping, stopping, or changing (e.g. in RA, a DAS38 score of >5.1 may suggest eligibility for new therapies or intensifying treatment).
- Evaluation of patient outcomes against recognized standards of care/guidelines in management (e.g. comparing patient populations against the national average expected outcomes). Includes aspects of benchmarking or audit.

A further key factor for clinicians to consider is that in many cases specific disease activity tools will be predefined by national organizations such as NICE who stipulate access to specific drugs based upon set criteria. These criteria sometimes include disease activity tools. Clinical application and fulfilling disease criteria may result in two disease activity tools being used, with different specific benefits in understanding disease activity. For example;

- *Systemic Lupus Erythematosus Disease Activity Index (SLEDAI)*. This tool has a list of 24 items: 16 are clinical (e.g. seizure, psychosis), eight of the items are laboratory results (e.g. urinalysis, blood complement levels). The items are then scored on whether they were present or absent in the previous 10 days. Organ involvement is weighted and depending upon the organ involvement the score is multiplied by four (e.g. kidneys) or by eight (e.g. central nervous system). Global scores for disease activity are calculated. Scores range from 0 to 105 with a scores >25 rare.
- *The British Isles Lupus Assessment Group (BILAG) Index* measures disease activity in different organs/systems. It comprises eight systems and the score is calculated for each system dependent on clinical features—new, worse the same, or improving in the last 4 weeks.

For further examples of tools measuring clinical indicators,  see pp. 605–608.

Further reading

Gordon C, Sutcliffe N, Skan J, et al. (2003). Definition and treatment of lupus flares measured by the BILAG Index. *Rheumatology* 43:1372–9.

Lam GKW, Petri M (2005). Assessment of systemic lupus erythematosus. *Clin Exp Rheumatol* 23 Suppl 39:S120–32.

Example of tools measuring clinical indicators

Systemic lupus erythematosus

- *The British Isles Lupus Assessment Group index* (Hay et al., 1993)[1]: this tool assesses 86 clinical signs, symptoms, and laboratory measures across eight areas (mucocutaneous, neurological, musculoskeletal, cardiovascular and respiratory, vasculitis, renal, haematological, and general aspects). Shown to be valid, reliable, and sensitive to change. Scoring is based upon the physicians' intention to treat with each system or organ being scored separately—the scoring is based upon changes seen and whether they are new, worse, better, the same, or improving from the previous assessment. Basic haematology and renal function determine scores of the different systems. It categorizes disease states into five different levels from A to E. With level A being the highest level of disease activity. A computer-scoring package is available as it is complex to score.

Ankylosing spondylitis

- *The Bath Ankylosing Spondylitis Metrology Index (BASMI)*: a clinical assessment tool measuring spinal mobility. Aggregate score is 0–10 using the variables in Table 20.2 (https://nass.co.uk/healthcare-professionals/resources-for-health-professionals/).

Examples of disease impact tools (disease specific)

Arthritis (general tool covering 'arthritis')

- *The Arthritis Impact Measurement Scales (AIMS-2)®* (Meenan et al. 1980)[2]: the AIMS contains 57 items with 12 subscales measuring function, social life, pain, work, tension and mood, satisfaction, and prioritization questions.

Rheumatoid arthritis

- *The Rheumatoid Arthritis Impact of Disease (RAID) score* (Gossec et al. 2011)[3]: the RAID score is a short and simple questionnaire assessing seven most important domains of impact of RA from the patient's perspective. The domains assessed are pain, functional capacity, fatigue,

Table 20.2 BASMI assessment tool

Measurement	Score 0	Score 1	Score 2
Tragus to wall	<15 cm	15–30 cm	>30 cm
Lumbar flexion (modified Schobert test)	>4 cm	2–4 cm	<4 cm
Cervical rotation	>70°	20–70°	<20°
Lumbar side flexion	>10 cm	5–10 cm	<5 cm
Intermalleolar distance	>100 cm	70–100 cm	<70 cm

physical and emotional well-being, quality of sleep, and coping. Each item has a numerical rating scale from 0 to 10. Different weightings are applied to each item and the total RAID score ranges from 0 to 10, with 10 indicating the worst status. The RAID has been adapted into >70 languages.

Osteoarthritis

- *The Western Ontario McMaster Universities Arthritis Index (WOMAC)* (Bellamy et al. 1988)[4]: a popular tool that has undergone several revisions and changes during its development. It is valid, reliable, and sensitive to change and uses three subscales with 24 items to assess pain, function, and stiffness in knee and hip OA. This can be scored using either a 5-point Likert scoring system (none, mild, moderate, severe, extreme) or 100 mm VAS.

The AIMS and WOMAC could be supported by measures specifically for the condition or joint affected, such as the Oxford Hip Score (OHS).

Knee and hip assessment tools

- *The Oxford Knee Score and the Oxford Hip Score* (Dawson et al. 1998[5] and Dawson et al. 1996[6]): these tools have 12 questions. The OHS covers pain and disability experienced over the past 4 weeks. Each item has five response categories. The responses are formatted as a Likert scales.

Ankylosing spondylitis

In arthritis, the two commonly used and validated tools are:

- *The Bath Ankylosing Spondylitis Functional Index (BASFI)*. A patient-completed tool assessing perceived functional ability. It comprises 10 questions each with 10 cm VAS assessing 10 aspects of functional ability in people with AS.
- *The Bath Ankylosing Spondylitis Disease Activity Index (BASDAI)*. Patient-completed tool with six components (fatigue, spinal pain, joint pain and enthesis, together with morning stiffness and severity of stiffness). Each item is a 10 cm VAS except morning stiffness is measured in duration of time from 0 to >2 hours.
  - The scores are added for questions 1–4; this is then combined with the mean scores of questions 5 and 6 (duration of morning stiffness and severity of stiffness) to give a score out of 50. Then multiply by 2 and divide by 10 to get the BASDAI score.

Low back pain

- *The Roland and Morris Disability Questionnaire (RDQ)* (Roland and Morris, 1983)[7]: a self-report, self-completed questionnaire to assess degree of functional ability. 24 items were modified from the Sickness Impact Profile (SIP).
  - Quick and easy to understand, complete and score (🔗 https://www.csp.org.uk)

References

1. Hay E, Bacon P, Gordon C, et al. (1993). The BILAG index: a reliable and valid instrument for measuring clinical disease in systemic lupus erythematosus. *Q J Med* 86:447–58.
2. Meenan R, Gertman P, Mason J (1980). Measuring health status in arthritis. The arthritis impact measurement scales. *Arthritis Rheum* 23:146–52.
3. Gossec L, Paternotte S, Aanerud GJ, et al. (2011). Finalisation and validation of the rheumatoid arthritis impact of disease score, a patient-derived composite measure of impact of rheumatoid arthritis: a EULAR initiative. *Ann Rheum Dis* 70:935–42.
4. Bellamy N, Buchanan WW, Goldsmith CH, et al. (1988). Validation study of WOMAC: a health status instrument for measuring clinically important patient relevant outcomes to antirheumatic drug therapy in patients with osteoarthritis of the hip or knee. *J Rheumatol* 15:1833–40.
5. Dawson J, Fitzpatrick R, Murray D, et al. (1998). Questionnaire on the perceptions of patients about total knee replacement. *J Bone Joint Surg Br* 80:63–9.
6. Dawson J, Fitzpatrick R, Carr A, et al. (1996). Questionnaire on the perceptions of patients about total hip replacement. *J Bone Joint Surg Br* 78:185–90.
7. Roland M, Fairbank J (2000). The Roland-Morris Disability Questionnaire and the Oswestry Disability Questionnaire. *Spine (Phila Pa 1976)* 25:3115–24.

Examples of domain- and disease-specific measures

Domain specific

Fatigue

- *The Functional Assessment of Chronic Illness Therapy (FACIT)* (Cella 1997)[1]: the FACIT contains a collection of health-related quality of life questionnaires targeted to the management of chronic illness. 27 items compiled and divided into four primary quality of life domains: physical well-being, social/family well-being, emotional well-being, and functional well-being. Initially developed for cancer but has been validated in a number of conditions including RA. Can be administered or be patient completed. FACIT enables a tailored assessment using the most relevant questions. Completion usually takes about 10–15 min.

Pain

- *VAS single item tool*: a VAS uses a horizontal or vertical line measuring 10 cm (100 mm) in length. The VAS scale uses verbal descriptors of 'no pain' at one end and 'pain as bad as it could be' at the other end (➔ see Fig. 9.1, p. 311).

Function (Functional disability)

- *Health Assessment Questionnaire-Disability Index (HAQ-DI)* (Fries 1980[2]; Bruce and Fries 2003[3]): HAQ-DI is probably the most widely used tool in rheumatology to assess physical function (disability) in clinical and research contexts. The questionnaire is self-administered by the patient and covers eight categories: (1) dressing and grooming, (2) rising, (3) eating, (4) walking, (5) hygiene, (6) reach, (7) grip, (8) common daily activities. The items are a 4-point scale ranging from: without any difficulty (score 0), with some difficulty (score 1), much difficulty (score 2), and unable to do (score 3). In addition, respondents are asked to indicate whether they use additional help (person) or aids are needed (e.g. special utensils). See Fig. 20.2.
- If additional help or aids are required, the score is adjusted to a maximum score of 3 for the area, e.g. if the question on hygiene was ticked as 'with some difficulty' yet the additional box at the end of the section is also ticked as using a bath seat, the new score for hygiene would be a maximum score of 3. A simple scoring system attributes the scores. Patients need to complete at least six items to have a meaningful score. Raw scores ranges from 0 (minimum) to 24 (maximum). This is divided by 8 to get a HAQ-DI score of 3 for maximum disability. It is quick to complete and score and frequently used as part of a battery of tools in research trials (http://www.aramis.standard.edu).
- HAQ-DI was validated for use in the UK population by Kirwan and Reeback.[4]

HEALTH ASSESSMENT QUESTIONNAIRE (HAQ)

Date: ☐☐☐☐☐☐☐☐ Patient Name: ☐

Please tick the one response which best describes your usual abilities over the past week

	Without ANY difficulty	With SOME difficulty	With MUCH difficulty	UNABLE to do
1. DRESSING and GROOMING				
Are you able to:				
a. Dress yourself, including tying shoelaces and doing buttons?	☐	☐	☐	☐
b. Shampoo your hair?	☐	☐	☐	☐
☆ **2. RISING**				
Are you able to:				
a. Stand up from an armless straight chair?	☐	☐	☐	☐
b. Get in and out of bed?	☐	☐	☐	☐
3. EATING				
Are you able to:				
a. Cut your meat?	☐	☐	☐	☐
b. Lift a full cup or glass to your mouth?	☐	☐	☐	☐
c. Open a new carton of milk (or soap powder)?	☐	☐	☐	☐
4. WALKING				
Are you able to:				
a. Walk outdoors on flat ground?	☐	☐	☐	☐
b. Climb up five steps?	☐	☐	☐	☐

PLEASE TICK ANY AIDS OR DEVICES THAT YOU USUALLY USE FOR ANY OF THESE ACTIVITIES:

Cane (W) ☐ Walking frame (W) ☐ Built-up or special utensils (E) ☐

Crutches (W) ☐ Wheelchair (W) ☐ Special or built-up chair (A) ☐

Devices used for dressing (button hooks, zipper pull, shoe horn) ☐

Other (specify)..

PLEASE TICK ANY CATEGORIES FOR WHICH YOU USUALLY NEED HELP FROM ANOTHER PERSON:

Dressing and Grooming ☐ Eating ☐

Rising ☐ Walking ☐

☆ Subscale – example of an Activities subscale

ID. ☐☐☐☐☐☐☐☐

For office use only

Fig. 20.2 Health Assessment Questionnaire.

References

1. Cella D, Yount S, Sorensen M, et al. (2005). Validation of the Functional Assessment of Chronic Illness Therapy Fatigue Scale relative to other instrumentation in patients with rheumatoid arthritis. *J Rheumatol* 32:811–9.
2. Fries JF, Spitz P, Kraines RG, et al. (1980). Measurement of patient outcome in arthritis. *Arthritis Rheum* 23:137–45.
3. Bruce B, Fries JF (2003). The Stanford Health Assessment Questionnaire: dimensions and practical applications. *Health Qual Life Outcomes* 1:20.
4. Kirwan JR, Reeback JS (1986). Stanford Health Assessment Questionnaire modified to assess disability in British patients with rheumatoid arthritis. *Br J Rheumatol* 25:206–9.

Assessment tools measuring psychological aspects

Anxiety and depression

- *Hospital Anxiety and Depression (HAD)* (Zigmond and Snaith, 1983)[1]: the HAD is a 14-item, one-page questionnaire which is self-administered by the patient. It measures two domains, depression (seven items) and generalized anxiety (seven items). The HAD is a useful tool in hospital, outpatients, and the community settings. It is easy to complete, score, and interpret. Each subscale has cut-off points to indicate 'within the normal range', or in a 'mildly', 'moderately', or 'severely' disordered state (https://www.gl-assessment.co.uk).

Helplessness

- *Arthritis Helplessness Index* (Stein et al., 1988)[2]: this questionnaire uses six categories for scoring (strongly agree to strongly disagree). This is a 15-item questionnaire. Scores range from 5 to 30. The higher the score, the higher the helplessness.

Self-efficacy

- *The Arthritis Self-Efficacy Scale (ASES)* (Lorig et al., 1989)[3]: this is a 20-item questionnaire which is self-completed by the patient. It has three subscales; self-efficacy pain, self-efficacy function, and self-efficacy other symptoms. The tool uses a number of VASs which are totalled and averaged to give a score. The higher scores indicate high levels of self-efficacy.
- *The Rheumatoid Arthritis Self-Efficacy scale (RASE)* (Hewlett et al., 2001)[4]: the RASE is a disease-specific, 28-item questionnaire which is self-administered by patient. It measures task-specific self-efficacy for the initiation of self-management and related behaviours. The score ranges from 28 to 140, with high scores indicating greater self-efficacy. Two items are shown as examples in Table 20.3.

Attitude

- *The Rheumatoid Attitude Index (RAI)* (Nicassio et al., 1985)[5]: this tool explores beliefs related to helplessness (e.g. actions do not affect outcomes). A self-reporting questionnaire focusing on learned helplessness and was originally developed from the Arthritis Helplessness Index (AHI).

Changes in knowledge following educational intervention

- *Patient Knowledge Questionnaire for OA (PKQ-OA)* (Hill and Bird, 2007)[6]: patient-completed questionnaire to identify level of knowledge and use of self-management techniques. Studies have also demonstrated the validity of this tool for measuring knowledge in early RA. The tool comprises 16 multiple choice questions with 30 correct answers. PKQ-OA is easy to read, complete, and interpret.

Table 20.3 Example of the RA self-efficacy tool

- We are interested in finding out what things you believe you *could* do to help you with your arthritis
- We want to know what you think you *could* do, even if you are not actually doing it at the moment. Please tick one column for each question
- Do you believe you *could* do these things to help you with your arthritis?

	Strongly disagree	Disagree	Neither disagree nor agree	Agree	Strongly agree
I believe I *could* use relaxation techniques to help with pain					
I believe I *could* use my joints carefully (joint protection) to help with pain					

Adapted with permission from Tugwell P, Shea B, Boers M, et al. (eds) (2003). *Evidence Based Rheumatology*. Copyright John Wiley & Sons Limited, Chichester, UK.

References

1. Zigmond AS, Snaith RP (1983). The hospital anxiety and depression scale. *Acta Psychiatr Scand* 67:361–70.
2. Stein MJ, Wallston KA, Nicassio PM (1988). Factor structure of the Arthritis Helplessness Index. *J Rheumatol* 15:427–32.
3. Lorig K, Chastain RL, Ung E, et al. (1989). Development and evaluation of a scale to measure perceived self-efficacy in people with arthritis. *Arthritis Rheum* 32:37–44.
4. Hewlett S, Cockshott Z, Kirwan J, et al. (2001). Development and validation of a self-efficacy scale for use in British patients with rheumatoid arthritis (RASE). *Rheumatology* 40:1221–30.
5. Nicassio PM, Wallston KA, Callahan LF, et al. (1985). The measurement of helplessness in rheumatoid arthritis. The development of the arthritis helplessness index. *J Rheumatol* 12:462–7.
6. Hill J, Bird H (2007). Patient knowledge and misconceptions of osteoarthritis assessed by a validated self-completed knowledge questionnaire (PKQ-OA). *Rheumatology (Oxford)* 46:796–800.

Chapter 21

Specialist nursing support: The role and nurse prescribing

The nurse specialist role

The role of the rheumatology nurse specialist (RNS) initially developed from research nurse roles. Today, many nurses working in rheumatology have developed their roles through an interest in the specialty. Increasingly, RNSs are expected to have obtained a specialist qualification, usually at degree or masters level. In addition, clarity about the role and responsibilities of the RNS are usually underpinned by documented competencies or a framework for practice that outlines their role. The RNS role involves the following components (➲ see also Chapter 23, 'Nurse-led clinics', pp. 629–638):

Advanced nursing practice

Patient assessment and delivery of care

Act as an advocate and provide chiefly nurse-led outpatient services and act as a specialist resource for health professionals in a range of care settings. Nurse-led care often includes:

- Review of patients using a holistic approach to assess treatment issues, ADLs, pain, disease activity, psychological status, coping styles, social circumstances, and employment issues.
- Advanced level of knowledge/competencies and autonomous clinical decision-making and negotiating a plan of care and disease management with the patient.
- Extended roles such as prescribing and administering joint injections.
- Coordinating referrals to the MDT.

Educator

Apply a patient-centred approach to ascertain the patient's knowledge, beliefs, and perceptions of their condition and treatment options. Signpost the patient to voluntary and support agencies. Also:

- Provides relevant written information to support education given.
- Provides patient (and carer) education and facilitates development of patient self-management. This may be delivered either as formal (group) or informal (individual) sessions and may be in collaboration with the MDT or community services.
- Engages in teaching all HCPs in the clinical setting and in universities.
- Develops the role of junior nurses and works with them to enhance their learning opportunities.
- Acts as an expert resource in the clinical setting with opportunistic teaching of clinical care aspects of specialism.

Leadership and management role

- Day-to-day management of the rheumatology nursing service.
- Considers succession planning and sustainability of services.
- Line management, clinical supervision, and assessment of competency for a team of nurses.
- Integral and collaborative member of the MDT.
- Acts as a role model for nurses and supports nursing development.
- Responsibility for clinical governance.
- Providing strategic direction for the trust and incorporating user patient involvement in rheumatology service development.

Research and audit role

Research studies are increasingly being undertaken and published by RNSs and along with audit, both are important to demonstrate:

- Quality and safety of care given.
- Access to treatment and adherence to specific guidance (e.g. organizations such as NICE).
- Introduction of service change.
- Health outcome and cost-effectiveness.

Nurse specialist—extended roles

Many nurse specialists have extended their roles with formal training, achieving practice base competencies and practice development. The rationale for role expansion is to provide a complete package of care for patients and this has taken place in the following areas of practice:

- A full and thorough physical assessment of patients to include examination of joints, heart, abdomen, and lungs, and performing DASs.
- Assessment and management of co-morbid conditions such as hypertension, coronary heart disease, hypercholesterolaemia, osteoporosis, and diabetes.
- Consulting with patients, taking a history, and determining a management plan.
- Prescribing drug treatment and titration of therapy.
- Provision of IA and soft tissue injections.
- Referral and communicating with medical and surgical colleagues regarding the patient's management.
- Ordering and interpreting a range of imaging and blood investigations.

In addition, a key component of the RNS role is that of ensuring that a proactive patient-centred approach is applied to management:

- Rapid access to care and treatments to optimize patient outcomes.
- Proactive review and assessment to review efficacy of treatment.
- Empowering patients to undertake informed shared decisions about their care and adhere to treatment.
- Adherence to guidelines particularly of new therapies to ensure open and transparent access to treatments.
- Ensure that symptom control is achieved to the satisfaction of the patient.
- Enable opportunities for patients to participate in research trials.

Further reading

Read C (2015). Time for some advanced thinking: the benefits of specialist nurses. *HSJ* 27 Feb Suppl. https://www.hsj.co.uk/downloads/workforce-supplement-the-benefits-of-specialist-nurses/5082712.article

Scottish Government (2012). A toolkit supporting the development of advanced nursing practice and an AHP advanced practice education and development framework (musculoskeletal). http://www.advancedpractice.scot.nhs.uk

Nurse prescribing

In 1989, the Crown Report proposed that nurse prescribing would improve patient care. In 2006, UK legislation enabled nurses, once they had undertaken training, qualified, and registered as an independent nurse prescriber, to prescribe the full range of medications according to their knowledge and competencies. The details of the development of nurse prescribing has been outlined by Beckwith and Franklin.[1]

The principles of nurse prescribing are:

- Improved patient access to medicines and subsequent improvements in health outcome.
- Better use of the doctors, nurses, and the patient's time.
- Clarification of professional responsibilities.
- Improved patient safety by fewer drug interactions and serious adverse events
- This includes ensuring that all HCPs involved in the patient's care are aware of any prescribed medications and treatment plans made, including patient review.
- Framework of that includes regular audit of prescribing practice, continued professional development, and prescribing updates.
- Reduction in costs as nurses can only prescribe generically.

Since May 2006, nurses with an English National Board (ENB) V300 qualification can act as independent and/or as supplementary prescribers.

Methods of nurse prescribing

Independent nurse prescribing

The nurse prescriber takes legal responsibility for the clinical assessment of the patient, arriving at a diagnosis for the condition to be treated, the management of that condition, the decision to prescribe, and the suitability of the prescription.[2] Nurse prescribers are entitled to prescribe drugs independently from the entire *BNF* but some employing authorities may ask for an approval to practice form that limits the range of drugs prescribed in the specialist area of practice.

Supplementary prescribing

Is a voluntary agreement between a nurse prescriber and a doctor or dentist facilitated by drawing up an agreed clinical management plan (CMP) in conjunction with the patient. There is no identified formulary or restrictions on the type of medical conditions that can be treated within supplementary prescribing. CMPs clearly set out a framework that the supplementary prescriber can use in daily practice.

The clinical management plan

A variety of CMPs exist.[3] The CMP must provide detail on:

- Guidelines, protocols, publications, and best evidence supporting the prescribing practice.
- A schedule setting out when the patient should be reviewed by the supplementary and independent prescribers.
- The process for reporting adverse drug reactions.
- The date from which the CMP became effective.

- The CMP, if not lapsed, should be reviewed at 1 year; this is an ideal opportunity for nurses working with patients who have a LTC to review them and their medication.
- The condition(s) to be treated and a single aim of treatment. A term to cover a wide patient group may be preferable, e.g. using the term 'inflammatory arthritis' thus enabling the nurse to prescribe for a variety of conditions, e.g. AS, RA, CTD, etc. Likewise, the aim of treatment could be 'To control inflammation and limit the progression of the disease'.
- A list of medications that are to be prescribed—defined by class, e.g. NSAID, or by named drug, e.g. diclofenac.

References

1. Beckwith S, Franklin P (2011). *Oxford Handbook of Nurse Prescribing for Nurses and Allied Health Professionals*, 2nd edn. Oxford: Oxford University Press.
2. Royal Pharmaceutical Society (2016). *A Competency Framework for all Prescribers: Prescribing Framework*. London: The Royal Pharmaceutical Society. ℘ https://www.rpharms.com
3. Drennan V, Goodman C (eds) (2014). Medicines management and nurse prescribing. In: *Oxford Handbook of Primary Care and Community Nursing*, 2nd edn, pp. 125–42. Oxford: Oxford University Press.

The nurse prescriber: managing drug interactions

Patients with arthritis often have other co-morbid conditions, may be elderly, and are usually taking several drugs at any one time which makes drug interactions more likely. It is therefore essential that nurse prescribers identify and avoid use of concomitant drugs that are likely to cause the patient harm. Nurses must be aware of the pharmacokinetics and pharmacodynamics of the drugs and check the SPC and *BNF*.

Adverse event reporting

A nurse prescriber must complete a full nursing assessment on the patient. The nurse should be aware of potential drug interactions and the risks specifically related to the patient's current medications and individual co-morbidities or other risk factors. In the event of an adverse event the nurse should:

- Report it via the yellow card reporting scheme found in the *BNF* to the Committee on Safety of Medicines or report to the Medicines Healthcare products Regulatory Agency.[1]
- Report the details in the patient's medical records.
- Notify the Medicines Management Committee within their organization.
- Make colleagues in their department and hospital trust aware.
- Report it to the pharmacovigilance department of the drug company whose product is alleged to have caused the adverse event.

Therapies unlicensed—exceptions that apply

A supplementary prescribing arrangement needs to be in place to support nurse prescribing of:

- Controlled drugs.
- Unlicensed drugs.
- Off-label drugs, such as using a licensed drug for an unlicensed indication, e.g. amitriptyline prescribed for neuropathic pain instead of at higher doses for depression.
- A clinical trials certificate—enables unlicensed and off-label drugs to be prescribed independently.

Reference

1. Medicines Healthcare Products Regulatory Agency: https://www.gov.uk/government/organisations/medicines-and-healthcare-products-regulatory-agency

Further reading

Beckwith S, Franklin P (2011). *Oxford Handbook of Nurse Prescribing for nurses and Allied Health Professionals*, 2nd edn. Oxford: Oxford University Press.

Ledingham J, Gullick N, Irving K, et al. (2017). BSR and BHPR guidelines for the prescription and monitoring of non-biologic disease-modifying anti-rheumatic drugs. *Rheumatology (Oxford)* 56:865–8.

Nurse specialists: rapid access and early arthritis clinics

Rapid access to specific services (such as early arthritis clinics) has developed to ensure patients get prompt early diagnosis and rapid aggressive treatment. National audits in the UK have shown a strong correlation between nurse staffing levels and compliance with treatment standards (e.g. initiation of treatment within 6 weeks). In addition, rapid access enables improved access for patients with severe side effects, e.g. breathing difficulties with suspicion of suspected pneumonitis or gross knee effusion and suspicion of septic arthritis, can access rapid referral.

Principles of monitoring

Monitoring does not just refer to the blood testing schedule for DMARDs but should incorporate a holistic assessment of the patient. A typical monitoring visit should involve the following actions:

- Review of medical records, treatment plans, and current health status of patient. Considers joint assessment and expected treatment response.
- The DMARD treatment and monitoring plans. Dose escalation/cessation of treatment in accordance with local, regional, or national guidelines.
- Monitoring of overall disease status taking into consideration drug therapies and patient issues/diagnosis.
- Inflammatory markers (ESR/CRP) to assess disease activity.
- Review of other systems evaluating weight, blood, urine, and physical examination function, e.g. renal and liver profiles and blood pressure. Consider results in the context of treatment plan, health status, and issues indicating referral or review of treatment.
- Identify side effects such as rash, nausea, diarrhoea, mouth ulcers, headache, dyspnoea, cough, hair loss, signs of infection, and bruising or bleeding.
- Adherence to monitoring time frames and identify appropriate steps in treatment pathway, e.g. reduction in monitoring frequency.
- Support and advise patients on symptom control, e.g. short-term use of NSAIDs and analgesics while waiting for DMARDs to become effective.
- Document information on blood monitoring and educate the patient about the values and results.
- Joint changes or damage that may indicate prompt referral, e.g. presence of nodules, rashes, wasted muscles, or flexion deformities requiring referral or review of treatment.
- Identify any educational opportunities or gaps in the patient's knowledge and provide education tailored to the patient's needs.
- Provide first point of contact for patients, e.g. access to telephone advice line and reasons to contact the nursing service.
- Document fully all decisions made, actions taken, and information given, and convey this information in writing to the GP and patient.

Further reading

British Society for Rheumatology (2016). *National Clinical Audit for Rheumatoid and Early Inflammatory Arthritis: 2nd Annual Report 2016*. London: HQIP, BSR.

Ledingham J, Gullick N, Irving K, et al. (2017). BSR and BHPR guidelines for the prescription and monitoring of non-biologic disease-modifying anti-rheumatic drugs. *Rheumatology (Oxford)* 56:865–8.

Chapter 22

Patient's perspective

What patients want from a rheumatology service

Rheumatology pathways and guidelines are very clinically and medically focused but those living with an incurable condition such as inflammatory arthritis need a more holistic approach. Holistic care should consider the individual, their social circumstances, and their individual needs, while offering guidance that is tailored and includes support and education for lifestyle adaptations, access to support, and opportunities to learn self-management skills. These approaches will enable them to develop coping strategies which foster emotional as well as physical well-being and achieve outcomes that are valued by the patient. Speaking as a person with RA for some 39 years but chiefly as chief executive of a national patient organization for some 18 years, patients have some specific needs:

What patients want and need from healthcare

- IJDs, including RA, PsA, and axial spondyloarthropathies, are all 'red flag' conditions and patients suspected to have any of these conditions, or an undifferentiated inflammatory arthritis, should be fast-tracked direct to a consultant rheumatologist in a specialist care setting. Current quality standards (RA) in the UK require patients to be referred within 3 working days to a rheumatology service.
- For those presenting with back pain, OA, or fibromyalgia, they should be seen by a musculoskeletal triage service and rapidly referred to the most appropriate service.
- HCPs who can provide expert advice or signpost to key resources.
- Once diagnosed, continuity of care with HCPs who have knowledge of their condition and who can provide advice, e.g. access to prompt telephone advice from a specialist nurse. Ensuring patients have the telephone number for the nurse-led helpline is key.

Specialist teams need to be an advocate for their patients

It is key that specialist teams recognize the patients and their individual needs so they can guide them through the early steps in their journey through the healthcare system. Initially, people do not know what they don't know. In many cases, although they present with pain and are worried, they may not, however, be totally prepared for disease-modifying drugs and regular assessments. Despite many campaigns, there remains a lack of awareness amongst the general population in the UK of the seriousness of inflammatory arthritis. People often delay seeking help, believing their symptoms will get better and ∴ GPs should not delay referring patients while they await blood test or X-ray results. They need to understand why they are being referred to a consultant-led MDT, the make-up of that team, and how and when to access the different HCPs within the team.

It can be very helpful at these early stages if patients are signposted to patient organizations, which have the resources to spend time explaining why learning to self-manage well is an important part of their treatment pathway. Those who embrace the concept generally do better than those who do not.

The cornerstone of care

It is the nurse specialist who is the cornerstone for patient support and education and can often make referrals to other members of the team. This is partly due to them being the one accessible member of the team who maintains continuity of care, unlike, for example, junior doctors, who may only see the patient once or twice. In surveys done by NRAS, what repeatedly comes top of the list for patients is the ability to access care and treatment when they need it. This is particularly important during time of flare when often an individual's own coping mechanisms fail. People respond differently to the overwhelming challenges they face and ∴ tailored information based upon the patient's preferences is vital. If patients are poorly advised, treat to target approaches fail to be effectively implemented. Patients need to be fully informed and appropriately supported in order to commit wholeheartedly to treatment. Continuity of care is highly valued by patients and plays a key role in achieving the best outcomes for patients. Patient organizations can play a vital role in supporting the patient but also the specialist teams by optimizing emotional support, and offering professionally endorsed information on a wide range of topics while being a 'knowledgeable, listening ear'.

Further reading

BSR (2016). *National Clinical Audit for Rheumatoid and Early Inflammatory Arthritis: 2nd Annual Report, 2016*. London: BSR, HQIP. ☞ https://www.hqip.org.uk/resource/rheumatoid-and-early-inflammatory-arthritis-2nd-annual-report-2016/#.XShngOtKiM8

NICE (2018). Diagnosis and management of rheumatoid arthritis and clinical review. Evidence C: treat to target (NG100). ☞ https://www.nice.org.uk/guidance/ng100/evidence/evidence-review-c-treattotarget-pdf-4903172320

NRAS. Immunisation for people with rheumatoid arthritis. ☞ https://www.nras.org.uk/immunisation-for-people-with-rheumatoid-arthritis-

The role of the nurse in supporting patients

Not every patient contact can be with a specialist in MSCs. Yet there are many opportunities when nurses will see patients in clinic, on the ward, or simply having an investigation, when they may be asked to provide some advice about their MSC. Nurses in all care settings who may not have extensive knowledge of MSCs should consider how they adequately signpost patients to the relevant support, including patient organizations. Fully endorsed patient organizations offer useful resources that support the information and guidance given in specialist units.

Fully endorsed patient organizations play a vital role in healthcare and have a wealth of resources including:

- Helplines offering practical help and emotional support.
- Informative websites.
- Chat rooms and online forums.
- Trained telephone volunteers who provide 1:1 peer support
- Patient information documents that are written in lay terms (for examples, see 'Further reading' at the end of this section).
- Advice on how and where to seek specialist services.
- Information for patients about social issues such as workplace issues, family relationships, and lifestyle.

Historically, 1° care nurses or healthcare support workers carried out blood monitoring for people with IJD but had little training in latest evidence-based treatment. The nurse specialist became the key first point of contact when patients needed guidance. Nurses in 1° care should direct the patient to the nurse-led helpline for a medical or drug-related query if they are unable to answer it or to a patient organization for emotional support or general information. Equally, specialist nurses do not always have adequate time or resources to provide extra care for those who need more emotional support. Working with patient organizations and building links to enable patients to access buddy systems and other means of support ∴ provide vital resources that often can be offered in the community for a number of LTCs.

Community nurses may visit elderly, frail patients with LTCs in their homes who have rheumatological conditions. They will have established links with the GPs, the specialist units, and the MDTs so they can feed back on any issues requiring specialist input.

Further reading

NRAS. Immunisation for people with rheumatoid arthritis. 🔗 https://www.nras.org.uk/immunisation-for-people-with-rheumatoid-arthritis-

NRAS. 'Newly diagnosed pack'—for those recently diagnosed with RA: 🔗 https://www.nras.org.uk/publications/new2ra-pack

Getting the best out of a clinic appointment

People approach an outpatient clinic appointment very differently but it's important for them to understand that by proactively ensuring that they get the best out of their visit, it can make a significant difference to their emotional and physical well-being, as well as long-term outcomes.

Doctors and other HCPs have their own agendas and things they need to discuss, whether this is an initial diagnostic appointment or a routine follow-up visit. Therefore, their agenda will dominate unless the patient ensures that what matters most to them or is concerning them is also discussed. In order for the patient to get the best out of their appointment, they have a role to play in using the time allocated for the appointment efficiently.

Patient organizations have extensive information and resources to help patients plan for their visit and this is another good reason to ensure that you signpost patients to relevant patient organizations at an early stage.

For example, NRAS resources include advice on how best to plan for a clinic appointment. Recommendations for the patient include:

- Preparation: think through what you want to get out of the appointment and write your questions down, with the most important ones at the top of the list. Use the list to make sure you don't forget anything and ask the nurse or doctor to go through it with you. It can include things such as 'concern about your job', 'planning for pregnancy', 'family demands you may be struggling with', 'getting a flu jab in winter'—it doesn't just have to be about symptoms or medication.
- Be honest, not brave. A clinic appointment is not the time to use the words 'I'm fine', if you're not. It can be hard to be honest with HCPs about your pain or concerns. But your team needs to know the real picture. Take a look at the information 'Behind the Smile' videos on the NRAS website (🖱 https://www.nras.org.uk/behind-the-smile).
- Be precise. Some people find it helps to keep a diary of how they are and what they can (and can't) do each day or week. There are also booklets about fatigue and diaries to record fatigue. See 'Further reading' at the end of this section.
- Make a list of all your medications (past and present) and take a copy with you which you can give to the doctor or nurse. It can save a lot of time instead of trying to remember this information. If you have a booklet with your blood monitoring results, take that too, although a lot of hospitals now have blood and imaging results on line within the hospital and shared with local GPs.
- Always ask if you don't understand. It's fine to keep on asking until you understand the explanation.
- Think about taking a partner, other family member, or friend with you, especially if you are making decisions about your care. Many people find it useful to have another pair of ears as there is a lot to take in! A partner or friend can take notes and support you after the consultation when you're digesting what's been said and thinking things through.

It helps the patient enormously to have a good understanding of the HCPs who make up their rheumatology team. Your patient needs peace of mind to be able to get on with their life and this comes from having a team they can trust. People can self-manage much better when they know who they can rely on for ongoing care and swift support when they are finding things difficult and their own coping skills run out.

If a patient can get to know who's who and how the health system works in their area, they will be better placed to get the support they need. MDTs vary from area to area and country to country, so it is important that the patient finds out from their specialist nurse or consultant who is available and if there is a nurse-led helpline they can call when in need.

Measuring 'patient activation' (how engaged patients are with their care) is something which has originated in the US and is taking hold in the UK and elsewhere. In order for HCPs to tailor shared decision-making during consultations, they need to be able to understand how much knowledge the patient has as well as how much they want to engage in their care. Shared decision-making is not a 'one-size-fits-all' process! To do this, it's possible to administer a patient activation questionnaire to gauge where the patient is on a scale of 1–4 where 1 is not at all engaged and 4 is moving towards becoming an expert patient. To find out more about this—visit ☞ https://www.england.nhs.uk/ourwork/patient-participation/self-care/patient-activation/.

Further reading

Apps developed for patients—see NRAS website: ☞ https://www.nras.org.uk
'Know your DAS' app: M https://www.nras.org.uk/know-your-das-mobile-app
'Rheumabuddy' app: ☞ https://www.nras.org.uk/rheumabuddy-an-app-to-help-you-live-better-with-ra-and-jia

Taking control: understanding the disease and managing care

What is supported self-management?

Active self-management is about using a set of skills that can be learned, rather than just relying on what health experts, such as doctors and allied HCPs, can offer the individual living with a LTC such as RA. It's also about approaching the challenges and burden that living with an incurable health condition such as RA brings, in a helpful and constructive way. It really is a crucial part of someone's care, and their attitude to their condition and how they decide to embrace it, or not, will affect their longer-term outcomes. The word 'supported' in this phrase is also crucially important because it means getting the right help to learn new skills and ways of coping rather than leaving the patient struggling on their own, trying to work out how best to help themselves or the team taking absolute control without considering the patient's perspective. That's where patient organizations support the person *and their healthcare team* as well as their families. Self-management works best when there is the right support at the right time delivered in a tailored way to suit the individual.

Why is it important?

It's important because people who are effective at self-managing generally have a better quality of life and better disease outcomes.

That makes a big difference to the individual living with the disease but it also benefits family and friends, work colleagues, the NHS, and wider society. Patient organizations are a key resource. Ultimately, people with LTCs will probably interact with their specialist team a few times in a year, but the problems they can experience continue daily throughout their lives. Challenges can present outside hospital appointment times.

In practice, supported self-management is about being able to manage the disease, treatments, and day-to-day life in the best possible and most realistic way to suit an individual's lifestyle. It's not about ignoring or denying a health condition, nor is it about allowing that condition to dominate someone's life, rather it offers a more constructive way of living that has been shown to improve long-term outcomes. What this means is that by having a helpful understanding of the condition, being able to recognize and manage the emotional and physical impact, and being able and willing to make adaptations to lifestyle and the approach to doing things, people can take back control of their life and get into the driving seat again.

When someone has a condition like RA, they're already managing it in lots of ways, but there are also specific skills people can gain and, as a result, have more confidence and knowledge. Becoming a good self-manager takes time and practice; it's rather like learning any other skill, such as driving a car. With the right skills and a positive approach, which NRAS can help with, individuals can become effective self-managers who feel confident to make the decisions and changes which can affect their own health in a positive way.

Further reading

NRAS (2018). 'Living Better with RA Pack' for people with existing/longer standing disease: https://www.nras.org.uk/publications/living-better-with-ra-pack; NRAS 'Emotions, Relationships and Sexuality': https://www.nras.org.uk/publications/emotions-relationships-and-sexuality

Chapter 23

Nurse-led clinics

Demonstrating the value of the nurse specialist

Introduction

The work of specialist nurse in LTCs is complex and can be hard to articulate to non-nurses and sometimes nurse leaders. Over the last few years the complexity of the work has ↑. As new drugs such as biologics have become more common, nurse specialists have tended to take on the day-to-day management of caring for these patients.

The value of specialist nursing to patients

The quality of care given by nurse specialists is consistently valued by patients. Having an accessible professional who can make complex clinical decisions and deliver care is key to this satisfaction. Another component is the enablement of self-care, helping newly diagnosed patients navigate the journey from fear to confidence.

The value of specialist nursing to employers and commissioners of services

Specialist nursing services ↑ efficiency and proactively manage care. They understand the end-to-end patient journey and often work hard to improve it. They understand when a patient is most at risk and they have to be more vigilant, e.g. when starting new therapies. It is through managing care and clinical acumen that they avoid unnecessary use of emergency care and often ↓ the length of stay. They are a safe and consistent workforce and a good return on investment. Specialist nurses also ensure clinical standards are met for many services and offer on-the-ground expertise.

The value of specialist nursing to the profession

Specialist nursing offers a career path that allows development and maintains contact with the patient by giving direct clinical care. The work of specialist nurses offers mentorship and learning opportunities to students and colleagues who are caring for patients with complex conditions. Many specialist nurses provide consultation services to other professionals such as GPs.

➲ See 'Nurse specialist roles: value for money?', pp. 637–638.

Further reading

Apollo Nursing Resource—a resource for specialist nurses: https://www.apollonursingresource.com

Ndosi M, Lewis M, Hale C, et al. (2014). The outcome and cost-effectiveness of nurse-led care in people with rheumatoid arthritis: a multicentre randomised controlled trial *Ann Rheum Dis* 73:1975–82.

Competencies and frameworks

Introduction

The work of specialist nurses is complex and in LTCs practice can vary widely. Most nurse specialists are proactive case managers and also have specific knowledge and skills around their particular field of practice. This has meant inconsistency in the way that competency frameworks have developed in the specialist nursing community in the UK.

Frameworks for practice: a UK perspective

In the UK, each country has its own guidance for specialist advanced practice and each has taken a different policy position. Scotland developed the Advanced Practice Toolkit in 2005 which has been a consistent way to develop practice. Wales and Northern Ireland issued guidance and England now has the Advanced Practice Framework, though at the time of writing this chapter (2018) the implementation has focused on deficits in the medical workforce rather than specialist advanced practice. With a focus on a more medical model, the clinical nurse specialist faces an additional challenge.

From a UK wide perspective, the RCN have issued various documents over the years but the most recent (2018) is a series on Advanced Level Practice. Section 2 contains competencies for advanced practice.

Rheumatology

Competency and capability frameworks specifically in rheumatology seem to be focused on areas such as biologics. The RCN rheumatology nursing forum published their fourth edition of *Assessing, Managing and Monitoring Biologic Therapies for Inflammatory Arthritis* in 2017 which is focused on a specific area of practice but comprehensively covers many areas of specialist practice such as safety.

In 2018, Skills for Health developed the Musculoskeletal Core Competencies Framework which is a multiprofessional framework. Although not aimed at a specialist audience, it covers many clinical domains such as patient-centred care and assessment, investigation, and diagnosis which could contribute to succession planning in the specialist nursing community.

Around the world, other groups have developed frameworks for practice. In the US, the American Nurses Association recognized rheumatology specialist nursing in 2012 defining a scope of practice which was published in 2013.

Further reading

American Nurses Association (2013). Rheumatology nursing: scope and standards of practice. ↗ https://www.nursingworld.org/~4add7e/globalassets/catalog/book-toc/rheumatology-nursing-scp--stds_toc.pdf

American Association of Advanced Nurse Practitioners: ↗ http://www.aanp.org/

Association of Advanced Practice Educators (UK): ↗ http://www.aape.org.uk

Canadian Centre for Advanced Practice Nursing Research: ↗ http://fhs.mcmaster.ca/ccapnr

Department of Health and Social Care (2010). Advanced level nursing: a position statement. ↗ https://www.dh.gov.uk/en/Publicationsandstatistics/Publications/PublicationsPolicyAndGuidance/DH_121739

Health Education England (2017). Multiprofessional framework for advanced clinical practice in England. https://hee.nhs.uk/sites/default/files/documents/HEE%20ACP%20Framework.pdf

NHS Scotland. Advanced nursing practice toolkit. http://www.advancedpractice.scot.nhs.uk

NHS Wales. Framework for advanced nursing, midwifery and allied health professional practice in Wales. http://www.nwssp.wales.nhs.uk/i-need-help-with-introducing-advanced-pr

Royal College of Nursing (2017). *Assessing, Managing and Monitoring Biologic Therapies for Inflammatory Arthritis: RCN Guidance for Rheumatology Practitioners*, 4th edn. London: RCN. https://www.rcn.org.uk/professional-development/publications/pdf-005579

Royal College of Nursing (2018). Advanced level practice. https://www.rcn.org.uk/professional-development/publications/pub-006894

Skills for Health (2018). Musculoskeletal core capabilities framework. http://www.skillsforhealth.org.uk/images/projects/msk/Musculoskeletal%20framework.pdf?s=form

What is nurse-led care?

Nurse-led care is a holistic approach to care, taking account of patients' physical, psychological, social, and spiritual needs.

Patients seen in nurse-led clinics usually have received their diagnosis and the initial treatment plan by the rheumatologist. The setting of nurse-led care is in a rheumatology outpatient clinic and on telephone advice lines.

Examples of nurse-led care activities include:

- Patient assessments.
- Patient education and training.
- Monitoring for disease activity, disease impact, effectiveness of therapies, and side effects.
- Ordering and reviewing investigations.
- Recommending escalation or changes in treatment.
- Supporting self-management.
- Counselling.
- Annual review for patients in low disease state or remission.
- Health promotion.

Given the holistic nature of rheumatology nursing, nurse-led care also involves coordination of the overall care of the patient. This may include:

- Referring patients and facilitating the interdisciplinary team care.
- Communication with 1° care.
- Communication with other agencies such as social care, work, and transport.

Further reading

Bala SV, Forslind K, Fridlund B, et al. (2018). Person-centred care in nurse-led outpatient rheumatology clinics: Conceptualization and initial development of a measurement instrument. *Musculoskeletal Care* 16:287–95.

Bech B, Primdahl J, van Tubergen A et al (2019). 2018 Update of the EULAR recommendations for the role of the nurse in the management of chronic inflammatory arthritis. *Ann Rheum Dis* 1–8. doi:10.1136/annrheumdis-2019-215458

Wong FKY, Chung LCY (2006). Establishing a definition for a nurse-led clinic: structure, process, and outcome. *J Adv Nurs* 53:358–69.

Clinical effectiveness

Effectiveness of an intervention is defined as the extent to which it produces a desired outcome under ordinary circumstances. In other words, an intervention is effective if it works in normal settings.

Nurse-led care can be considered as a complex intervention. Complex interventions are said to have several interacting components. This complexity makes it difficult to evaluate their effectiveness.

Nurse-led care has the following interacting components:

- Clinical activities.
- Supportive activities.
- Care coordination.

All these interact with the following factors:

- Education and experience of the practitioner in rheumatology.
- Practitioner's additional skills such as prescribing, joint injections, imaging, and motivational interviewing.
- Setting of care (outpatient clinic, telephone advice lines, or community-based care).

The evidence for nurse-led care has been established using randomized controlled trials (RCTs) and systematic reviews. RCTs are the best primary studies to provide the evidence for effectiveness. Most RCTs of nurse-led care effectiveness have been pragmatic, conducted in the outpatient clinics or telephone advice lines thus examining nurse-led care as it occurs in the clinic and comparing patient outcomes with those seen in the traditional clinics run by the rheumatologist.

Early RCTs conducted in the UK showed that the outcomes of a rheumatology nurse-led clinic were at least similar to those obtained in rheumatologists' clinics. The outcomes evaluated were disease activity, morning stiffness, fatigue serenity, pain, physical function, and satisfaction with care.

Later RCTs of higher quality and systematic reviews of effectiveness established the evidence for nurse-led care in RA. The most robust evidence exists in the management of RA because this is the most prevalent inflammatory arthritis.

Research supports the evidence for nurse-led care in patients with both active disease and those with low disease activity or in remission. In addition, clinical care is compounded by the risk for co-morbidities which must be assessed and addressed together with disease activity.

Nurse-led care: RA disease activity

Nurse-led care has been shown to be effective in managing RA disease activity. Patients with early and established disease have seen their disease activity ↓ under nurse-led care.

The current management of disease activity includes early referral and diagnosis, early commencement of treatment, intensive treatment, and a treat to target approach. The aim of RA treatment is to achieve a state of remission or low disease activity. Keeping the patient at a state of sustained remission limits the damage caused by chronic inflammation and the associated risk for co-morbidities.

Disease activity is controlled mainly by pharmacological means. It is likely that nurse-led care achieves this by tight control of the RA and promoting adherence with treatment.

Nurse-led care: disease impact

Even when disease activity is controlled, many patients may continue to be affected by the impact of the disease on their lives. RA impacts may include pain, functional disability, fatigue, sleep problems, and lack of coping. Non-pharmacological interventions are required to address the disease impact in RA and other MSCs.

Pain

Current evidence supports the effectiveness of nurse-led care in managing pain in inflammatory arthritis and in OA. Nurses are likely achieving this by holistic assessment which includes assessing pain and recommending effective analgesia. In their role of coordinating care, clinical nurse specialists can refer to specialist pain services and physiotherapy for pain that is difficult to manage.

Functional disability

There is also good evidence of nurse-led care effectiveness in reducing physical disability or improving physical function. Most studies assessing this outcome used the Health Assessment Questionnaire as an outcome measure, ∴ the improvement meant ability to perform the activities of daily living. Referral for occupational therapy may be needed to improve physical function.

Fatigue

Fatigue is common in RA, affecting a large proportion of patients. It has a multifactorial cause and is multimodal in nature. Nurse-led clinics have been shown to be effective at reducing fatigue intensity. Previous studies assessed fatigue intensity using a VAS. More evidence is required to support the effectiveness of nurse-led care in managing different subdomains of fatigue.

Coping with disease

Several factors are involved to enable coping with a chronic disease. One of the most important factors is self-efficacy, the belief in one's capability to manage their condition. Nurse-led care has been shown to improve patients' self-efficacy and coping with their rheumatic disease.

Emotional well-being

While nurses address psychosocial issues in people with MSCs, it is been difficult to capture all aspects of support that patients receive. The research evidence available is based on specific symptoms of anxiety and depression.

Nurse-led care: safety

All studies have shown that nurse-led care is safe and acceptable to patients. Patients under nurse-led care are not likely to have higher disease activity than those under rheumatologist-led care. This applies to any other safety measures assessed in clinical trials settings such as out-of-range blood results, admissions to hospital, visits to the ED, and death. The evidence is strong for both patients with active disease and those in remission or with low disease activity.

Nurse-led care: other outcomes

Research supports the evidence for nurse-led care in terms of other outcomes of interest for patients, such as access to service, satisfaction with care, quality of life, and social–emotional communication.

Supporting self-management

A great deal of what happens in rheumatology nurse-led clinics involves patient education and enabling/supporting self-management of the disease and its impact. Self-management is the individual's ability to manage the symptoms, treatment regimens, physical and psychosocial consequences, and lifestyle changes inherent in living with a chronic condition.

Patients with MSCs need support to develop skills to manage disease-specific needs, engage with resources/services, and live with chronic illness. Needs-based patient education delivered by nurses has been shown to improve patients' self-efficacy. Qualitative evidence suggests that nurse-led care which is holistic in nature has patient involvement at its core and this helps to strengthen patients' ability to self-manage their disease.

References

Barlow J, Wright C, Sheasby J, et al. (2002). Self-management approaches for people with chronic conditions: a review. *Patient Educ Couns* 48:177–87.

de Thurah A, Esbensen BA, Roelsgaard IK, et al. (2017). Efficacy of embedded nurse-led versus conventional physician-led follow-up in RA: a systematic review and meta-analysis. *RMD Open* 3:e000481.

Garner S, Lopatina E, Rankin JA, et al. (2017). Nurse-led care for patients with RA: a systematic review of the effect on quality of care. *J Rheumatol* 44:757–65.

Koksvik HS, Hagen KB, Rødevand E, et al. (2013). Patient satisfaction with nursing consultations in a rheumatology outpatient clinic: a 21-month RCT in patients with inflammatory arthritides. *Ann Rheum Dis* 72:836–43.

Ndosi M, Lewis M, Hale C, et al. (2014). The outcome and cost-effectiveness of nurse-led care in people with rheumatoid arthritis: a multicentre randomised controlled trial. *Ann Rheum Dis* 73:1975–82.

Primdahl J, Sørensen J, Horn HC, et al. (2014). Shared care or nursing consultations as an alternative to rheumatologist follow-up for RA outpatients with low disease activity—patient outcomes from a 2-year RCT. *Ann Rheum Dis* 73:357–64.

Nurse specialist roles: value for money?

Cost-effectiveness is a technical term but can be defined simply as the gains in health relative to the costs of different health interventions. The evidence supporting the cost-effectiveness of nurse-led care has been based on its ability to produce desirable clinical outcomes at a lower cost relative to the traditional physician-led care.

Proving your worth

In the UK, nurse specialists have become an integral member of the MDT in many fields of practice, but particularly in the care of those with LTCs. However, nurse specialists are often seen as an expensive resource by hospital authorities, who are frequently struggling to meet financial challenges and are vulnerable to cost-saving initiatives. Nurse specialists' work is relatively autonomous compared to that of ward-based nurses and is not part of routine ward work; they manage a caseload of patients (who are usually outpatients) and liaise frequently with 1° care teams.

There are challenges in providing evidence of the value for money based upon evidence from routine clinical practice. Demonstrating the value of the complexities of the nurse specialist role relies upon sophisticated data collection similar to the data collected on consultant activities.

So, there are critical issues that nurse specialists should be mindful of in understanding their role, value for money for the healthcare system, and ensuring transparency of their activities. Consider:

- What data do the hospital authorities collect about your regular activities (e.g. nurse clinics)?
- What activities do you undertake that data are not collected about? Is there a way of collecting appropriate evidence to demonstrate the nurse specialist contribution? For example, outcomes of patients following the use of a telephone advice line.
- How do you contribute to better patient outcomes across the hospital? For example, do you provide an expert resource for nurses caring for patients with specific conditions?
- Do the patients you support benefit from your expertise in specific ways—e.g. educational sessions, coordinating care with 1° care teams on behalf of the patient, etc.
- Critically appraise your role and compare with other LTC nurse specialist roles—explore data capture and good practice examples to share.

Note: Apollo Nursing Resource provides a practical tool for capturing the value of nurse specialist roles.[1]

Although the work of specialist nurses is complex, there are a number of things that can be done to support the evidence and demonstrate the value of rheumatology nursing:

- Keep a log of caseload numbers and the proportion of patients who require complex care, e.g. symptom control, psychosocial care, or self-management support.
- Check if you can set up a way for your employer to record your activity, e.g. a correctly coded electronic health record.

- Draw up a job plan that shows the complexity of your work, not just where you are.
- Don't oversimplify your work by using phrases with managers such as 'advice and support' to describe your work—reflect its complexity in everything you say and write. Be clear about the evidence base for your work. The national guidance or evidence-based recommendations are good examples.
- Engage with leadership.

Patients with LTCs highly value the support nurse specialists offer. In the UK, when financial crises have forced threats to nurse specialist roles, patient organizations have rallied in their support, particularly as continuity of care is highly valued by patients with LTCs. In the past, patient organizations published papers making the case for nurse specialists in cancer, rheumatology, multiple sclerosis, and respiratory diseases.

Reference

1. Apollo Nursing Resource. Job planner. https://www.apollonursingresource.com/job-planner/

Further reading

Larsson I, Fridlund B, Arvidsson B, et al. (2015). A nurse-led rheumatology clinic versus rheumatologist-led clinic in monitoring of patients with chronic inflammatory arthritis undergoing biological therapy: a cost comparison study in a randomised controlled trial. *BMC Musculoskelet Disord* 16:354.

Ndosi M, Johnson D, Young T, et al. (2016). Effects of needs-based patient education on self-efficacy and health outcomes in people with RA: a multicentre, single blind, RCT. *Ann Rheum Dis* 75:1126–32.

Sørensen J, Primdahl J, Horn HC, et al. (2015). Shared care or nurse consultations as an alternative to rheumatologist follow-up for RA outpatients with stable low disease-activity RA: cost-effectiveness based on a 2-year randomized trial. *Scand J Rheumatol* 44:13–21.

Watson RA, Mooney J, Barton G, et al. (2015). The outcome and cost-effectiveness of nurse-led care in the community for people with RA a non-pragmatic study. *BMJ Open* 5:e007696.

Chapter 24

Public health awareness

Health systems and global health

The United Nations (UN) combined with the WHO in 1948 to work collaboratively with the aim of promoting and protecting health worldwide.

International initiatives to improve global health have resulted in some positive outcomes, e.g. the global mortality rates across all ages have ↓ in the last five decades and deaths from communicable diseases have largely ↓. In 2015, the UN set 17 sustainable development goals to transform our world.[1]

However, there remain disparities across the world in terms of health outcomes, particularly in the poorer countries. Non-communicable diseases (NCDs) are a leading cause of death globally and were responsible for 68% of the world's deaths in 2012; 40% of premature deaths were in those under the age of 70. Low- and middle-income countries bear 86% of the burden of premature deaths from NCDs. In addition, inequality deepens poverty and ↑ the inequity in access to healthcare and ultimately gaps in health outcomes. The social determinants of health are a significant factor in improving health outcomes and recommended reading and sources of information can be found in the references and further reading lists in this chapter. See Fig. 24.1.

WHO aims to reduce the global burden of NCDs, seeing it is a vital step in sustainable development. The WHO global NCD action plan has set objectives and targets for the prevention and control of NCDs.[2] The targets include:

- A 25% ↓ in risk of premature mortality from cardiovascular disease, cancer, diabetes, and chronic respiratory disease.
- At least a 10% relative reduction in harmful use of alcohol.
- A 10% relative reduction in the prevalence of insufficient physical activity.
- A 30% relative reduction in mean population intake of salt/sodium.
- A 25% relative reduction in the prevalence of current tobacco use in persons aged >15 years.
- A 25% relative reduction in the prevalence of raised blood pressure.
- Halting the ↑ in diabetes and obesity.
- At least 50% of eligible people to receive drug therapy and counselling (including glycaemic control) to prevent heart attacks and strokes.
- An 80% availability of the affordable basic technologies and essential medicines, including generics, required to treat major NCDs in both public and private facilities.

To achieve global health goals, governments need to define the patterns of different conditions, and the ways in which conditions develop, spread, or evolve. Governments must constantly monitor and improve the health of their nation and this involves short-term and long-term strategic plans together with financial commitments so that resources will positively impact health outcomes.

Key areas may include healthcare systems available for all (from birth to the grave), while considering infrastructures that individuals need to live safe healthy lives. These systems need to undertake strategies to reduce or eradicate communicable diseases, as well as to make provision for those

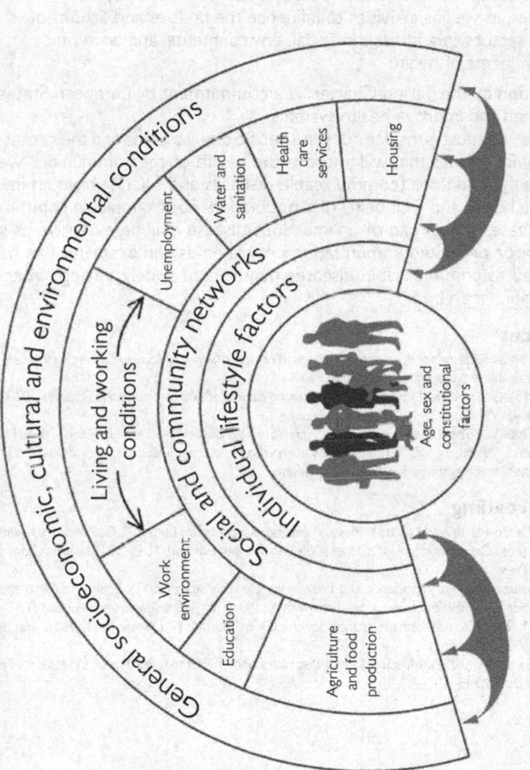

Fig 24.1 The main determinants of health.

Reprinted from Dahlgren G, Whitehead M. (1991). 'Policies and Strategies to Promote Social Equity in Health'. Stockholm, Sweden: Institute for Futures Studies. https://www.iffs.se/policies-and-strategies/

who are disabled, frail, elderly, or have an acute condition or NCD (e.g. heart disease). The following European Union commitment encapsulates the principles:

> Within the political and institutional framework of each country, a health system is the ensemble of all public and private organizations, institutions and resources mandated to improve, maintain or restore health. Health systems encompass both personal and population services, as well as activities to influence the policies and actions of other sectors to address the social, environmental and economic determinants of health.

This definition by the Tallinn Charter[3] is a commitment by European States to strengthen and improve health systems.

As HCPs, we must consider not just specific disease areas and their treatment but wider issues that will improve the health of the communities we serve. Health conditions (communicable diseases and NCDs) have an impact on the health and well-being of a population. For example, in communicable diseases the spread of an infectious disease may be extensive as a result of poor or limited immunization programmes and problems can be perpetuated as communicable diseases may spread widely through international traffic/travel.

References

1. United Nations. Sustainable development goals. https://www.undp.org/content/undp/en/home/sustainable-development-goals.html
2. WHO (2013). *Global Action Plan for the Prevention and Control of Noncommunicable Diseases 2013–2020*. Geneva: WHO.
3. WHO (2008). *The Tallinn Charter: Health Systems for Health and Wealth*. Copenhagen: WHO. http://www.euro.who.int/en/publications/policy-documents/tallinn-charter-health-systems-for-health-and-wealth

Further reading

Barrero LH, Caban-Martinez AJ (2015). Musculoskeletal disorders. In: Detels R, Gullliford M, Karim QA, et al. (eds) *Oxford Textbook of Global Public Health*, 6th edn, pp. 1046–59. Oxford: Oxford University Press.

GBD 2016 Disease and Injury Incidence and Prevalence Collaborators (2017). Global, regional and national incidence, prevalence and years lived with disability for 328 diseases and injuries for 195 countries, 1990–2016: a systematic analysis for the Global Burden of Disease Study 2016. *Lancet* 390:1211–59.

Storheim K, Swart JA (2014). Musculoskeletal disorders and the Global Burden of Disease study. *Ann Rheum Dis* 73:949–50.

Public health and the role of the nurse

The WHO defines public health as 'the art and science of preventing disease, prolonging life and promoting health through the organized efforts of society'.

In recent years, the nurse's role has been increasingly recognized as playing a vital part in helping to meet the needs of patients with NCDs. The WHO Global Action Plan[1] describes the need to improve prevention and control of NCDs as countries experience a rising demand for healthcare partly due to the growing elderly and chronic disease populations.

The nurse fulfils the criteria of 'making every contact count',[2] providing services for all while considering the inter-relationship between all the other healthcare services and resources available. Nurses caring for patients may use various aspects of their expertise in different ways to achieve the WHO public health aims. A nurse strives to support patients, restoring their health, while also empowering them to participate in society and continuing their normal ADLs. Each of these interventions is part of a strategic approach that is part of an overall public health challenge, something that nurses are well placed to respond to as they have a good understanding of the community they serve.[3]

Nurses, as the largest HCP workforce, are in a good position to work across all key areas and offer support for prevention and control for NCDs. As such, the vision of the International Council of Nurses is to build the capacity and capability of the nursing professional to support the global plans to prevent, control, and manage NCDs in all care settings.[4]

Barriers to investing in nurse education and training as well as the slow pace of legislative changes to enable nurses to undertake more advanced roles has historically meant the full potential of nursing has not always been optimized. Investment in nursing development lags behind the needs of society and has often restrained the role of nurses in developing countries. The WHO has recognized the need to optimize nursing roles in NCDs.

Nurses should recognize these potential changes and be ready to optimize evidence-based examples of good practice that can improve health outcomes. Sharing good practice internationally can be rewarding not only in terms of patient outcomes but also job satisfaction. Recent initiatives such as 'Nursing Now' are resulting in collaborations across the world to raise the profile of nurses and the potential development opportunities.[5] (➲ Also see Chapter 21, 'Specialist nursing support: the role and nurse prescribing', Chapter 21, p. 618; ➲ Chapter 23, 'Nurse-led clinics', pp. 629–638.)

Where MSCs occur, they tend to last longer and add complexities to individuals who already have other co-morbidities. The additional important factor is that there is now an ↑ recognition that nurses provide a patient-centred and holistic approach that empowers and informs patients at the same time as undertaking disease assessments.[4]

HCPs in all fields of practice can play an important role in improving health outcomes. There are many opportunities for HCPs to influence people's perceptions of health and disease management while ultimately improving health outcomes.

For example;

- Encouraging changes in behaviour.
- Education about health conditions and how to self-manage.
- Acting as an advocate and advisor on where to seek further guidance on vaccinations, smoking cessations, physical exercise, and dietary changes.

Moving forward

Within the US, Australia, and the European region, nurses have advanced their practice for many years with nurse-led clinics which are now integral to many NCDs including rheumatology services. Advanced practitioners or specialist nurses undertake a holistic approach to assessing, managing, and treating patients with MSCs. Many manage a caseload of patients with more stable disease, monitor disease and bloods, and carry out annual reviews to manage other co-morbidities (e.g. cardiovascular risks, lifestyle and behavioural risks, osteoporosis, etc.)

These initiatives continue to spread across the world and evidence across the Asia Pacific region show that nurses are increasingly taking on additional training to enhance their support to patients with MSCs using a chronic disease management approach.[6–8]

References

1. WHO (2013). *Global Action Plan for the Prevention and Control of Noncommunicable Diseases 2013–2020*. Geneva: WHO.
2. Bennett V (2012). Every nursing contact counts for improving public health. *Nurs Times* 108:7.
3. International Council of Nursing. Health policy consultation document, May 2017. ℜ http://www.icn.ch
4. Royal College of Nursing (2016). *Nurses 4 Public Health. Promote, Prevent and Protect: The Value and Contribution for Nursing to Public Health in the UK. Final Report.* London: RCN.
5. WHO. Nursing Now Campaign. ℜ http://www.who.int/hrh/news/2018/nursing_now_campaign/en/
6. Chew LC, Yee SL (2013). The rheumatology monitoring clinic in Singapore—a novel advanced practice nurse/pharmacist led clinic. *Proc Singapore Healthc* 22:48–55.
7. Kondo A (2012). Advanced practice nurses in Japan: education and related issues. *J Nurs Care* S5:004.
8. Wu XJ, Zhang L (2014). Enhancing the nursing discipline and developing nursing science in China. *Int J Nurs Sci* 1:323–9.

Further reading

Acheson D (1988). *Public Health in England. The Report of the Committee of Inquiry into the Future Development of the Public Health Function*. London: HMSO.

RCN—search for Public Health: ℜ http://www.rcn.org.uk

Musculoskeletal conditions: non-communicable diseases

Musculoskeletal conditions include a number of health conditions that can affect the muscles, bones, tendons, ligaments, and nerves. As a group, MSCs are responsible for 21.3% of the YLDs and are the second most common cause of disability worldwide with low back pain being the most frequently reported for YLDs. MSCs have been shown to have an impact upon quality of life, ability to work, and are expensive (in 2009, the world spent a total of US$5.97 trillion in health-related expenses for MSCs.) There is now an ↑ interest in MSCs in health policy terms as MSCs are estimated to have increased by 45% from 1990 to 2010. These figures may be partly attributed to the growing elderly populations (OA) and obesity.

Examples of MSC include:

- OA.
- Back pain.
- Osteoporosis.
- RA.
- Seronegative spondyloarthropathies such as PsA and AS.
- Crystal arthropathies, e.g. gout.
- CTDs

The worldwide occurrence of MSCs can partly be attributed to four risk factors. Obesity, ageing, and the ↑ in trauma (road traffic collisions) and work-related injuries (e.g. low back pain). Factors that feed into these are changes in diet and sedentary lifestyle/lack of physical activity (linked to obesity).

Pain is the predominant feature of many MSCs and may limit function and independence, particularly if untreated and if they coexist with other health conditions (e.g. diabetes or cardiovascular disease).

MSCs are increasingly seen as expensive in health terms. Some factors that have influenced this include:

- Days lost from work (e.g. low back pain), particularly in middle- and high-income countries.
- Use of resources as ~20% of regular 1° care consultations are related to MSCs.
- Growing elderly and chronic disease populations with OA requiring an ↑ number of knee or hip replacements.

Although there are no specific targets for MSCs, there are targets that address the needs of those with MSCs: physical activity, access to affordable technologies and medicines, as well as the reduction in co-morbidities linked to many MSCs such as diabetes, cardiovascular disease, and respiratory disease. MSCs occur more frequently than many other conditions and tend to last longer and impact other co-morbidities, such as cardiovascular disease or obesity where functional issues such as joint pain will prevent exercise.

Globally, low back pain is one of the five leading causes of YLDs. MSCs and cardiovascular disease were the most important causes of YLDs in older age groups. Socioeconomic status and major NCD risk factors are robustly associated with loss in physical functioning in early to more advanced years of life.

In the twenty-first century, global health challenges continue and, in many ways, have become more complex:

- Rising healthcare costs as result of improved drug therapies and technological/treatment options—there are now ↑ costs as well as an ↑ population of chronic NCDs.
- Years have been added to life but not always quality of life, leading to ↑ long-term healthcare needs. The growing elderly and chronic disease populations are now the focus for strategic healthcare planning, particularly for the richer, more developed nations. Generally, an ↑ in age and survival rates is accompanied by an ↑ in health and social care costs.
- International travel and movement of populations add additional challenges to health surveillance and monitoring.
- ↑ urbanization with rapid changes to some communities.

➲ See Chapter 1, 'Musculoskeletal conditions', p. 4–6.

Further reading

Barrero LH, Caban-Martinez AJ (2015). Musculoskeletal disorders. In: Detels R, Gullliford M, Karim QA, et al. (eds) *Oxford Textbook of Global Public Health*, 6th edn, pp. 1046–59. Oxford: Oxford University Press.

GBD 2016 Disease and Injury Incidence and Prevalence Collaborators (2017). Global, regional and national incidence, prevalence and years lived with disability for 328 diseases and injuries for 195 countries, 1990–2016: a systematic analysis for the Global Burden of Disease Study 2016. *Lancet* 390:1211–59.

Versus Arthritis (2018). State of musculoskeletal health 2018. [Arthritis and other musculoskeletal conditions in numbers.] ℘ https://www.versusarthritis.org/media/12349/state-fo-msk-report-2018.pdf

WHO (2013). *Global Action Plan for the Prevention and Control of Noncommunicable Diseases 2013–2020*. Geneva: WHO.

Index

Tables, figures and boxes are indicated by an italic *t*, *f* and *b* following the page number.

A

D

E

F

I

K

L

M

N

O

P

S